Adjunctive Rehabilitation Approaches to Oncology

Editor

ANDREA L. CHEVILLE

PHYSICAL MEDICINE AND REHABILITATION CLINICS OF NORTH AMERICA

www.pmr.theclinics.com

Consulting Editor
SANTOS F. MARTINEZ

February 2017 • Volume 28 • Number 1

ELSEVIER

1600 John F. Kennedy Boulevard • Suite 1800 • Philadelphia, Pennsylvania, 19103-2899

http://www.theclinics.com

**PHYSICAL MEDICINE AND REHABILITATION CLINICS OF NORTH AMERICA Volume 28, Number 1
February 2017 ISSN 1047-9651, ISBN 978-0-323-49673-5**

Editor: Lauren Boyle
Developmental Editor: Donald Mumford

Reprints. For copies of 100 or more of articles in this publication, please contact the Commercial Reprints Department, Elsevier Inc., 360 Park Avenue South, New York, NY 10010-1710. Tel.: 212-633-3874; Fax: 212-633-3820; E-mail: reprints@elsevier.com.

Physical Medicine and Rehabilitation Clinics of North America (ISSN 1047-9651) is published quarterly by Elsevier Inc., 360 Park Avenue South, New York, NY 10010-1710. Months of issue are February, May, August, and November. Business and Editorial Offices: 1600 John F. Kennedy Blvd., Suite 1800, Philadelphia, PA 19103-2899. Customer Service Office: 3251 Riverport Lane, Maryland Heights, MO 63043. Periodicals postage paid at New York, NY and additional mailing offices. Subscription price per year is $288.00 (US individuals), $560.00 (US institutions), $100.00 (US students), $210.00 (Canadian individuals), $737.00 (Canadian institutions), $210.00 (Canadian students), $210.00 (foreign individuals), $737.00 (foreign institutions), and $210.00 (foreign students). Foreign air speed delivery is included in all *Clinics* subscription prices. All prices are subject to change without notice. **POSTMASTER:** Send address changes to *Physical Medicine and Rehabilitation Clinics of North America*, Customer Service Office: Elsevier Health Sciences Division, Subscription Customer Service, 3251 Riverport Lane, Maryland Heights, MO 63043. **Customer Service: 1-800-654-2452 (US). From outside of the United States, call 314-447-8871. Fax: 314-447-8029. E-mail: JournalsCustomer Service-usa@elsevier.com (for print support); JournalsOnlineSupport-usa@elsevier.com (for online support).**

Physical Medicine and Rehabilitation Clinics of North America is indexed in *Excerpta Medica, MEDLINE/ PubMed (Index Medicus), Cinahl,* and *Cumulative Index to Nursing and Allied Health Literature.*

Contributors

CONSULTING EDITOR

SANTOS F. MARTINEZ, MD, MS
Diplomate of the American Academy of Physical Medicine and Rehabilitation,
Certificate of Added Qualification Sports Medicine, Assistant Professor, Department of
Orthopaedics, Campbell Clinic Orthopaedics, University of Tennessee, Memphis,
Tennessee

EDITOR

ANDREA L. CHEVILLE, MD, MSCE
Professor and Research Chair, Department of Physical Medicine and Rehabilitation;
Medical Director, Care Experience Program, Center for the Science of Health Care
Delivery, Mayo Clinic, Rochester, Minnesota

AUTHORS

CATHERINE M. ALFANO, PhD
American Cancer Society, Inc, Atlanta, Georgia

ARASH ASHER, MD
Health Sciences Associate Clinical Professor at the University of California Los Angeles,
Department of Physical Medicine and Rehabilitation, Samuel Oschin Comprehensive
Cancer Institute at Cedars-Sinai Medical Center, Health Sciences, University of California
Los Angeles, Los Angeles, California

ANJALI BHAGRA, MBBS
Associate Professor, Department of General Internal Medicine, Mayo Clinic, Rochester,
Minnesota

JENNIFER CAMP, MD
Department of Physical Medicine and Rehabilitation, Carolinas Rehabilitation, Charlotte,
North Carolina

FRANCESCO CARLI, MD, MPhil
Department of Anesthesia, McGill University Health Centre, Montreal, Quebec, Canada

ANDREA L. CHEVILLE, MD, MSCE
Professor and Research Chair, Department of Physical Medicine and Rehabilitation;
Medical Director, Care Experience Program, Center for the Science of Health Care
Delivery, Mayo Clinic, Rochester, Minnesota

CHRISTIAN M. CUSTODIO, MD
Associate Attending, Rehabilitation Medicine Service, Department of Neurology, Memorial
Sloan Kettering Cancer Center; Associate Professor, Division of Rehabilitation Medicine,
Weill Cornell Medicine, New York, New York

LIANE S. FELDMAN, MD
Department of Surgery, McGill University Health Centre, Montreal, Quebec, Canada

JACK B. FU, MD
Department of Palliative, Rehabilitation and Integrative Medicine, University of Texas MD Anderson Cancer Center, Houston, Texas

GAIL L. GAMBLE, MD
Department of Physical Medicine and Rehabilitation, Mayo Clinic, Rochester, Minnesota

ANN GAMSA, PhD
Department of Anesthesia, McGill University Health Centre, Montreal, Quebec, Canada

LYNN H. GERBER, MD
University Professor, George Mason University, Fairfax; Director of Research, Department of Medicine, Inova Fairfax Medical Campus, Falls Church, Virginia

CHELSIA GILLIS, MSc, RD
Department of Anesthesia, McGill University Health Centre, Montreal, Quebec, Canada

SEAN GILMAN, MD
Department of Medicine, McGill University Health Centre, Montreal, Quebec, Canada

HONG GUO, MD, PhD
Department of Digestive Diseases, Xinqiao Hospital, The Third Military Medical University, Chongqing, China

YING GUO, MD
Department of Palliative, Rehabilitation and Integrative Medicine, University of Texas MD Anderson Cancer Center, Houston, Texas

NICOLE HANRAHAN, MD
Cancer Rehabilitation Fellow, MedStar National Rehabilitation Network, Washington, DC

BRADFORD HIRSCH, MD
Flatiron Health, New York, New York

MARY JURISSON, MD
Assistant Professor, Department of Physical Medicine and Rehabilitation, Mayo Clinic, Rochester, Minnesota

THOMAS P. LIONE, DO
Department of Physical Medicine and Rehabilitation; Resident Physician, PGY-3, Hofstra Northwell School of Medicine, Manhasset, New York

SUSAN MALTSER, DO
Division Chief, Cancer Rehabilitation; Assistant Professor, Department of Physical Medicine and Rehabilitation, Hofstra Northwell School of Medicine, Manhasset, New York

ANDREA McKEE, MD
Department of Radiation Oncology, Lahey Hospital and Medical Center, Burlington, Massachusetts

KAREN MUSTIAN, PhD, MPH, ACSM
University of Rochester Medical Center, Rochester, New York

LYNN J. PALMER, PhD
Corrona Research Foundation, Albany, New York

TERRENCE M. PUGH, MD
Department of Physical Medicine and Rehabilitation, Carolinas Rehabilitation, Charlotte, North Carolina

VISHWA S. RAJ, MD
Division of Rehabilitation Medicine, Levine Cancer Institute; Department of Physical Medicine and Rehabilitation, Carolinas Rehabilitation, Charlotte, North Carolina

KATHRYN J. RUDDY, MD, MPH
Associate Professor, Department of Oncology, Mayo Clinic, Rochester, Minnesota

LISA MARIE RUPPERT, MD
Assistant Attending, Department of Neurology, Rehabilitation Medicine Service, Memorial Sloan Kettering Cancer Center; Assistant Professor, Division of Rehabilitation Medicine, Weill Cornell Medical College, New York, New York

CELENA SCHEEDE-BERGDAHL, PhD
Department of Kinesiology and Physical Education, McGill University, Montreal, Quebec, Canada

KI Y. SHIN, MD
Department of Palliative, Rehabilitation and Integrative Medicine, University of Texas MD Anderson Cancer Center, Houston, Texas

JULIE K. SILVER, MD
Department of Physical Medicine and Rehabilitation, Spaulding Rehabilitation Hospital, Harvard Medical School, Charlestown, Massachusetts

SEAN ROBINSON SMITH, MD
Assistant Professor and Medical Director of Cancer Rehabilitation, Department of Physical Medicine and Rehabilitation, University of Michigan, Ann Arbor, Michigan

DANIELA L. STAN, MD
Assistant Professor, Department of General Internal Medicine, Mayo Clinic, Rochester, Minnesota

NICOLE STOUT, DPT, CLT-LANA
Rehabilitation Medicine Department, National Institutes of Health, Clinical Center, Bethesda, Maryland

MICHAEL D. STUBBLEFIELD, MD
Medical Director for Cancer Rehabilitation, Kessler Institute for Rehabilitation, Department of Physical Medicine and Rehabilitation, West Orange, New Jersey

SHI-MING TU, MD
Department of Genitourinary Medical Oncology, University of Texas MD Anderson Cancer Center, Houston, Texas

MARY M. VARGO, MD
Associate Professor, Physical Medicine and Rehabilitation; Staff Physician, MetroHealth Medical Center, Case Western Reserve University, Cleveland, Ohio

KERRI WINTERS-STONE, PhD
School of Nursing, Knight Cancer Institute, Oregon Health & Science University, Portland, Oregon

ERIC WISOTZKY, MD
Director of Cancer Rehabilitation, MedStar National Rehabilitation Network; Assistant Professor of Rehabilitation Medicine, Georgetown University School of Medicine, Washington, DC

RAJESH YADAV, MD
Department of Palliative, Rehabilitation and Integrative Medicine, University of Texas MD Anderson Cancer Center, Houston, Texas

DAVID S. ZUCKER, MD, PhD
Swedish Cancer Institute, Swedish Medical Center, Seattle, Washington

Contents

> The relevance of cancer rehabilitation as a public health issue grows
> steadily as cancer incidence, survival, and mean patient age increase. Re-
> ported rates of physical impairment and disability are already high, prior to
> the anticipated influx of aged cancer survivors. Despite the high prevalence
> of cancer-related disablement, treatment rates, even for readily remediable
> physical impairments, are as low as 1–2%. In addition to low referral rates,
> a challenge to patient-centric cancer rehabilitation is a fractured system
> that requires multiple visits to a range of specialists to address even a sin-
> gle issue, and cancer survivors generally have several. Effective solutions
> must acknowledge the limited cancer rehabilitation clinical work force
> and its clustering in tertiary centers, as well as the lack of consensus
> regarding the essential and effective components of a cancer rehabilitation
> program. A number of models of cancer rehabilitation service delivery have
> been developed, but, as yet, none have been empirically validated. This pa-
> per describes these models and proposes a taxonomy for stratifying the
> needs of cancer survivors. Modalities used to preserve or restore function
> among survivors range from simple, relatively intuitive activities to com-
> plex, integrated programs that include diagnostic and multi-modal phar-
> macological, manual, and even procedural interventions. Criteria for
> determining a survivor's needs across this spectrum are proposed, and
> the role of the physiatrist as a vital advocate and champion discussed.

> Acute care is usually associated with disease progression, treatments
> for cancer, and medical comorbidities. Patients with cancer may
> develop sudden functional deficits that require rehabilitation. Some of
> these patients benefit from acute rehabilitation, others benefit from
> subacute rehabilitation. After acute rehabilitation, continuous care for
> these patients has not been well described. Three studies are presented
> to demonstrate that cancer rehabilitation is a continuous process.
> Rehabilitation professionals should know how to detect fall risk, monitor
> symptoms, and render symptom management. Patients with cancer

As cancer evolves from a terminal illness to a chronic medical condition, so too does the view of clinical services. Palliative care and physical medicine and rehabilitation (PM&R) will increase in acceptance because they provide a valuable resource. The overarching theme is improving cancer-related symptoms or treatment-related side effects, improving patient health-related quality of life, lessening caregiver burden, and valuing patient-centered care and shared decision making. Managing symptom burden may improve therapy participation/performance. PM&R and palliative care departments are well-equipped to develop patient-centered care protocols, and could play an important role in developing a universal measure of performance status.

This review by a 10-member panel of experts in surgical prehabilitation addresses processes that may improve oncologic care. Surgical prehabilitation is the process on the continuum of care that occurs between the time of cancer diagnosis and the beginning of surgical treatment. The panel focused on the current state-of-the-science and recommended future research that would help to identify the elements that enhance preoperative physical, nutritional, and psychological health in anticipation of surgery, mitigate the burden of disease, facilitate the return of patient health status to baseline values, decrease postoperative morbidity, and reduce health care costs.

Cancer-related fatigue (CRF) is commonly reported by patients with cancer before, during, and after treatment. It is a persistent sense of tiredness that interferes with function, is distressing, and requires monitoring and, possibly, treatment. Fatigue assessment requires objective measures and self-reports, such as Functional Assessment of Cancer Therapy–Fatigue. Significant contributors to CRF include anemia, pain, insomnia, depressive symptoms, and elevated BMI. Elevated inflammatory cytokines, diabetes mellitus, cortisol, and cellular dysregulation have been associated with CRF. None is causal. Effective treatments include correction of other medical problems, especially anemia, cognitive behavioral therapy, exercise, modafinil, and corticosteroids for short-term use.

impairment: involvement of the skin/fascial and cardiopulmonary organ systems, as well as steroid-induced myopathy and bone and joint destruction.

Deconstructing Postmastectomy Syndrome: Implications for Physiatric Management

Eric Wisotzky, Nicole Hanrahan, Thomas P. Lione, and Susan Maltser

Postmastectomy pain syndrome is a common sequela of breast cancer treatment that can lead to impairments and limited participation in work, recreational, and family roles. Pain can originate from multiple anatomic sites. A detailed evaluation to determine the specific cause or causes of pain will help guide the clinician to successfully manage this pain syndrome. There are many available treatments, but more evidence is needed for the efficacy of rehabilitation, pharmacologic, and nonpharmacologic therapy. There is evidence for some effective treatments to prevent this syndrome, but, here also, more research is needed.

Rehabilitation Strategies and Outcomes of the Sarcoma Patient

Sean Robinson Smith

Sarcomas are a relatively rare cancer that, depending on the location, can cause significant neuromusculoskeletal dysfunction and require rehabilitation interventions to reduce pain, restore function, and improve quality of life. This review focuses on sarcoma subtypes that frequently cause these complications: bony and soft tissue sarcomas leading to limb salvage or amputation, desmoid tumors, and malignant peripheral nerve sheath tumors. Rehabilitation approaches and outcomes are discussed, as well as considerations for childhood sarcoma survivors transitioning to adulthood.

Alternative Exercise Traditions in Cancer Rehabilitation

Kathryn J. Ruddy, Daniela L. Stan, Anjali Bhagra, Mary Jurisson, and Andrea L. Cheville

Alternative exercise traditions (AETs) such as Pilates, yoga, Tai Chi Chuan, Qigong, and various forms of dance offer the potential to improve diverse outcomes among cancer survivors by reducing adverse symptoms and mood disorders, and by enhancing function. Additionally AETs have emerged as a potential means to address deficits in current disease-focused care delivery models which are marked by prevalent under-treatment of symptoms and physical impairments. Relative to therapeutic exercise in allopathic models, many AETs are comparatively affordable and accessible. AETs have the further potential to simultaneously address needs spanning multiple domains including social, physical, and psycho-emotional. AETs additionally offer the salient benefits of promoting integrated whole body movement and concurrently enhancing strength, coordination, balance, posture, flexibility, and kinesthetic awareness. Despite AETs' benefits, compelling concerns leave many clinicians ambivalent and reluctant to endorse or even discuss them. One issue is the extensive heterogeneity across and even within specific AETs. An additional concern is that the one-size-fits-many nature of AET group classes undermines an instructor's capacity to individualize dose, type, frequency, and intensity, which are cornerstones of effective therapeutic exercise. Inconsistencies in AET practitioner expertise and certification, as well as the extent of practitioner familiarity with vulnerabilities unique to cancer populations, may also be problematic. At this juncture, an extensive literature of inconsistent quality that spans diverse cancer populations frustrates efforts to precisely determine the effect size of any specific AET in improving a specific outcome; Although systematic reviews and meta-analyses have concluded that AETs have beneficial effects, they consistently identify a high risk of bias in a majority of trials related to a lack of blinding, poor allocation concealment, small sample sizes, and incomplete outcome data.

With numerous advancements in early detection and multimodal therapy, cancer has become a chronic disease. As the number of cancer survivors continues to increase, physiatrists and other neuromuscular disease specialists are more likely to encounter individuals with residual impairments, disabilities, and/or handicaps resulting from cancer or related treatments. The patient with cancer is especially prone to injury directed at the peripheral nervous system at multiple anatomic levels. Electrodiagnosis is an invaluable tool in the evaluation of neuromuscular disorders in this patient population.

PHYSICAL MEDICINE AND REHABILITATION CLINICS OF NORTH AMERICA

FORTHCOMING ISSUES

May 2017
Traumatic Brain Injury
Blessen C. Eapen and David X. Cifu,
Editors

August 2017
Pelvic Pain
Kelly Scott, *Editor*

November 2017
Promoting Health and Wellness in the Geriatric Patient
David A. Soto-Quijano,
Editor

RECENT ISSUES

November 2016
Regenerative Medicine
Santos F. Martinez, *Editor*

August 2016
Outpatient Ultrasound-Guided Musculoskeletal Techniques
Evan Peck, *Editor*

May 2016
Concussion in Sports
Scott R. Laker, *Editor*

February 2016
Running Injuries
Michael Fredericson and Adam Tenforde,
Editors

RELATED INTEREST

Hematology/Oncology Clinics of North America, June 2016 (Vol. 30, Issue 3)
Transfusion Medicine
Jeanne E. Hendrickson and Christopher A. Tormey, *Editors*

VISIT THE CLINICS ONLINE!
Access your subscription at:
www.theclinics.com

Foreword

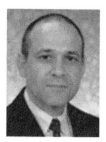

Santos F. Martinez, MD, MS
Consulting Editor

Physical medicine and rehabilitation provides care for a wide array of disorders requiring the clinician to at times have chameleon-like qualities.

Rehabilitation oncology is composed of such a diversity of challenges and clinical syndromes as to intimidate many nonsubspecialty physicians. Many of us are in facilities and practices that have limited exposure to this population, which makes it difficult to develop an expertise. We are certainly in gratitude to Dr Cheville for bringing these topics to the forefront to serve as a resource for expanding our base of knowledge.

I am also in gratitude to Carmen and other such cancer survivors, who inspire us on a daily basis with their courage and fortitude to meet and surpass the many hardships on the road to recovery. There are many players behind the scenes providing support and at times just basic necessities (eg, Ronald McDonald House Charities) that certainly also play an important part in our rehabilitation team.

Santos F. Martinez, MD, MS
American Academy of Physical Medicine
and Rehabilitation
Campbell Clinic Orthopaedics
Department of Orthopaedics
University of Tennessee
Memphis, TN 38104, USA

E-mail address:
smartinez@campbellclinic.com

Phys Med Rehabil Clin N Am 28 (2017) xiii
http://dx.doi.org/10.1016/j.pmr.2016.10.002
1047-9651/17/© 2016 Published by Elsevier Inc.

pmr.theclinics.com

Preface

Cancer Rehabilitation: Forging Consensus

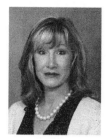

Andrea L. Cheville, MD, MSCE
Editor

This issue of *Physical Medicine and Rehabilitation Clinics of North America* represents an attempt to provide an overview of current cancer rehabilitation. Its timing could not be more opportune as the last ten years have seen a rapidly growing recognition of its importance, an unprecedented incorporation of its practices into clinical care, and the establishment of an increasing number of training programs.

This growth has been accompanied by a maturation of our field and a growing presence at national meetings and in the medical literature. In addition, a number of themes/concepts are emerging that are shaping our thinking about how we treat cancer and provide our services. Among these are the potential role of prehabilitation; the complementary natures of rehabilitation and palliative care; the growth of cancer survivorship awareness; and, not least, the impact of governmental policy. Advances outside our field influence, and will continue to influence, our care as well. Notably, patient-reported outcomes (PROs) have gained such acceptance that the systematic collection of patients' perceptions of the benefits of their care is now required by payers, policymakers, and advocacy groups. Similarly, the mandated and growing presence of electronic health records (EHRs) provides an unmatched opportunity to evaluate the function of cancer populations over time with minimal incremental effort and resources.

Unfortunately, while the last decade has seen a large growth in the provision of cancer rehabilitation services, this growth has not been matched by a comparable intensification of our research activities. As a consequence, uncertainty regarding the effectiveness of different treatment elements impacts an ever-increasing number of patients as well as the acceptance of our efforts by our colleagues. The heart of this problem is that we lack the infrastructure that will allow us to generate, much less effectively translate, findings into routine clinical practice. For example, the evidence base for strength and aerobic training in cancer populations has grown largely through the efforts of exercise physiologists, yet these advances have not spurred their routine

Phys Med Rehabil Clin N Am 28 (2017) xv–xvi
http://dx.doi.org/10.1016/j.pmr.2016.10.001
1047-9651/17/© 2016 Published by Elsevier Inc.

pmr.theclinics.com

availability to the patient. In effect, there are two breakdowns in the process: (1) we lack the research base necessary to further the development of our field, and (2) even when knowledge is available, we lack the means to translate it effectively to clinical care.

Such deficits are no longer tenable in light of the growing impact of cancer and its treatment on the patient, the caregiver, and society. The old adage was, "Care delayed is care denied." Since we know that function lost in the later stages of cancer is seldom recovered, our new adage might be "care delayed is function lost."

The limited number of large-scale cancer rehabilitation trials and observational studies underway makes it unlikely that our evidence base will improve markedly over the next five years. The growing importance of PROs and EHRs will be beneficial, but the bulk of their impact will be in the future. As a result, there is a pressing need for an authoritative, interdisciplinary consensus sponsored by the appropriate credentialing bodies, professional societies, consumer groups, and payers that leverages the best of clinical experience with the best available evidence. The consensus should highlight not only which cancer rehabilitation services should be universally available but also the most problematic gaps in evidence and training.

The caliber and diversity of the contributing authors in this issue are extraordinary. The distribution of their thoughts over the gamut of cancer rehabilitation should not only be useful for the reader but it is hoped will also serve as fodder and support for this needed consensus.

Andrea L. Cheville, MD, MSCE
Department of Physical Medicine
and Rehabilitation
Care Experience Program
Center for the Science of Health Care Delivery
Mayo Clinic
200 First Street Southwest
Rochester, MN 55905, USA

E-mail address:
cheville.andrea@mayo.edu

Cancer Rehabilitation

An Overview of Current Need, Delivery Models, and Levels of Care

Andrea L. Cheville, MD, MSCE[a],*, Karen Mustian, PhD, MPH[b],
Kerri Winters-Stone, PhD[c], David S. Zucker, MD, PhD[d],
Gail L. Gamble, MD[a], Catherine M. Alfano, PhD[e]

KEYWORDS

- Cancer rehabilitation • Delivery models • Levels of care

KEY POINTS

- Reported rates of cancer-related physical impairment and disability are currently high and expected to increase, but treatment rates, even for readily remediable physical impairments, remain as low as 1% to 2%.
- A limited clinical workforce has cancer rehabilitation training and these individuals are largely clustered in tertiary centers giving rise to access barriers.
- There is a need to clarify the scope of cancer rehabilitation by identifying its critical and effective components so that these can be made available to all survivors across diverse care settings.
- Currently, no accreditation, reimbursement, or designation criteria require institutions to provide high-quality cancer rehabilitation services.
- Models of cancer rehabilitation service delivery have been developed, but, as yet, none has been empirically validated.

SCOPE OF THE ISSUE

The relevance of cancer rehabilitation as a public health issue grows steadily as cancer incidence, survival, and mean patient age increase.

Epidemiology

Per latest estimates, 15.5 million cancer survivors currently reside in the United States.[1] This figure includes patients presumed cured and those with active disease.

[a] Department of Physical Medicine and Rehabilitation, Mayo Clinic, 200 First Street SW, Rochester, MN 55905, USA; [b] University of Rochester Medical Center, Department of Surgery, 601 Elmwood Avenue, Rochester, NY 14642, USA; [c] School of Nursing, Knight Cancer Institute, Oregon Health & Science University, 3181 S.W. Sam Jackson Park Road, Portland, OR 97239-3098, USA; [d] Swedish Cancer Institute, Swedish Medical Center, 1101 Madison, Suite 200, Seattle, WA 98104, USA; [e] American Cancer Society, Inc, 250 Williams Street NW, Atlanta, GA 30303, USA
* Corresponding author.
E-mail address: Cheville.andrea@mayo.edu

Phys Med Rehabil Clin N Am 28 (2017) 1–17
http://dx.doi.org/10.1016/j.pmr.2016.08.001
1047-9651/17/© 2016 Published by Elsevier Inc.

In less than 10 years, the US prevalence of cancer survivorship, similarly defined, will approach 20 million, and current estimates do not account for increased responsiveness achieved with biological agents, precision medicine, and the expansion of screening programs.[2] The advancing age of the US population will contribute not only to increased prevalence but also to an increased burden of disability among cancer survivors.[2,3] Older cancer survivors have increased rates of multimorbidity, premorbid disablement, and cancer treatment–related toxicity.[4,5] It is expected that by 2020 approximately three-quarters of cancer survivors will be age 65 or older.[3]

Reported rates of physical impairment and disability are already high, prior to the anticipated influx of aged cancer survivors. Efforts to systematically describe rates of physical impairments have highlighted differences across survivorship populations. For example, 20% of childhood compared with 53% of adult-onset cancer survivors report limitations in their functioning,[6] and as many as two-thirds of breast cancer survivors experience 1 or more long-term adverse sequelae (eg, fatigue, lymphedema, pain, and contractures).[7] As expected, rates of physical impairment increase among patients with metastatic cancer. In a cohort of 163 patients receiving treatment of stage IV breast cancer, 92% endorsed at least 1 physical impairment, and the mean number of impairments per patient was 3.3.[8] The presence of physical impairments reduces quality-of-life (QOL) and participation in work, family, and society. Additionally, the presence of impairments and related disability radically increase health care utilization.[9]

Despite the high prevalence of cancer-related disablement, treatment rates, even for readily remediable physical impairments, are as low as 1% to 2%.[10] The reasons for the decades-long persistence of undertreatment are complex and multifold. Low detection, documentation, and referral rates in oncology practices are an important factor.[10] Systemic issues, however, for example, shortages of oncologists[11] and primary care practitioners,[12] that constrain attention directed beyond cancer treatment, also contribute. The United States increasingly struggles to meet the complex and varied needs of its rapidly expanding cancer survivor population. Advocates have proposed both de facto operationalized and novel models for cancer rehabilitation that range from a discrete focus on singular impairments to a more holistic scope that encompasses survivors' physical, psychological, vocational, and social capabilities.[13]

A challenge to integrated, comprehensive and patient-centric cancer rehabilitation is the currently fractured system that requires multiple visits to a range of specialists spanning different disciplines to address even a single issue, and cancer survivors generally have several. A similar challenge has been highlighted by Bruera and Hui[14] in palliative care. Cancer survivors, irrespective of their disease or treatment status, have limited fiscal and energetic resources. Their support systems are often overtaxed and frayed. Even were there an adequately trained and geographically dispersed clinical workforce, the travel, temporal, and monetary demands of current fee-for-service care delivery structures would pose formidable access barriers. Although the raw ingredients for a reconceptualization of medical practice and reimbursement are present in the Affordable Care Act, it may take decades to have a meaningful impact on the legacy of fee-for-service reimbursement on the delivery of multidisciplinary supportive care.[15] This situation highlights the vital need to meet as many needs as possible with a 1-stop shop, near-term solution. Physiatrists with their diagnostic, prescriptive, educational, and advocacy capabilities are poised to play a vital role.

This article proposes a skeletal taxonomy for stratifying the needs of cancer survivors, examines models of cancer rehabilitation that are de facto operational and others that remain largely theoretic, and highlights important considerations in developing pragmatic, near-term solutions to cancer survivors' pressing need for function-directed care.

Needed First Steps

Any effective solution to the challenge of meeting cancer survivors' disparate rehabilitation needs must acknowledge the alarmingly limited clinical workforce with cancer rehabilitation training and that such clinicians are largely clustered in tertiary centers where fewer than 15% of patients receive their cancer care.[16] In addition to training more providers in cancer rehabilitation, the provider shortage underscores the need to explore strategies that neutralize personnel and geographic barriers. Legislative, infrastructural, and technological support for telemedicine has increased, and trials are currently under way to determine the comparative effectiveness of tele-rehabilitation for cancer-related symptoms and disablement. A complementary approach to extending the reach of limited cancer rehabilitation specialists is the empowerment and support of nonspecialist clinicians to detect and treat threats to survivors' functionality. Guidelines, print materials, and Web-based resources for the management of even common cancer-related impairments are, however, currently limited. As discussed later, survivors find travel and copayments burdensome.[17] It may, therefore, be most patient-centric to address their primary rehabilitation issues through the local providers that address their primary and cancer-directed care and restrict physiatric consultations for problems that have not responded to first-line therapy or occur in complex and morbid individuals. For this to occur, however, it is essential that physiatrists and specialty-trained cancer therapists work to enable primary providers and oncological care teams, which should include varied types of highly qualified allied health professionals to provide first-line rehabilitative interventions.

If cancer rehabilitation is to advance, there is also a critical need to forge consensus regarding its scope. No one argues that cancer survivors have staggeringly complex needs spanning physical, vocational, and sexual domains, to name a few. A majority of survivors endorse 1 or more of the following: fatigue, cognitive dysfunction, pain, neuropathies, balance problems, mobility issues, lymphedema, bladder and bowel problems, stoma care, dysphonia and other communication difficulties, dysphagia, and psychosocial problems.[18,19] This heterogeneity is compounded by treatments of these issues that may require diverse modalities, including conventional allopathic and alternative treatments. **Fig. 1** displays potential components of a comprehensive cancer rehabilitation program — in addition to the generally accepted medical management of impairments and comorbidities that degrade function — suggested during a summit held at the National Institutes of Health in 2015 and recently described in the *Archives of Physical Medicine and Rehabilitation*.[20] The scope in **Fig. 1** reflects the diverse disciplines and therapeutic approaches currently allied to cancer rehabilitation. An alarming corollary of this breadth, because a minority of survivors currently receive even rudimentary cancer rehabilitation, is that services can only reliably and democratically be provided that fall within an aggressively constrained scope. Therefore, an initial minimalist approach emphasizing access over breadth seems reasonable. Rigorous constraint need not be fixed and should evolve over time as capacity increases. At present, however, identifying survivors' most pressing and prevalent needs, determining which evidence-based treatments effectively mitigate them, and establishing a conservative but doable structure for delivering these treatments, are logical first steps.

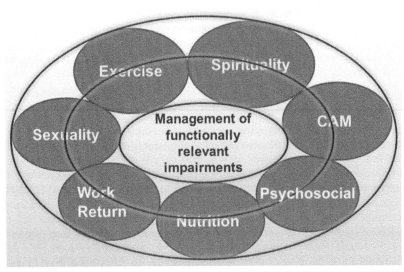

Fig. 1. Potential components of a comprehensive cancer rehabilitation program. CAM, complementary and alternative medicine.

Uncertainty regarding the roles of different disciplines in providing cancer rehabilitation services is, in part, a consequence of scope ambiguity. In addition to physiatrists, physical, occupational, recreational, and speech therapists; athletic trainers; exercise physiologists; and nurses routinely provide function-oriented care. Some oncological clinicians also extend their practices to encompass dimensions of care, such as lymphedema and fatigue management. National efforts from the American Society of Clinical Oncology and the American Cancer Society are beginning in 2016 to better coordinate and deliver care for people with cancer. In the past, however, limited consensus has been forged regarding disciplinary roles in cancer rehabilitation and needed patterns of interdisciplinary referrals and interface. As a result, idiosyncratic and institution-specific patterns of care delivery have developed. These generally reflect clinician skills and interest, and institutional emphases, for example, allogeneic bone marrow transplantation. This diversity of delivery patterns reinforces role ambiguity and sustains a lack of clarity regarding the essential components of a cancer rehabilitation program. For example, the MD Anderson Cancer Center rehabilitation program focuses on its imbedded inpatient acute rehabilitation facility,[21,22] whereas the Memorial Sloan Kettering Cancer Center's is more outpatient directed. Although institutional differences are inevitable and often positive, emerging organically from unique institutional strengths to meet the needs of specific populations, they have had the unfortunate effect of perpetuating cancer rehabilitation's nebulous components and boundaries. Consequently, oncological trainees, for example, medical, radiation, and surgical oncologists, have not had the opportunity to learn practice patterns that integrate rehabilitation services in a manner that generalizes across care settings.

Because many cancer rehabilitation interventions are nonurgent and negotiated, patient preferences play a central role. Several findings warrant mention. First, whereas a majority of cancer survivors do not discuss exercise or their functionality with either their primary or oncological care teams,[23–25] they prefer that oncologists initiate discussions about exercise and make appropriate referrals.[25] This preference has been noted across different institutions and survivor populations.[26] Second, survivors desire the continuous delivery of exercise-related information, particularly as it relates to their cancer, beginning early in the course of their treatment with appropriate adaptation as they complete or change treatments and, ultimately, as some enter long-term disease-free survivorship.[27] Third, up to two-thirds of patients with late-stage cancer express ambivalence or disinterest in receiving rehabilitation services despite high rates of disability and related distress.[28] Last, some cancer survivors have limited understanding of the dose, type, and frequency of exercise required to achieve symptom relief and functional improvement, with many maintaining that their usual daily activities offer sufficient rigor.[26] These issues highlight the critical importance of educational initiatives targeting patients and providers to screen for impairments that may make independent exercise unsafe without rehabilitation interventions and to clarify the benefits of integrating activity enhancement and rehabilitative service provision in conventional cancer care.

What Stakeholders Say — Mixed Messages

The number of large-scale, high profile, cancer-related organizations, both federal and private, that endorse the importance of cancer rehabilitation is simultaneously reassuring and disheartening, the latter because although over the last decade, the National Comprehensive Cancer Network, National Cancer Institute (NCI), American Society of Clinical Oncology, and American Cancer Society have all increasingly emphasized the functional needs of survivors, no accreditation, reimbursement, or designation criteria require institutions to provide high-quality cancer rehabilitation services. Strikingly, the NCI's mission statement states that it "...coordinates the National Cancer Program, which conducts and supports ... rehabilitation from cancer..." Yet, the NCI does not require or recommend that its comprehensive cancer centers provide their patients with rehabilitation services.

There are several important exceptions to this general trend. First, the American College of Surgeons stands out with its Commission on Cancer mandating that, for cancer center accreditation, institutions must ensure the availability of rehabilitation services.[29] Although this is laudable and the only such mandate, it does not go far enough because it does not require on-site or coordinated delivery of cancer rehabilitation services as a standard part of cancer care. Second, in 2014, the Commission on Accreditation of Rehabilitation Facilities International (CARF) introduced accreditation standards for cancer rehabilitation specialty programs. This specialty accreditation can be applied to hospitals, health care systems, outpatient clinics, and community-based programs. Although availability of the new CARF accreditation may not incentivize institutions, it represents a vital first step as a formal effort to enumerate the essential components of a cancer rehabilitation program. Three provider certification programs have also been developed. The Survivorship Training and Rehabilitation program, a commercial entity, offers therapist training that may lead to institutional Survivorship Training and Rehabilitation certification. The American College of Sports Medicine developed a certifying examination for cancer exercise trainers.[30] The American Physical Therapy Association recently developed oncology certification for physical therapists, although administration of the first certification examination is not anticipated until Spring 2019. As yet, the outcome and utilization implications of practitioner or institutional certification are not known.

PROPOSED MODELS FOR THE DELIVERY OF CANCER REHABILITATION SERVICES

Several different models of cancer rehabilitation service delivery have been developed, some only in theory and others operationalized in the absence of theoretic frameworks. In the models described later, attention is paid to their assumptions regarding cancer rehabilitation workforce availability, reimbursement structures, referring providers' (mostly oncologic clinicians) receptivity and bandwidth, patient burden, and implementation constraints related to geography and built environment. Soberingly, none has been empirically tested. The need for empiricism becomes more urgent as available resources and stakeholder appetites contract due to the skyrocketing costs of disease-directed cancer care and as cancer patients become progressively older and more functionally impaired.[31]

Prospective Surveillance Model

In the prospective surveillance model (PSM), rehabilitation begins at diagnosis with a multidimensional, comprehensive assessment, usually conducted preoperatively, which is followed by serial, scheduled follow-up visits with a specialized provider.[32] Evaluation at the time of diagnoses establishes patients' baseline functioning and identifies individuals with preexisting conditions who are potentially predisposed to developing toxicities and impairments. In this manner it is akin to the comprehensive geriatric assessment that has been proposed as a critical initial element of caring for aged cancer patients. The PSM recommends a comprehensive function-focused evaluation that includes history taking regarding function-limiting symptoms, previous function-degrading injuries, and current exercise patterns as well as a physical examination with expanded musculoskeletal and neurologic components. Although not explicitly enumerated in the PSM, objective performance testing (eg, Timed Up and Go test) and patient-reported outcome (PRO)-based measures for symptoms, receptivity to exercise, and function may be used to detect meaningful change during follow-up visits.[33,34]

The PSM specifies ongoing surveillance with repeated visits to a specialized provider. The intent of the follow-up visits is to monitor for treatment toxicities and impairments and to administer appropriate and timely treatment as required. Follow-up visits afford the treatment team the opportunity to ensure resolution of problems over time and to promote wellness through general activity enhancement, stress management, and healthy eating.

Published experience with the PSM is restricted to a case series of 196 breast cancer survivors treated at the Walter Reed National Military Medical Center in Bethesda, Maryland.[35] Reports suggest that the PSM may reduce lymphedema incidence and accelerate recovery of shoulder range of motion, although the absence of a comparator group makes it impossible to isolate benefit attributable to the PSM.[35,36] In the National Naval Medical Center's implementation of the PSM, expert cancer rehabilitation physical therapists evaluated patients preoperatively and 3, 6, 9, and 12 months after surgery. Reports did not describe the number, type, or treatment of physical impairments that were detected through the PSM. An important aspect was the use of an optoelectrical volumeter (Perometer, JUZO®, USA) to measure arm volumes at all visits. A 3% relative increase in the volume of the arm ipsilateral to the breast cancer triggered the prescription of a compression garment. The practice was credited with reducing lymphedema incidence, although a larger study failed to replicate these results.[37]

In discussing the pros and cons of the PSM, a distinction must be drawn between how the model was implemented at the Walter Reed National Military Medical Center, the approach with a degree of empirical validation, and how the model was described in a supplement to the journal *Cancer*.[32] The latter was nonprescriptive regarding provider types or roles, and enlarged the scope of the model to encompass wellness activities and domains of survivorship care that do not fall exclusively within the purview of rehabilitation, for example, bone health, fatigue management, and so forth. Perhaps the most salient and positive attribute of both PSM versions is the comprehensive baseline functional assessment. This assessment is feasible through established care delivery and reimbursement structures as a conventional visit to a physiatrist, physical therapist, or other allied health specialist. The general physical therapy (PT) workforce is distributed with sufficient breadth to ensure patient access in all but the most remote areas. Standardization could be achieved by conditioning reimbursement on the completion of designated forms, in a manner similar to work capacity evaluation. Serial follow-up assessments to detect important changes are also a positive attribute of the PSM. An evidence base to determine how such follow-ups should occur or where thresholds for interventions should be set is, however, lacking. Having patients visit a physical therapist 4 times over the course of a year solely for screening may not represent optimal resource allocation.[38] Such visits may not be reimbursed by select payers and, for patients whose payers place an annual cap on PT visits, may consume limited visits with nontherapeutic activities. Travel and copayments are also an issue. For high-risk patients, however, the cost and inconvenience may be justified. Current iterations of the PSM do not risk-stratify patients or adjust the nature and timing of their follow-up activities accordingly. Emerging technologies may offer strategies for the cost-sensitive and patient-centric implementation of the PSM. For example, functional status and symptom burden can be assessed remotely through the use of electronic PROs and/or motion sensors. Additionally, Web-based educational strategies have been used to instruct providers in the conduct follow-up assessments and to assist generalist physiatrists and therapists in cancer survivor-directed assessments.

The PSM, even if adapted to be less costly and more patient-centric, does not adequately address the rehabilitation needs of large subgroups of cancer survivors, notably those with liquid tumors and recurrent or metastatic disease. The PSM was developed for patients with stages 0 to III breast cancer and, as implemented at the Walter Reed National Military Medical Center, designed to detect and address the typical impairments associated with breast cancer surgeries and radiation therapy. As a consequence, it may be too intensive for patients with in situ tumors and not intensive enough for patients with advanced cancers or undergoing highly morbid treatments.

Triggered Rehabilitation Referral by Procedures, Diagnoses, or Threshold Scores

A common approach to patient selection for cancer rehabilitation services is linking referrals to specific diagnoses or procedures, that is, criteria that place them in high-needs categories. This approach differs from the PSM because baseline evaluations or follow-up screenings by rehabilitation clinicians are not systematically imbedded in cancer care. At the Mayo Clinic (Rochester, Minnesota) all patients who have undergone an axillary, inguinal, or cervical lymph node dissection are referred for a PT or occupational therapy (OT) evaluation. This evaluation is frequently a patient's only visit to the therapist and includes functional screening, education, and provision with compression garments as required. Follow-up PT/OT visits or referral to a physiatrist occurs at the discretion of the treating therapist. Some institutions have used diagnoses rather than procedures as triggers for rehabilitation referrals: patients who develop chronic graft-versus-host disease, symptomatic bone metastases, and so forth. Another approach to identifying high risk patients is the use of imbedded screening during oncology appointments. An NCI-supported symptom monitoring study conducted at Northwestern University used this approach to screen for symptoms as well as disablement.[39] The approach was positively received by both providers and patients. The Collaborative Care to Preserve Performance in Cancer (COPE) Trial, also NCI-supported, uses remote patient-reported outcome–based monitoring via interactive voice recognition or a Web-based interface to screen patients with advanced-stage cancer for functional deficits who may require rehabilitation services.[40] COPE results are anticipated in the spring of 2017.

Established Rehabilitation Care Delivery Pathways

A majority of cancer survivors are hospitalized at some point after their diagnoses, and hospital-based systems for the detection and treatment of disability can serve cancer populations extremely well. A notable drawback of this delivery approach is that hospital-based rehabilitation services are generally focused on patients who have sustained acute, traumatic, or ischemic injuries with resulting major physical impairments, as in the cases of traumatic brain injury, spinal cord injury, and stroke. When cancer causes a similarly acute functional decline, affected patients are, in general, reliably identified and appropriately treated through well-established mechanisms and pathways. Research suggests that most cancer-related disablement occurs through insidious processes driven by an accumulation of mild-moderate physical impairments and adverse symptoms that ultimately overwhelm a patient's reserves and compensatory mechanisms.[41]

The International Classification of Functioning, Disability and Health

The International Classification of Functioning, Disability and Health (ICF) is more a taxonomy of conditions and impairments with the capacity to degrade function than a model for rehabilitation service delivery. Nevertheless, it offers a framework against which the breadth of a cancer rehabilitation program may be gauged. The ICF is familiar to many rehabilitation clinicians, in particular those engaged in research but is little known outside the confines of rehabilitation medicine. This is a notable drawback in cancer rehabilitation, because discourse between medical, surgical, and rehabilitation clinicians is crucial to optimizing care delivery. To date, efforts to apply the ICF to cancer rehabilitation have taken 2 forms: (1) mapping of ICF impairments onto patient-rated and clinician-rated functional measures[42] and (2) assembling core cancer-specific sets of ICF codes using modified Delphi methodology.[43,44] Neither approach has had a significant impact on clinical practice. Future application of the ICF to cancer rehabilitation will require consideration of the distinguishing characteristics of cancer-related disablement, namely the critical role of adverse symptoms and treatment toxicities. These factors tend to be far more heterogeneous and dynamic than other determinants of disability and may be underemphasized in the ICF, which emerged from more linear conceptualization of impairment, disability, and handicap.[45]

Center-based Programs

Despite obvious parallels between the acute disablement after a major cardiac or pulmonary event and the profound fatigue and weakness that may attend cancer treatment, the development of center-based reconditioning programs for patients after cancer treatment, similar to cardiac and pulmonary rehabilitation, has been limited. Numerous research studies conducted by Kerry Courneya's (Edmonton, California),

Lis Adamsen's (Copenhagen, Denmark), and Lee Jones' (New York, New York) research teams involving diverse cancer populations in all disease stages have established that patients with cancer make aerobic and strength gains similar to demographically matched, well populations. Due to the lack of an established reimbursement mechanism, however, similar programs are not available to cancer survivors in the United States.

A program pioneered in the McGill University Health Centre (Montreal, Quebec, Canada), enrolled patients both presumed disease-free and with advanced-stage cancer into an incremental aerobic conditioning and strength training center–based program enhanced with psychological services and nutritional counseling. Descriptions of the program's outcomes[46–48] suggest that patient satisfaction as well as functional and symptomatic improvements was high. Unfortunately, the approach has not gained traction. A comprehensive, interdisciplinary QOL-directed program delivered to patients receiving radiation to treat late-stage cancer was validated in 2 randomized controlled trials and shown to reduce hospitalizations while concurrently increasing the proportion of patients who completed their planned anticancer therapies.[49] Again, due to the lack of an established reimbursement mechanism, the program has not transitioned from research to pragmatic clinical implementation.

Exercise for Rehabilitation and Fitness

Robust evidence supports models of care that imbed structured exercise during and after cancer treatment to mitigate toxicity and optimize function.[50–53] Such models are somewhat discipline agnostic in that clinicians ranging from nurses to exercise physiologists have delivered effective interventions. Exercise has the established ability to ameliorate both physical and psychological toxicities, including objective parameters, such as sarcopenia, weakness, and weight gain.[54–78] Additionally, diverse exercise approaches have been well studied in cancer populations, including walking, weight lifting, yoga, and tai chi.[61,72,79] Many of these approaches have been validated as means to improve PROs, such as QOL, sleep quality, function, mood, and fatigue. Proponents of exercise for cancer survivors emphasize the need to individualize programs by accommodating physical and psychological side effects, targeting specific outcomes, and considering patient preferences.

Proponents of exercise as integral to cancer care emphasize that a majority of patients with cancer are deconditioned at cancer diagnosis. Many become more so during treatment, often to the point of frailty, leading to lower levels of aerobic fitness, muscle strength and endurance, and overall physical activity after cancer treatment.[80] Survivors often do not resume pretreatment activity levels without intervention,[24,81,82] and many require clinical interventions directed to their treatment-related impairments prior to commencing or concurrent with exercise training. Unfortunately and despite advocacy, models that integrate exercise have not been pragmatically operationalized in routine cancer care. In contrast, waning physical activity is often reinforced by advice received from clinicians to limit activity, particularly when patients are older, fatigued, or experiencing other toxicities and side effects.[4,83–87] Mounting evidence suggests that regular and moderate to high levels of exercise may be effective in secondary cancer prevention.[88,89] Because most survivors have difficulty engaging in enough exercise, however, to lower their risk of recurrence, it is imperative that conversations from providers about the importance of exercise are initiated at diagnosis and incorporated into care plans.

LEVELS OF CANCER REHABILITATION

Virtually all modalities used to preserve or restore function among patients with cancer range from simple, relatively intuitive activities that a majority of patients can perform independently with generic guidance to more complex, integrated programs that include diagnostic and multimodal pharmacologic, manual, and even procedural interventions. The former may solely require well-designed patient education materials, whereas the latter may require acute rehabilitation at an inpatient facility. **Fig. 2** illustrates the incremental levels of specialization and resource intensity that characterize cancer rehabilitation.

Several factors determine at which point along this continuum of complexity and specialization a given patient's treatment should fall. First, context is a principal consideration. Patients who are receiving aggressive anticancer therapies, have concerning comorbidities, or have cognitive, social, symptom, or psychological characteristics likely to interfere with their rehabilitation should enter this continuum at the level of collaborative specialist/physician-direct care. Patients requiring diagnostic work-up, pharmacologic management, or coordination of care across medical specialties require physician oversight. Second, therapeutic goals may range from basic, for example, restore a low level of community ambulation, to sophisticated and precise, for example, restore a female breast cancer survivor at high risk of lymphedema to competitive power lifting. Goals that require specific type, dose, and frequency of

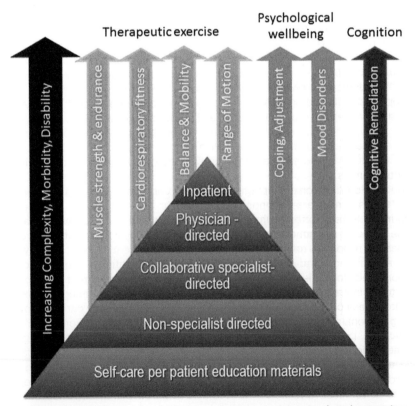

Fig. 2. The incremental levels of specialization and resource intensity that characterize cancer rehabilitation.

therapeutic exercise are generally most successfully pursued with specialist oversight. Third, high impairment severity and multiplicity also indicate a need for specialist and physician oversight. For example, after axillary surgery for breast cancer, many patients recover functional shoulder mobility with direction and encouragement to perform simple flexibility activities, often provided through print materials. Some patients, however, develop function-limiting adhesive capsulitis, whereas others may have milder range of motion restrictions but additional chemotherapy-induced impairments, for example, neuropathy, sarcopenia, and fatigue. For such patients with severe or multiple impairments, rehabilitation outcomes may be enhanced with specialist-directed treatment. Last, treatment refractoriness is an important driver to higher levels of specialization and physician involvement because it may reflect diagnostic uncertainty. This may occur when cancer fatigue persists, absent other causes, despite the provision of guideline-concordant care, or when swelling attributed to lymphedema does not reduce with decongestive therapy. In such cases, review of treatment by a specialist-directed and physician-directed diagnostic work-up may be indicated.

It is neither patient-centric, cost-sensitive, nor frankly even possible with current workforce limitations to refer all patients to cancer rehabilitation specialists to diagnose impairments and assign levels of need, as has been advocated by the PSM. Unfortunately, levels of need are not determined in routine oncology practice either. Oncology training programs do not instruct clinicians in these levels or the means to reliably refer patients for care along the continuum of specialization. Receiving little modeling or guidance in the means to direct patients to needs-matched rehabilitation, many oncology clinicians are ill equipped to triage patients. Cancer centers, having received no mandate to ensure patient access to care along the cancer rehabilitation continuum, have remained effectively mute and inactive. This situation must change, but change is unlikely in the absence of physician champions. Hence, there is a critical need for focused, consistent, and goal-directed advocacy on the part of cancer rehabilitation physiatrists that includes engaging and partnering with oncology and therapy colleagues.

A CALL TO ACTION

Physiatrists are uniquely positioned to expand cancer rehabilitation's accessibility and scope. Their qualifications stem from experience leading and coordinating multidisciplinary teams to realize patient-specific functional goals through highly individualized programs.[90] Physiatrists' holistic scope of practice has required them to play the diverse roles of diagnostician, educator, proceduralist, coach, and advocate, all of which are needed to comprehensively address the functional needs of cancer survivors. Addressing the pressing functional needs of cancer patients in a coordinated, team-oriented, and patient-centric way, however, will require physiatrists to adopt and promote a systems-based approach. Relying on nonphysiatrist stakeholders to recognize the value of cancer rehabilitation, develop service lines for basic services (eg, patient education), and refer patients to physiatrists for complex medical rehabilitation services has simply not worked, as attested by the alarming and persistently low rates of rehabilitation service utilization.[8,41,91] Low levels of physiatric involvement in developing seamless service delivery across the full spectrum of cancer rehabilitation have stymied its maturation and democratic expansion to provide survivors with a consistent access to effective services.

A forward-thinking reconceptualization of current service delivery requires shedding of constraints imposed by fee-for-services reimbursement and faith that by expanding and endorsing nonphysician dimensions of cancer rehabilitation, physiatric practices will be enhanced rather than undermined. Costly physiatric care should be reserved for complex, challenging, or nonresponding cases that potentially require pharmacologic, psychological, and procedural interventions. This is to say that physiatrists have a unique niche in the spectrum of cancer rehabilitation—although overlapping those of therapists and oncology clinicians, it is unequivocally distinct. Cancer rehabilitation physiatrists will be better able to practice at the top of their licenses by encouraging and training other providers and therapists on the team to complementarily practice at the top of their licenses as well. By executing the steps needed to expand cancer rehabilitation in a democratic manner, physiatrists will increase their bandwidth to fulfill the roles they sought and trained for, and the health care system will better meet the needs of the growing number of people living with and beyond cancer.

REFERENCES

1. Cancer Treatment & Survivorship Facts and Figures 2016-2017. 2016. Available at: http://www.cancer.org/acs/groups/content/@research/documents/document/acspc-048074.pdf. Accessed August 15, 2016.
2. de Moor JS, Mariotto AB, Parry C, et al. Cancer survivors in the United States: prevalence across the survivorship trajectory and implications for care. Cancer Epidemiol Biomarkers Prev 2013;22:561–70.
3. Parry C, Kent EE, Mariotto AB, et al. Cancer survivors: a booming population. Cancer Epidemiol Biomarkers Prev 2011;20:1996–2005.
4. Bellizzi KM, Mustian KM, Palesh OG, et al. Cancer survivorship and aging: moving the science forward. Cancer 2008;113:3530–9.
5. Avis NE, Deimling GT. Cancer survivorship and aging. Cancer 2008;113: 3519–29.
6. Stubblefield MD, Schmitz KH, Ness KK. Physical functioning and rehabilitation for the cancer survivor. Semin Oncol 2013;40:784–95.
7. Schmitz KH, Stout NL, Andrews K, et al. Prospective evaluation of physical rehabilitation needs in breast cancer survivors: a call to action. Cancer 2012;118: 2187–90.
8. Cheville AL, Troxel AB, Basford JR, et al. Prevalence and treatment patterns of physical impairments in patients with metastatic breast cancer. J Clin Oncol 2008;26:2621–9.
9. Chang S, Long SR, Kutikova L, et al. Estimating the cost of cancer: results on the basis of claims data analyses for cancer patients diagnosed with seven types of cancer during 1999 to 2000. J Clin Oncol 2004;22:3524–30.
10. Cheville AL, Beck LA, Petersen TL, et al. The detection and treatment of cancer-related functional problems in an outpatient setting. Support Care Cancer 2009; 17:61–7.
11. Erikson C, Salsberg E, Forte G, et al. Future supply and demand for oncologists: challenges to assuring access to oncology services. J Oncol Pract 2007;3: 79–86.
12. Salsberg E, Grover A. Physician workforce shortages: implications and issues for academic health centers and policymakers. Acad Med 2006;81:782–7.
13. Alfano CM, Ganz PA, Rowland JH, et al. Cancer survivorship and cancer rehabilitation: revitalizing the link. J Clin Oncol 2012;30:904–6.
14. Bruera E, Hui D. Integrating supportive and palliative care in the trajectory of cancer: establishing goals and models of care. J Clin Oncol 2010;28:4013–7.

15. Ridgely MS, de Vries D, Bozic KJ, et al. Bundled payment fails to gain a foothold In California: the experience of the IHA bundled payment demonstration. Health Aff 2014;33:1345–52.

16. NCI Community Cancer Centers Program Pilot: 2007-2010. Available at: http://ncccp.cancer.gov/Media/FactSheet.htm. Accessed August 29, 2010.

17. Kale HP, Carroll NV. Self-reported financial burden of cancer care and its effect on physical and mental health-related quality of life among US cancer survivors. Cancer 2016;122:283–9.

18. Stubblefield MD, O'Dell MW, editors. Cancer rehabiliation principles and practice. New York: Demos Medical Publishing; 2009.

19. Silver JK, Baima J, Mayer RS. Impairment-driven cancer rehabilitation: an essential component of quality care and survivorship. CA Cancer J Clin 2013;63:295–317.

20. Stout NL, Silver JK, Raj VS, et al. Towards a National Initiative in Cancer Rehabilitation: Recommendations from a Subject Matter Expert Group. Arch Phys Med Rehabil 2016. [Epub ahead of print].

21. Shin KY, Guo Y, Konzen B, et al. Inpatient cancer rehabilitation: the experience of a national comprehensive cancer center. Am J Phys Med Rehabil 2011;90:S63–8.

22. Grabois M. Integrating cancer rehabilitation into medical care at a cancer hospital. Cancer 2001;92:1055–7.

23. Jones LW, Courneya KS. Exercise discussions during cancer treatment consultations. Cancer Pract 2002;10:66–74.

24. Mustian KM, Griggs JJ, Morrow GR, et al. Exercise and side effects among 749 patients during and after treatment for cancer: a University of Rochester Cancer Center Community Clinical Oncology Program Study. Support Care Cancer 2006;14:732–41.

25. Yates JS, Mustian KM, Morrow GR, et al. Prevalence of complementary and alternative medicine use in cancer patients during treatment. Support Care Cancer 2005;13:806–11.

26. Cheville AL, Dose AM, Basford JR, et al. Insights into the reluctance of patients with late-stage cancer to adopt exercise as a means to reduce their symptoms and improve their function. J Pain Symptom Manage 2012;44:84–94.

27. Sprod LK, Peppone LJ, Palesh OG, et al. Timing of information on exercise impacts exercise behavior during cancer treatment (N=748): A URCC CCOP protocol. J Clin Oncol 2010;28(15):9138.

28. Cheville A, Rhudy L, Basford J, et al. How receptive are patients with late stage cancer to rehabilitation services and what are the sources of their resistance? Arch Phys Med Rehabil 2016. [Epub ahead of print].

29. Commission On Cancer. The commission on cancer's (CoC) cancer program standards: ensuring patient-centered care. Chicago: American College of Surgeons; 2016.

30. American College of Sports Medicine. ACSM's guidelines for exercise testing and prescription. 8th edition. Philadelphia: Lippincott Williams & Wilkins; 2016.

31. Zafar SY, Abernethy AP. Financial toxicity, Part I: a new name for a growing problem. Oncology 2013;27:80–1, 149.

32. Stout NL, Binkley JM, Schmitz KH, et al. A prospective surveillance model for rehabilitation for women with breast cancer. Cancer 2012;118:2191–200.

33. Cheville AL, Yost KJ, Larson DR, et al. Performance of an item response theory-based computer adaptive test in identifying functional decline. Arch Phys Med Rehabil 2012;93:1153–60.

34. Hahn EA, Devellis RF, Bode RK, et al. Measuring social health in the patient-reported outcomes measurement information system (PROMIS): item bank development and testing. Qual Life Res 2010;19:1035–44.

35. Stout Gergich NL, Pfalzer LA, McGarvey C, et al. Preoperative assessment enables the early diagnosis and successful treatment of lymphedema. Cancer 2008;112:2809–19.

36. Springer BA, Levy E, McGarvey C, et al. Pre-operative assessment enables early diagnosis and recovery of shoulder function in patients with breast cancer. Breast Cancer Res Treat 2010;120:135–47.

37. Specht MC, Miller CL, Russell TA, et al. Defining a threshold for intervention in breast cancer-related lymphedema: what level of arm volume increase predicts progression? Breast Cancer Res Treat 2013;140:485–94.

38. Cheville AL, Nyman JA, Pruthi S, et al. Cost considerations regarding the prospective surveillance model for breast cancer survivors. Cancer 2012;118:2325–30.

39. Cella D, Choi S, Garcia S, et al. Setting standards for severity of common symptoms in oncology using the PROMIS item banks and expert judgment. Qual Life Res 2014;23:2651–61.

40. Collaborative targeted case management in improving functional status in patients with stage III-IV cancer. Clinicaltrials.gov. 2012. Available at: https://clinicaltrials.gov/ct2/show/NCT01721343?term=cheville&rank=3. Accessed January 29, 2015.

41. Cheville AL, Kornblith AB, Basford JR. An examination of the causes for the underutilization of rehabilitation services among people with advanced cancer. Am J Phys Med Rehabil 2011;90:S27–37.

42. Gilchrist LS, Galantino ML, Wampler M, et al. A framework for assessment in oncology rehabilitation. Phys Ther 2009;89:286–306.

43. Glaessel A, Kirchberger I, Stucki G, et al. Does the Comprehensive International Classification of Functioning, Disability and Health (ICF) Core Set for Breast Cancer capture the problems in functioning treated by physiotherapists in women with breast cancer? Physiotherapy 2011;97:33–46.

44. Brach M, Cieza A, Stucki G, et al. ICF core sets for breast cancer. J Rehabil Med 2004;121–7.

45. Nagi S. Disability concepts revisited: implication for prevention. In: Pope A, Tarlov A, editors. Disability in America: toward a national agenda for prevention. Washington, DC: Institute of Medicine; Division of Health Promotion and Disease Prevention; National Academy Press; 1991. p. 309–27.

46. Gagnon B, Murphy J, Eades M, et al. A prospective evaluation of an interdisciplinary nutrition-rehabilitation program for patients with advanced cancer. Curr Oncol 2013;20:310–8.

47. Eades M, Murphy J, Carney S, et al. Effect of an interdisciplinary rehabilitation program on quality of life in patients with head and neck cancer: review of clinical experience. Head Neck 2013;35:343–9.

48. Chasen MR, Bhargava R. A rehabilitation program for patients with gastroesophageal cancer–a pilot study. Support Care Cancer 2010;18(Suppl 2):S35–40.

49. Cheville AL, Alberts SR, Rummans TA, et al. Improving adherence to cancer treatment by addressing quality of life in patients with advanced gastrointestinal cancers. J Pain Symptom Manage 2015;50:321–7.

50. Winters-Stone KM, Dobek JC, Bennett JA, et al. Skeletal response to resistance and impact training in prostate cancer survivors. Med Sci Sports Exerc 2014;46:1482–8.

51. Schmitz KH, Courneya KS, Matthews C, et al. American College of Sports Medicine roundtable on exercise guidelines for cancer survivors. Med Sci Sports Exerc 2010;42:1409–26.

52. Jones LW, Demark-Wahnefried W. Diet, exercise, and complementary therapies after primary treatment for cancer. Lancet Oncol 2006;7:1017–26.

53. Winters-Stone KM, Beer TM. Review of exercise studies in prostate cancer survivors receiving androgen deprivation therapy calls for an aggressive research agenda to generate high-quality evidence and guidance for exercise as standard of care. J Clin Oncol 2014;32:2518–9.

54. Demark-Wahnefried W, Clipp EC, Morey MC, et al. Lifestyle intervention development study to improve physical function in older adults with cancer: outcomes from Project LEAD. J Clin Oncol 2006;24:3465–73.

55. Morey MC, Snyder DC, Sloane R, et al. Effects of home-based diet and exercise on functional outcomes among older, overweight long-term cancer survivors: RENEW: a randomized controlled trial. JAMA 2009;301:1883–91.

56. Campo RA, Agarwal N, LaStayo PC, et al. Levels of fatigue and distress in senior prostate cancer survivors enrolled in a 12-week randomized controlled trial of Qigong. J Cancer Surviv 2014;8:60–9.

57. Winters-Stone KM, Leo MC, Schwartz A. Exercise effects on hip bone mineral density in older, post-menopausal breast cancer survivors are age dependent. Arch Osteoporos 2012;7:301–6.

58. Cormie P, Galvao DA, Spry N, et al. Can supervised exercise prevent treatment toxicity in patients with prostate cancer initiating androgen-deprivation therapy: a randomised controlled trial. BJU Int 2015;115:256–66.

59. Winters-Stone KM, Lyons KS, Dobek J, et al. Benefits of partnered strength training for prostate cancer survivors and spouses: results from a randomized controlled trial of the Exercising Together project. J Cancer Surviv 2016;10(4):633–44.

60. Winters-Stone KM, Dieckmann N, Maddalozzo GF, et al. Resistance exercise reduces body fat and insulin during androgen-deprivation therapy for prostate cancer. Oncol Nurs Forum 2015;42:348–56.

61. Sprod LK, Fernandez ID, Janelsins MC, et al. Effects of yoga on cancer-related fatigue and global side-effect burden in older cancer survivors. J Geriatr Oncol 2015;6:8–14.

62. Sprod LK, Mohile SG, Demark-Wahnefried W, et al. Exercise and cancer treatment symptoms in 408 newly diagnosed older cancer patients. J Geriatr Oncol 2012;3:90–7.

63. Sprod LK, Janelsins MC, Palesh OG, et al. Health-related quality of life and biomarkers in breast cancer survivors participating in tai chi chuan. J Cancer Surviv 2012;6:146–54.

64. Sprod LK, Palesh OG, Janelsins MC, et al. Exercise, sleep quality, and mediators of sleep in breast and prostate cancer patients receiving radiation therapy. Community Oncol 2010;7:463–71.

65. Janelsins MC, Peppone LJ, Heckler CE, et al. YOCAS(c)(R) yoga reduces self-reported memory difficulty in cancer survivors in a nationwide randomized clinical trial: investigating relationships between memory and sleep. Integr Cancer Ther 2016;15(3):263–71.

66. Janelsins MC, Davis PG, Wideman L, et al. Effects of Tai Chi Chuan on insulin and cytokine levels in a randomized controlled pilot study on breast cancer survivors. Clin Breast Cancer 2011;11:161–70.

67. Peppone LJ, Janelsins MC, Kamen C, et al. The effect of YOCAS(c)(R) yoga for musculoskeletal symptoms among breast cancer survivors on hormonal therapy. Breast Cancer Res Treat 2015;150:597–604.

68. Peppone LJ, Mustian KM, Janelsins MC, et al. Effects of a structured weight-bearing exercise program on bone metabolism among breast cancer survivors: a feasibility trial. Clin Breast Cancer 2010;10:224–9.

69. Kamen C, Heckler C, Janelsins MC, et al. A dyadic exercise intervention to reduce psychological distress among lesbian, gay, and heterosexual cancer survivors. LGBT Health 2015. [Epub ahead of print].

70. Mustian KM, Katula JA, Gill DL, et al. Tai Chi Chuan, health-related quality of life and self-esteem: a randomized trial with breast cancer survivors. Support Care Cancer 2004;12:871–6.

71. Mustian KM, Peppone L, Darling TV, et al. A 4-week home-based aerobic and resistance exercise program during radiation therapy: a pilot randomized clinical trial. J Support Oncol 2009;7:158–67.

72. Mustian KM, Sprod LK, Janelsins M, et al. Multicenter, randomized controlled trial of yoga for sleep quality among cancer survivors. J Clin Oncol 2013;31:3233–41.

73. Mustian KM, Katula JA, Zhao H. A pilot study to assess the influence of tai chi chuan on functional capacity among breast cancer survivors. J Support Oncol 2006;4:139–45.

74. Brown JC, Huedo-Medina TB, Pescatello LS, et al. Efficacy of exercise interventions in modulating cancer-related fatigue among adult cancer survivors: a meta-analysis. Cancer Epidemiol Biomarkers Prev 2011;20:123–33.

75. Irwin ML, Alvarez-Reeves M, Cadmus L, et al. Exercise improves body fat, lean mass, and bone mass in breast cancer survivors. Obesity 2009;17:1534–41.

76. Gleeson M, Bishop NC, Stensel DJ, et al. The anti-inflammatory effects of exercise: mechanisms and implications for the prevention and treatment of disease. Nat Rev Immunol 2011;11:607–15.

77. Tang M-F, Liou T-H, Lin C-C. Improving sleep quality for cancer patients: benefits of a home-based exercise intervention. Support Care Cancer 2010;18:1329–39.

78. Salmon P. Effects of physical exercise on anxiety, depression, and sensitivity to stress: a unifying theory. Clin Psychol Rev 2001;21:33–61.

79. Zeng Y, Luo T, Xie H, et al. Health benefits of qigong or tai chi for cancer patients: a systematic review and meta-analyses. Complement Ther Med 2014;22:173–86.

80. Gilliam LA, St Clair DK. Chemotherapy-induced weakness and fatigue in skeletal muscle: the role of oxidative stress. Antioxid Redox Signal 2011;15:2543–63.

81. Irwin ML, Crumley D, McTiernan A, et al. Physical activity levels before and after a diagnosis of breast carcinoma. Cancer 2003;97:1746–57.

82. Courneya KS, Friedenreich CM. Relationship between exercise pattern across the cancer experience and current quality of life in colorectal cancer survivors. J Altern Complement Med 1997;3:215–26.

83. Mustian KM, Sprod LK, Janelsins M, et al. Exercise recommendations for cancer-related fatigue, cognitive impairment, sleep problems, depression, pain, anxiety, and physical dysfunction: a Review. Oncol Hematol Rev 2012;8:81–8.

84. Mustian KM, Sprod LK, Palesh OG, et al. Exercise for the management of side effects and quality of life among cancer survivors. Curr Sports Med Rep 2009;8:325–30.

85. Mustian KM, Peppone LJ, Palesh OG, et al. Exercise and cancer-related fatigue. US Oncol 2009;5:20–3.

86. Mustian KM, Morrow GR, Carroll JK, et al. Integrative nonpharmacologic behavioral interventions for the management of cancer-related fatigue. Oncologist 2007;12(Suppl 1):52–67.
87. Bellizzi KM, Mustian KM, Bowen DJ, et al. Aging in the context of cancer prevention and control : perspectives from behavioral medicine. Cancer 2008;113: 3479–83.
88. Lahart IM, Metsios GS, Nevill AM, et al. Physical activity, risk of death and recurrence in breast cancer survivors: a systematic review and meta-analysis of epidemiological studies. Acta Oncol 2015;54:635–54.
89. Ballard-Barbash R, Friedenreich CM, Courneya KS, et al. Physical activity, biomarkers, and disease outcomes in cancer survivors: a systematic review. J Natl Cancer Inst 2012;104:815–40.
90. Lehmann JF, DeLisa JA, Warren CG, et al. Cancer rehabilitation: assessment of need, development, and evaluation of a model of care. Arch Phys Med Rehabil 1978;59:410–9.
91. Cheville AL, Shen T, Chang M, et al. Appropriateness of the treatment of fatigued patients with stage IV cancer. Support Care Cancer 2013;21:229–33.

Postacute Care in Cancer Rehabilitation

Ying Guo, MD[a],*, Jack B. Fu, MD[a], Hong Guo, MD, PhD[b], Jennifer Camp, MD[c], Ki Y. Shin, MD[a], Shi-Ming Tu, MD[d], Lynn J. Palmer, PhD[e], Rajesh Yadav, MD[a]

KEYWORDS

- Cancer • Rehabilitation • Symptom management • Outpatient • Function

KEY POINTS

- Symptom management is a crucial part of cancer rehabilitation.
- Cancer patients' functional status can change depending on their disease progression, treatment side-effect, and comorbidities.
- Postacute care cancer rehabilitation is a continuous process, requiring frequent monitoring, early detection of functional loss, management of symptoms, and adjustment of goals.

INTRODUCTION

The American Cancer Society estimated 1.6 million new diagnoses of cancer in 2015. With advances in cancer diagnosis and treatment, the 5-year survival rate for all cancers has increased from 49% (1975–1977) to 67% (2006–2012).[1,2] With such improvements in survival, cancer has become more a chronic disease. Cancer survivors can be defined as persons "living with a cancer diagnosis following primary cancer treatment through the end of life."[3,4] Older adults are much more likely to be diagnosed with cancer and this group already has a higher incidence of other medical comorbidities such as diabetes, stroke, arthritis, and obesity.

In the cancer treatment trajectory, many patients are cured of disease and are able to function normally in society again, although most patients, especially older patients, may experience fluctuations of function, with a trend of decline with cancer diagnosis and treatments.[5,6] This decline is due to cancer and its treatment, and it may result

[a] Department of Palliative, Rehabilitation and Integrative Medicine, University of Texas M D Anderson Cancer Center, 1515 Holcombe Boulevard, Unit 1414, Houston, TX 77030, USA; [b] Department of Digestive Diseases, Xinqiao Hospital, The Third Military Medical University, Chongqing, China; [c] Department of Physical Medicine and Rehabilitation, Carolinas Rehabilitation, Charlotte, NC, USA; [d] Department of Genitourinary Medical Oncology, University of Texas MD Anderson Cancer Center, Houston, TX, USA; [e] Corrona Research Foundation, Albany, NY, USA
* Corresponding author.
E-mail address: yguo@mdanderson.org

Phys Med Rehabil Clin N Am 28 (2017) 19–34
http://dx.doi.org/10.1016/j.pmr.2016.09.004
1047-9651/17/© 2016 Elsevier Inc. All rights reserved.

from pain, misalignment, contracture of joints, muscle atrophy, fatigue, peripheral neuropathy malnutrition, and other symptoms. These pathologic states lead to impairment of gait and poor balance.[5] The most common factors contributing to functional decline include asthenia, anorexia, pain, fatigue, depression, and anxiety. Asthenia is characterized by significant fatigue, both mental and physical, resulting in limited endurance, tiring easily, difficulty in initiating activity and maintaining concentration, and impaired memory.[7,8] Patients admitted to acute care hospitals due to medical or surgical reasons are likely to suffer from functional deficits and further decline. Rehabilitation can help survivors and patients with cancer with physical, psychosocial, and vocational functional limitations posed by the disease and treatments.[9–13] Some patients may require inpatient rehabilitation, whereas others require subacute rehabilitation, home health, or outpatient rehabilitation.

Studies have shown that inpatient rehabilitation can improve functional status.[14] However, the following questions remain unanswered:

1. Can functional gains achieved during inpatient rehabilitation be sustained in patients with cancer?
2. When encountering a patient with cancer, how should clinicians evaluate his or her risk for falling?
3. When patients with cancer are followed up in an outpatient rehabilitation clinic after acute care, what characteristics do these patients have, and what interventions can physiatrists offer?

This article presents the authors' research in functional status following acute inpatient rehabilitation, detection of fall risk in elderly patients with cancer, and functional needs and symptoms in the outpatient cancer survivor setting.

SUSTAINING FUNCTIONAL GAIN ACHIEVED DURING INPATIENT REHABILITATION

General weakness and asthenia due to cancer and its treatments are common.[14–16] Of patients who underwent inpatient rehabilitation, 40% to 50% did so because of deconditioning, asthenia, or general weakness.[11,17]

Inpatient rehabilitation has been shown to improve functional status in deconditioned patients with cancer,[13,17,18] yet no study has assessed whether these patients are able to maintain their functional level after discharge from inpatient rehabilitation. The objective of the authors' study was to assess whether patients with general weakness can maintain their functional status measured by the Timed Get-Up-and-Go (TGUG) test and timed 50-foot walk 4 weeks after discharge from acute rehabilitation or from a consult-based rehabilitation mobile team in a comprehensive cancer center.

Methods

This study was conducted at a National Cancer Institute (NCI) Comprehensive Cancer Center with Institutional Review Board approval. Subjects with cancer who underwent rehabilitation with an acute inpatient rehabilitation or a consult-based rehabilitation inpatient mobile team and were able to ambulate with or without an assistive device or assistance from another person were recruited and assessed within 3 days of discharge. These subjects were also reassessed at a 4-week follow-up visit.

The consult-based rehabilitation team (known as the mobile team) consists of a physiatrist, physical therapist, and occupational therapist, as well as a speech therapist when indicated. This mobile team serves a similar role as inpatient rehabilitation, providing 2 hours of therapy, with a goal to directly discharge patients from acute care to home. A similar model has been described at the Mayo Clinic.[19]

Patients who had other serious orthopedic conditions or active central nervous system (CNS) disease were excluded in this study.

Functional tests were performed with or without assistive devices, including

- TGUG, as previously described[20,21]
- 50-foot walk at fastest speed.[22]

Symptoms were assessed by the Edmonton Symptom Assessment System (ESAS).[23] Each subject received standard-of-care rehabilitation on discharge, which consisted of either home health, out-patient therapy, or a maintenance exercise program.

Statistical Analysis

Descriptive statistics were used to calculate demographic data. A Wilcoxon Two-Sample t-test (continuous or ordinal data) was used to compare the variable at baseline and 4 weeks later. Statistical analyses were performed using SAS version 9.2 (SAS Institute Inc, Cary, NC, USA). A P value less than .05 was considered statistically significant.

Results

Table 1 presents the characteristics of all participants at baseline. Twenty-four eligible subjects were enrolled in the study; 12 subjects returned for follow-up at 4 weeks after discharge. The remaining 12 subjects dropped out of the study. Reasons for failure to follow-up included: hospitalization (6), death (1), procedure (2), withdrawal (1), and no-show (2, they lived 204 and 430 miles from the cancer center, respectively).

Despite the high drop-out rate, the authors found that the remaining 12 subjects were able to maintain their functional status and even showed a trend of improvement on TGUG from 13.1 seconds (10.5, 26.3) at time of discharge to 10.0 seconds (8.1, 15.0) 4 weeks after discharge ($P = .07$) (**Table 2**).

RISK-FOR-FALL EVALUATION IN A PATIENT WITH CANCER

Falls in the elderly population are very common, affecting 30% to 60% of the population.[24] A cancer diagnosis further increases the risk of falls and related mortality in the elderly.[25] Falls can cause a significant amount of morbidity and mortality; 10% to 20% of falls result in injury, fracture, postfall anxiety syndrome, hospitalization, and/or death.[24–26] Many risk factors for falls have been identified, including environmental causes, history of prior falls, depression, dizziness or vertigo, drop attacks, confusion, postural hypotension, visual disorders, syncope, urinary incontinence, weakness, balance deficits, gait deficits, and cognitive impairment.[25,27,28] An awareness of risk factors for falls is not the same as having tool to assess the risk of falls. There is a need to develop a simple clinical tool to assess fall risk.

The authors conducted research in the elderly subjects with prostate cancer undergoing androgen deprivation therapy (ADT). This is a population with higher risk for fall when compared with those not receiving ADT or healthy controls.[29–31] They have a high rate of osteopenia or osteoporosis that can lead to hip fracture and other devastating outcomes.[32] Previously, there has been some effort to develop fall assessment tools, such as the TGUG test.[33,34] However, this tool is time-consuming and requires trained staff. This study used 2 simple questions[35] to determine the association with validated objective functional tests[34,36–40] and history of fall.

Table 1
Subject characteristics at baseline (n = 24)

Male (%)	10 (42)
Mean age, years (range)	68 (41–93)
Mean weight ± SD (kg)	85 ± 26
Mean height ± SD (cm)	173 ± 11
Body mass index ± SD	28 ± 8
Race	
White: Black: Hispanic	19:4:1
Tumor diagnosis	
Solid: hematological	20:4
ESAS score	Mean ± SD
Pain	2.8 ± 2.2
Fatigue	2.6 ± 2.6
Nausea	0.5 ± 1.5
Depression	0.8 ± 1.9
Anxiety	0.8 ± 2.1
Drowsiness	2.2 ± 2.9
Shortness of breath	1.4 ± 2.4
Appetite	3.3 ± 3.3
Sleep	3.0 ± 2.7
Feeling of Well being	3.4 ± 3.2
Hemoglobin	9.8 ± 0.9
TGUG (s)	22.7 ± 13.5
Timed 50-foot fastest speed (s)	22.8 ± 10.9

Abbreviation: SD, standard deviation.

Methods

After approval from the Institutional Review Board, the authors conducted a study of 34 subjects. The inclusion criteria consisted of male gender, age 65 years or older, diagnosis of prostate cancer, capability of ambulating with or without an assistive device and without assistance from another person, received ADT for at least 3 months with a response as measured by prostate-specific antigen, received chemotherapy within the last month, and English-speaking. Subjects with active CNS disease, such as clinically evident CNS metastases, leptomeningeal disease, dementia, or encephalopathy, were excluded.

Table 2
Comparison of functional tests at the time of discharge to 4 week postdischarge (n = 12)

	Time of Discharge		4 wk After Discharge		P (Mann-Whitney U)
TGUG (s)	13.10	(10.46, 26.3)	10.00	(8.07, 15.0)	.07
Timed 50-foot fastest speed (s)	16.70	(11.95, 24.5)	13.57	(10.69, 18.9)	.15

While visiting their oncologist in the genitourinary oncology clinic, the participants were asked to complete a series of questionnaires:

- Two simple questions (answered yes or no)
  1. "Do you have difficulty climbing stairs?"
  2. "Do you have difficulty climbing down stairs?"[35]
- Fall incidence and risk factors assessment
  1. How many falls had they experienced in the past year?
  2. Did they have difficulty with their vision?
  3. Did they have difficulty with urinary incontinence?

Barthel index

Using the validated Barthel index, the participants were asked 10 questions about their physical function and ability to complete activities of daily living (ADL). Subjects reported their ability for each function using a score of 0 (dependent), or 5 (needs some help but can do something alone), or 10 (independent). The Barthel index is the sum of the score ranging from 0 to 100, with 100 being the most independent level of function.[36,40]

Edmonton Symptom Assessment System

The ESAS scale measures 9 symptoms of pain, fatigue, nausea, depression, anxiety, drowsiness, shortness of breath, appetite, and sleep on a scale from 0 to 10, with 0 being the best and 10 being the worst.[23] In addition, overall feelings of well-being were rated from 0 to 10.

Functional tests

Timed Get-Up-and-Go test Subjects were asked to rise from a seated position from a chair 17 inches from the floor, walk 10 feet as quickly and as safely as possible, turn around, and return to the chair and sit again. The time was recorded for 3 consecutive tests and the average of the 3 was used for analysis.[20,21] A time greater than or equal to 10 seconds was associated with poorer balance, slower gait speed, and decreased functional capacity.[21]

Unipedal stance test Participants stood on their dominant leg without external support for as long as possible and the time was recorded (maximum of 30 seconds).[37,40] A unipedal stance test time of less than 30 seconds is associated with a history of falls.[37]

Grip strength analysis Grip strength was measured in kilograms in the dominant arm using the Jamar Hand Dynamometer (Lafayette Instrument Co, Lafayette, IN, USA) while the subject was in the seated position with elbow flexed. The best of 3 measures were recorded for analysis.[35,38,41] For elderly males ages 70 to 79 years, a grip strength 38 plus or minus 9 kg is considered normal.[41]

Statistical Analysis

Descriptive statistics were used to calculate demographic data. A Wilcoxon Two-Sample t-test (continuous or ordinal data) was used to compare the variables at baseline and 4 weeks later. Spearman rank correlation coefficients were calculated between the functional test and postural assessments. The Fisher exact test was used to test the association between TGUG greater than 30 seconds and hospital readmission within 1 month. Statistical analyses were performed using SAS version 9.2. A P value less than .05 was considered statistically significant.

Results

Thirty-four subjects met inclusion criteria and participated in the study. **Table 3** shows that the mean age of participants was 72.6 years. All of the subjects had stage 4 diseases and 91% had metastases to bone.

Table 4 shows that subjects who reported difficulty in climbing stairs had weaker grip ($P = .045$) and significantly longer TGUG times, with a median of 10.2 seconds versus 6.7 seconds in those subjects who reported no difficulty ($P = .002$). Subjects

Table 3
Subject demographics (number = 34)

	Mean ± SD
Age (y)	73 ± 4
Weight (kg)	86 ± 16
Height (cm)	173 ± 6
Body mass index (kg/m^2)	29 ± 5
Race	n (%)
White	26 (77)
African American	4 (12)
Hispanic	1 (3)
American Indian or Alaskan	3 (9)
Location of metastases	
Bone	31 (91)
Lymph nodes	21 (62)
Bladder	3 (9)
Rectum	1 (3)
Liver	5 (15)
Lung	4 (12)
Peritoneum	1 (3)
Abdominal wall	1 (3)
Mediastinum	1 (3)
Cancer treatment	
Receiving chemotherapy	34 (100)
Receiving androgen deprivation therapy	34 (100)
History of prostate surgery	16 (47)
History of radiation	20 (59)
Current medications	
Opioids	14 (41)
Beta blocker	10 (29)
Calcium channel blocker	5 (15)
Anticholinergic	13 (38)
Benzodiazepine	3 (8.9)
Antipsychotic	1 (2.9)
Medical comorbidities	
Hypertension	23 (67.7)
Leg claudication	0 (0)
Osteoarthritis	17 (50)

Table 4
Association between functional measures and subject's report of difficulty climbing and climbing down stairs

	Difficulty Climbing Stairs? Median (Range)			Difficulty Climbing Down Stairs? Median (Range)		
	Yes (n = 15)	No (n = 19)	P-Value	Yes (n = 10)	No (n = 24)	P-Value (NS = P>.05)
TGUG (s)	10.2 (6.2–1.8)	6.7 (4.7–10.4)	.002	12.9 (6.2–21.8)	6.8 (4.7–10.8)	.008
Unipedal stance (s)	2.6 (1–30)	5.99 (1.7–30)	NS	5.6 (1–30)	4.86 (1.4–30)	NS
Grip strength (kg)	32 (18–42)	38 (25–50)	.045	31 (18–48)	38 (25–50)	NS
Barthel index	95 (70–100)	95 (90–100)	NS	90 (70–100)	97.5 (90–100)	.004

Abbreviation: NS, not statistically significant.

who reported difficulty climbing down stairs had significantly longer TGUG times with a median of 12.9 seconds versus 6.8 seconds in those subjects who reported no difficulty (P = .008). These subjects also scored lower on the Barthel index (P = .004).

Table 5 shows the association of recalled falls in the past year with various risk factors.

Fall was associated with performance on the TGUG test, poorer feeling of well-being, reported difficulty climbing stairs, and reported difficulty climbing down stairs (P = .03, P = .006, P<.001, and P = .03, respectively).

Table 6 reveals the sensitivity, specificity, and positive predictive value of 3 tools (2 simple questions and TGUG >10 seconds) in identifying fall in elderly prostate cancer subjects in the past year. The sensitivity of a positive response to the question "Do you have difficulty climbing the stairs?" was highest (80%) among the 3 tools. The specificity of negative response to the question "Do you have difficulty climbing down the stairs?" was 89%. The positive predictive value of both questions was 80%, better than that of the TGUG greater than 10 seconds (75%).

PATIENT CHARACTERISTICS AND PHYSIATRIST INTERVENTIONS AFTER ACUTE CARE

After patients with cancer are discharged from acute care, their rehabilitation issues can be followed in an outpatient setting. This retrospective study described symptom burden, functional deficits, and physiatric interventions offered. Symptom and functional deficits in an ambulatory cancer rehabilitation clinic in short-term survivors (<5 years since diagnosis [YSD]) were compared with long-term survivors (≥5 YSD).

Methods

This study was conducted at an NCI Comprehensive Cancer Center. Institutional Review Board approval was obtained. Data for 200 consecutive subjects seen in an outpatient rehabilitation clinic in a tertiary cancer center between March 2 and June 24, 2009, were collected from electronic medical records databases.

As a routine practice, a registered nurse interviewed the subject, verified medication and reason for medication, used the ESAS to assess symptoms ranging from 0 (absence of symptom) to 10 (worst symptom),[23,42] and inquired whether the subject required assistance in several activities. Physiatrists then conducted interviews with

Table 5
Association of recalled falls in the past year and risk factors

	No Falls (n = 18)		≥1 Fall (n = 16)		P-Value
	Mean ± SD	Median	Mean ± SD	Median	(NS = P>.05).
Age (year)	72 ± 3	—	73 ± 6	—	NS
Body mass index (kg/m²)	30 ± 5	—	28 ± 4	—	NS
ESAS pain	0.5 ± 1.0	0	0.88 ± 2.31	0	NS
ESAS fatigue	2.1 ± 1.9	2	2.88 ± 2.50	2	NS
ESAS nausea	0.1 ± 0.3	0	0	0	NS
ESAS depression	0.2 ± 0.5	0	1.25 ± 2.32	0	NS
ESAS anxiety	0.5 ± 1.3	0	1.44 ± 1.97	0.5	NS
ESAS drowsiness	0.8 ± 1.5	0	2 ± 2.53	0.5	NS
ESAS shortness of breath	1.1 ± 2.1	0	1.69 ± 1.78	1.5	NS
ESAS appetite	1.9 ± 2.0	2	2.6 ± 2.3	2	NS
ESAS sleep	3.0 ± 2.5	2	3.6 ± 2.7	4	NS
ESAS well-being	1.7 ± 1.8	1	3.9 ± 2.1	4.5	.006
Barthel index	96.3 ± 27.3	95	92.1 ± 27.3	95	NS
TGUG test	7.4 ± 1.8	6.8	11.1 ± 4.9	9.9	.027
Unipedal stance	10.4 ± 11.7	4.7	9.0 ± 8.9	5.7	NS
Grip strength	36.8 ± 7.1	36.0	32.9 ± 8.7	34.5	NS
	N (%)				
Opioids	5 (28)		9 (56.3)		NS
Beta blockers	5 (28)		5 (31.3)		NS
Calcium channel blockers	3 (17)		2 (12.5)		NS
Anticholinergics	6 (33)		7 (44)		NS
Benzodiazepines	1 (6)		2 (12.5)		NS
Antipsychotics	0 (0)		1 (6)		NS
Hypertension	14 (78)		9 (56)		NS
Osteoarthritis	9 (50)		8 (50)		NS
Prostate surgery	6 (33)		10 (63)		NS
Radiation	10 (56)		10 (63)		NS
Answer yes to Q1	3 (17)		12 (75)		<.001
Answer yes to Q2	2 (11)		8 (50)		.03
Answer yes to Q1 and/or Q2	3 (17)		13 (81)		<.001

Q1: "Do you have difficulty climbing stairs?"
Q2: "Do you have difficulty climbing down stairs?"
  Abbreviation: NS, not statistically significant.

the patients, performed physical examinations, and provided rehabilitation interventions.

Statistical Analysis

Specific statistical tests involved the comparison of subject characteristics between the short-term survivors (<5 YSD) and long-term survivors (≥5 YSD) using t-test and the chi-squared test. Comparison of symptoms was based on ESAS scores using the Mann-Whitney U test; comparison of medication using the chi-squared test and Fisher exact test, comparison of function using the Fisher exact test, and a

Table 6						
Sensitivity, specificity, and positive predictive value for identifying falls in the past year						
		Number of Subjects		Sensitivity (% Fallers)	Specificity (% Nonfallers)	Positive Predictive Value
		No Fall	≥1 Fall			
Answer to Q1	Yes	3	12	12/16 (80%)	15/18 (83%)	12/15 (80%)
	No	15	4			
Answer to Q2	Yes	2	8	8/16 (50%)	16/18 (89%)	8/10 (80%)
	No	16	8			
TGUG ≥10 s	Yes	3	9	9/16 (56%)	14/17 (82%)	9/12 (75%)
	No	14	7			

Q1: "Do you have difficulty climbing stairs?"
Q2: "Do you have difficulty climbing down stairs?"

comparison of rehabilitation intervention between the 2 groups using the chi-squared test and the Fisher exact test. Associations between symptom burden and the symptoms addressed by a physiatrist, and association between symptoms and the listed medications subjects received were determined by univariate logistic regression. A P value of less than or equal to .05 was considered statistically significant. All tests were 2-tailed, and statistical analyses were performed with IBM SPSS Statistics, version 19.0 (SPSS, Chicago, IL, USA).

Results

Of the 208 subjects identified from the database, 200 met the criteria for study eligibility and 8 were excluded from analysis because they did not undergo symptom assessment. Subjects were divided into 2 groups according to YSD: group 1 less than 5 YSD and group 2 greater than or equal to 5 YSD.

Cancer survivor group comparison
Table 7 lists subject characteristics of the 2 groups.

Fig. 1A shows the comparison of symptom scores between the 2 groups. The median pain in long-term survivors was 4, significantly higher than 2 in the short-term survivors ($P = .048$). The symptoms that present with moderate severity (median ≥3) in both groups were fatigue, poor appetite, and poor sleep.

Fig. 1B compared the medications used for symptom management between the 2 groups.

Fig. 1C showed the comparison of percentage of the subjects whose activity needed assistance between the 2 groups.

Fig. 1D showed the comparison of rehabilitation intervention rendered by physiatrists.

DISCUSSION

After acute hospitalization due to acute medical events or surgical intervention, a patient with cancer is likely to present with functional decline. Some patients have minor decline and may benefit from outpatient therapies, home exercise, or home health therapy. Some patients require subacute rehabilitation in the skilled nursing facility or long-term acute care facility. Others require acute rehabilitation. After completing appropriate rehabilitation, patients returned to the community. The authors' research efforts attempted to answer the questions related to the postacute rehabilitation period.

Table 7
Characteristics of subjects in the short-term and long-term survivor groups

	<5 YSD (N = 133)	≥5 YSD (N = 67)
Age, mean (SD)	53.4 (16.9)	57.8 (15.6)
Female	63 (47.4)	40 (59.7)
Weight (kg), (mean [SD])	81.0 (22.2)	78.6 (21.9)
Height (cm), (mean [SD])	168.9 (10.5)	166.8 (11.1)
BMI, (mean [SD])	28.5 (8.3)	28.3 (8.1)
	N (%)	
Race		
Black	14 (10.5)	12 (17.9)
Hispanic	16 (12.0)	6 (9.0)
White	94 (70.7)	42 (62.7)
Other	9 (6.7)	7 (10.4)
Cancer treatment history		
Prior chemotherapy	75 (56.4)	44 (65.7)
Prior radiation therapy	74 (55.6)	44 (65.7)
Prior surgery	115 (86.5)	59 (88.1)
Treatment within 1 mo		
Chemotherapy	31 (23.3)	15 (22.4)
Radiation therapy	16 (12.0)	1 (1.5)
Surgery	8 (6.0)	5 (7.5)
Types of cancer		
Brain or spinal	42 (31.6)	15 (22.4)
Breast	14 (10.5)	18 (26.9)
Gastroenterological	12 (9.0)	5 (7.5)
Head & neck	10 (7.5)	4 (6.0)
Leukemia	9 (6.8)	3 (4.5)
Lung	7 (5.3)	3 (4.5)
Lymphoma	4 (3.0)	5 (7.5)
Melanoma	6 (4.5)	2 (3.0)
Prostate	3 (2.3)	2 (3.0)
Sarcoma	15 (11.3)	5 (7.5)
Other[a]	11 (8.3)	5 (7.5)
Recurrent	62 (46.6)	35 (52.2)

There were no statistically significant differences between the 2 groups (all *P*>.05).
  [a] Urogenital cancers other than prostate cancer, gynecologic cancer, other types of cancer, and multiple cancers.

In the authors' first study, at least 50% of the subjects who underwent inpatient rehabilitation or a consult-based rehabilitation intervention were able to maintain their functional level over 4 weeks of time after discharge. On discharge from the hospital, the mean TGUG of the 24 subjects was 23 seconds, much higher than the mean TGUG reported in a healthy elderly cohort (9.5 seconds in ages 70–90 years old)[43] and the prostate cancer outpatient nonfaller group (7.4 seconds). TGUG greater than 20 seconds was associated with a higher risk of early death (odds ratio 2.55, 95% CI 1.32–4.94).[44]

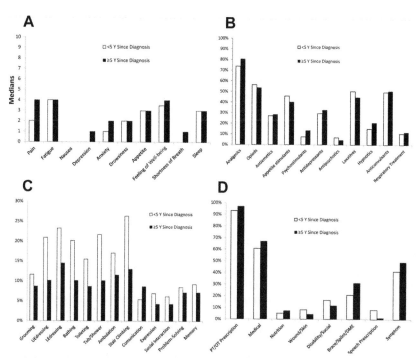

Fig. 1. (*A*) Median ESAS in the short-term (<5 YSD) and long-term survivor (≥5 YSD) groups. (*B*) Comparison of medications used for symptom management in the short-term (<5 YSD) and long-term survivor (≥5 YSD) groups. (*C*) Comparison of percentage of patients who required assistance for daily activities in short-term (<5 YSD) and long-term survivor (≥5 YSD) groups. (*D*) Rehabilitation interventions rendered by physiatrists in the short-term (<5 YSD) and long-term survivor (≥5 YSD) groups. PT/OT, physical therapy or occupational therapy. DME, durable medical equipment; LE, lower extremity dressing; UE dressing, upper extremity dressing.

Therefore, an average TGUG of 23 seconds in the study participants was an indication of frailty and high risk of fall, even after completing an acute rehabilitation program. Among the 12 subjects who completed the trial, a trend of improvement from mean TGUG (from 13 seconds at time of discharge to 10 seconds 4 weeks after discharge, $P = .07$) was seen. These results showed that functional gains can be maintained in at least 50% of these subjects for 4 weeks. In addition, these subjects had achieved good symptom control, with most symptoms with less than 3 mean score on discharge from the hospital. This finding is consistent with the authors' previous study, which demonstrated significant symptom improvement during in-patient rehabilitation.[45]

The authors' second study tried to identify the subjects who had high risk for falling in elderly subjects with prostate cancer who received both ADT and chemotherapy using 2 easy questions. In this subject group, self-reported difficulty in climbing stairs or climbing down stairs was associated with fall history and a poor performance on the TGUG test. The findings were consistent with previous findings in healthy elderly patients, in whom a time greater than 10 seconds on the TGUG test was associated with functional impairments.[46] The median TGUG in subjects who reported difficulty climbing and climbing down stairs was greater than 10 seconds. Subjects who did not report difficulty climbing and climbing down stairs had a median TGUG of 6.7 (range

4.7–10.4) and 6.8 (range 4.7–10.8) seconds, respectively. This result shows that the negative response to the 2 simple questions correlates with relatively normal TGUG.

Difficulty in climbing down stairs is associated with a lower score on the Barthel index. Although different scales were used, a previous study also showed an association between difficulty climbing down stairs and poorer ADL performance.[36] Decreased ADL performance has been shown to increase caregiver burden, causing some caregivers to decrease their work hours or quit their jobs to provide care for their loved ones.[35] A patient-reported difficulty climbing down stairs may serve as an indicator for ADL deficiencies in patients and a reminder for occupational therapy referral.

Given the high incidence of falls among subjects with prostate cancer (47% in the authors' study) and its potential severe consequences, a simple tool to screen fall risk is important. The responses to the 2 simple questions had a high sensitivity, specificity, and positive predictive value compared with the TGUG in identifying fall risk in the elderly patient with prostate cancer population. It can be used as a valuable screening tool for fall risk.

The authors' third study reviewed and compared the long-term survivor and short-term survivor on their symptoms and management rendered by physiatrists in an outpatient cancer rehabilitation clinic. This study is the first to describe in cancer rehabilitation, the symptom burden, and functional needs in short-term versus long-term survivors. It is also the first study to describe the multidimensional role of physiatrists in delivering cancer survivorship care. Findings reveal the extensive rehabilitation needs of the short-term and long-term cancer survivors. In both survivor groups, analgesic use was above 70% and opiate use was above 50% (see **Fig 1**B). Besides pain, the most prominent symptoms in both groups were fatigue, poor appetite, and poor sleep. These were consistent with a previous report.[47] In this study, greater than or equal to 3 pain intensity was associated with analgesic prescription and physiatrist's action to address the pain.

Fatigue, poor appetite, and insomnia greater than or equal to 3 were not associated with either medication targeting the symptoms, nor with physiatrist addressing the symptoms. Methylphenidate is the most studied pharmacologic agent for the treatment of cancer-related fatigue. It was prescribed for 10 out of 133 (8%) short-term survivors and 9 out of 67 (13%) long-term survivors, whereas 132 out of 200 (66%) total subjects had fatigue ratings of greater than or equal to 3. Appetite stimulants were prescribed for 61 (46%) short-term survivors and 27 (40%) long-term survivors. However, among those subjects with poor appetite ratings of greater than or equal to 3, only 51 out of 100 (51%) had appetite stimulants in their medication lists. These results indicate that these symptoms with moderate intensity were undertreated, which may be due to lack of effective and standardized treatment of these symptoms, lack of emphasis in symptom control, or patient's hesitation in taking additional medications. Recent research suggests that fatigue and anorexia may have similar mechanisms.[48] It is hoped that multifaceted therapy contributing to the fatigue-anorexia-cachexia symptom cluster will become available soon.[49] Hypnotics were prescribed for 20 (15%) short-term survivors and 14 (21%) long-term survivors, whereas 110 (56%) total subjects had poor sleep ratings of greater than or equal to 3. The authors' results are consistent with a previous report.[50] Sleep disorders have been reported to strongly correlate with fatigue[51] and depression[52] in cancer survivors, which could be related to increased inflammatory mediators.[53] Fatigue, poor appetite, and sleep disturbance, therefore, is a cluster of symptoms that deserves attention from the treating physicians. Many studies have shown the association between high symptom burdens with poor quality of life (QOL).[47,54–57] To improve the QOL of cancer survivors, it is clear that physiatrists need to increase their attention to symptoms, and continuously update their clinical skills for symptom management and aggressively treating symptoms.

Rehabilitation interventions rendered by physiatrists clearly demonstrated the emphasis on therapy (see **Fig 1**D). More than 90% of both short-term and long-term survivors needed physical therapy or occupational therapy (PT/OT) treatment. PT/OT prescriptions are highly specific, including a definition of the type, frequency, duration, and intensity of exercise[58] Deficits and goals are also clearly indicated. The second most frequent intervention by the physiatrist was related to medical issues. For example, patients with cancer are 4- to 7-fold more likely to develop venous thrombotic events compared with patients without cancer.[59] Anemia is more prominent in patients with cancer as well.[60] Autonomic dysfunction affects about 80% of patients with advanced cancer.[61,62] These conditions can directly affect patient symptoms and, therefore, may indirectly interfere with a physiatrist's rehabilitation intervention. The third-ranked intervention by the physiatrists was symptom management, which was rendered to more than 40% of cancer survivors in both groups. One-fourth (more than 20%) of rehabilitation interventions in both groups involved adaptive devices, such as prosthetics, orthotics, and durable medical equipment. Due to the aging process of survivors, recurrence or progression of the cancer, late effect of the cancer treatment, comorbidities, and functional impairments can exacerbate and present as new deficits that require new equipment, prosthetics, or orthotics. Following acute cancer rehabilitation, patients are often discharged with outpatient or home health therapies to continue work on additional functional goals over a longer period of time. Outpatient follow-up by a physiatrist is helpful to further maximize functional gains for the cancer survivors and those with active or quiescent disease. Ongoing adjustments in functional goals may be needed to account for changes in clinical status. In addition, symptom burden, particularly during activity, the aging process, changes in medical comorbidity, changes in medications, and late side effects from the cancer treatments, may lead to additional functional problems. A functional decline may herald clinical instability and may mean additional workup, as well treatments, in cancer survivors.

LIMITATIONS

First, the studies had small sample sizes. Second, the data are from a single institution. Third, there was a high drop-out rate (50%) in the first study. Out of the 12 drop-outs, 7 were medically fragile, resulting in a hospital readmission or death. This drop-out rate illustrates the intrinsic frailty of patients with cancer who required rehabilitation during their prior hospitalizations. Fourth, these subjects were followed for 4 weeks after discharge from acute rehabilitation in the first study. Future studies are needed to test whether functional gains can be maintained over a longer period.

SUMMARY

There were no significant differences in symptoms other than pain, medications for symptoms control. Daily activities required assistance and rehabilitation interventions. Patients with cancer and survivors of cancer may develop significant functional deficits during their acute hospital stay, which may be related to progression of disease, ongoing treatments, and medical comorbidities. For patients with more significant functional limitations, acute inpatient cancer rehabilitation may be recommended. The authors' study showed 50% of deconditioned patients with cancer can maintain functional level 4 weeks after discharge from acute inpatient rehabilitation. Multicenter and longer-duration studies are needed to assess whether the functional gains from inpatient cancer rehabilitation are sustainable.

Postacute care, short-term and long-term cancer survivors continue to have significant rehabilitation needs. High symptom burden adversely affects function and QOL.

Physiatrists who care for cancer survivors must be sensitive to changes in their functional status, and be skillful in symptom management and coordinating care with other health care providers to provide optimal resolution to stressors affecting their QOL.

For certain patients, the functional decline may be gradual and subtle. In those patient populations, screening tools to identify high-risk groups are needed. Two simple questions may be used as a valuable screening tool for fall in elderly patients with prostate cancer who received both ADT and chemotherapy. More study is needed to validate this tool in different oncologic patient populations.

REFERENCES

1. Cancer Facts & figures 2016. 2016.
2. Institute NC. Surveillance, epidemiology, and end results program [SEER] Stat Fact Sheets: All Sites. 2016.
3. Ganz PA, Casillas J, Hahn EE. Ensuring quality care for cancer survivors: implementing the survivorship care plan. Semin Oncol Nurs 2008;24(3):208–17.
4. Hellbom M, Bergelt C, Bergenmar M, et al. Cancer rehabilitation: a Nordic and European perspective. Acta Oncol 2011;50(2):179–86.
5. Loescher LJ, Welch-McCaffrey D, Leigh SA, et al. Surviving adult cancers. Part 1: Physiologic effects. Ann Intern Med 1989;111(5):411–32.
6. Welch-McCaffrey D, Hoffman B, Leigh SA, et al. Surviving adult cancers. Part 2: Psychosocial implications. Ann Intern Med 1989;111(6):517–24.
7. Bruera E, MacDonald RN. Asthenia in patients with advanced cancer. Issues in symptom control. Part 1. J Pain Symptom Manage 1988;3(1):9–14.
8. Watanabe S, Bruera E. Anorexia and cachexia, asthenia, and lethargy. Hematol Oncol Clin North Am 1996;10(1):189–206.
9. Movsas SB, Chang VT, Tunkel RS, et al. Rehabilitation needs of an inpatient medical oncology unit. Arch Phys Med Rehabil 2003;84(11):1642–6.
10. Fialka-Moser V, Crevenna R, Korpan M, et al. Cancer rehabilitation: particularly with aspects on physical impairments. J Rehabil Med 2003;35(4):153–62.
11. Guo Y, Persyn L, Palmer JL, et al. Incidence of and risk factors for transferring cancer patients from rehabilitation to acute care units. Am J Phys Med Rehabil 2008;87(8):647–53.
12. Ganz PA. The status of cancer rehabilitation in the late 1990s. Mayo Clin Proc 1999;74(9):939–40.
13. Marciniak CM, Sliwa JA, Spill G, et al. Functional outcome following rehabilitation of the cancer patient. Arch Phys Med Rehabil 1996;77(1):54–7.
14. Cheville AL. Cancer rehabilitation. Semin Oncol 2005;32(2):219–24.
15. Hoppe S, Rainfray M, Fonck M, et al. Functional decline in older patients with cancer receiving first-line chemotherapy. J Clin Oncol 2013;31(31):3877–82.
16. Guise TA. Bone loss and fracture risk associated with cancer therapy. Oncologist 2006;11(10):1121–31.
17. Cole RP, Scialla SJ, Bednarz L. Functional recovery in cancer rehabilitation. Arch Phys Med Rehabil 2000;81(5):623–7.
18. Tay SSLP, Ng YS. Poster 21: functional outcomes of cancer patients in an inpatient rehabilitation setting. Arch Phys Med Rehabil 2007;88(9):E15–6.
19. Sabers SR, Kokal JE, Girardi JC, et al. Evaluation of consultation-based rehabilitation for hospitalized cancer patients with functional impairment. Mayo Clin Proc 1999;74(9):855–61.
20. Mathias S, Nayak US, Isaacs B. Balance in elderly patients: the "get-up and go" test. Arch Phys Med Rehabil 1986;67(6):387–9.

21. Podsiadlo D, Richardson S. The timed "Up & Go": a test of basic functional mobility for frail elderly persons. J Am Geriatr Soc 1991;39(2):142–8.
22. Simmonds MJ. Physical function in patients with cancer: psychometric characteristics and clinical usefulness of a physical performance test battery. J pain symptom Manag 2002;24(4):404–14.
23. Bruera E, Kuehn N, Miller MJ, et al. The Edmonton Symptom Assessment System (ESAS): a simple method for the assessment of palliative care patients. J Palliat Care 1991;7(2):6–9.
24. Rubenstein LZ. Falls in older people: epidemiology, risk factors and strategies for prevention. Age Ageing 2006;35(Suppl 2):ii37–41.
25. Grossman MD, Miller D, Scaff DW, et al. When is an elder old? Effect of preexisting conditions on mortality in geriatric trauma. J Trauma 2002;52(2):242–6.
26. Stel VS, Smit JH, Pluijm SM, et al. Consequences of falling in older men and women and risk factors for health service use and functional decline. Age Ageing 2004;33(1):58–65.
27. Tromp AM, Pluijm SM, Smit JH, et al. Fall-risk screening test: a prospective study on predictors for falls in community-dwelling elderly. J Clin Epidemiol 2001;54(8): 837–44.
28. Stalenhoef PA, Diederiks JP, Knottnerus JA, et al. A risk model for the prediction of recurrent falls in community-dwelling elderly: a prospective cohort study. J Clin Epidemiol 2002;55(11):1088–94.
29. Bylow K, Dale W, Mustian K, et al. Falls and physical performance deficits in older patients with prostate cancer undergoing androgen deprivation therapy. Urology 2008;72(2):422–7.
30. Chan BK, Marshall LM, Winters KM, et al. Incident fall risk and physical activity and physical performance among older men: the osteoporotic fractures in men study. Am J Epidemiol 2007;165(6):696–703.
31. Terret C, Albrand G, Droz JP. Geriatric assessment in elderly patients with prostate cancer. Clin Prostate Cancer 2004;2(4):236–40.
32. Malcolm JB, Derweesh IH, Kincade MC, et al. Osteoporosis and fractures after androgen deprivation initiation for prostate cancer. Can J Urol 2007;14(3):3551–9.
33. Lee J, Geller AI, Strasser DC. Analytical review: focus on fall screening assessments. PM R 2013;5(7):609–21.
34. Overcash JA, Rivera HR Jr. Physical performance evaluation of older cancer patients: a preliminary study. Crit Rev Oncol Hematol 2008;68(3):233–41.
35. Verghese J, Wang C, Xue X, et al. Self-reported difficulty in climbing up or down stairs in nondisabled elderly. Arch Phys Med Rehabil 2008;89(1):100–4.
36. Sainsbury A, Seebass G, Bansal A, et al. Reliability of the Barthel Index when used with older people. Age Ageing 2005;34(3):228–32.
37. Hurvitz EA, Richardson JK, Werner RA, et al. Unipedal stance testing as an indicator of fall risk among older outpatients. Arch Phys Med Rehabil 2000;81(5): 587–91.
38. Rantanen T, Guralnik JM, Foley D, et al. Midlife hand grip strength as a predictor of old age disability. JAMA 1999;281(6):558–60.
39. Shumway-Cook A, Brauer S, Woollacott M. Predicting the probability for falls in community-dwelling older adults using the timed up & go test. Phys Ther 2000; 80(9):896–903.
40. Thomas JI, Lane JV. A pilot study to explore the predictive validity of 4 measures of falls risk in frail elderly patients. Arch Phys Med Rehabil 2005;86(8):1636–40.
41. Gunther CM, Burger A, Rickert M, et al. Grip strength in healthy Caucasian adults: reference values. J Hand Surg 2008;33(4):558–65.

42. Anderson KO. Assessment tools for the evaluation of pain in the oncology patient. Curr Pain Headache Rep 2007;11(4):259–64.

43. Herman T, Giladi N, Hausdorff JM. Properties of the 'timed up and go' test: more than meets the eye. Gerontology 2011;57(3):203–10.

44. Soubeyran P, Fonck M, Blanc-Bisson C, et al. Predictors of early death risk in older patients treated with first-line chemotherapy for cancer. J Clin Oncol 2012;30(15):1829–34.

45. Guo Y, Young BL, Hainley S, et al. Evaluation and pharmacologic management of symptoms in cancer patients undergoing acute rehabilitation in a comprehensive cancer center. Arch Phys Med Rehabil 2007;88(7):891–5.

46. Beauchet O, Fantino B, Allali G, et al. Timed up and go test and risk of falls in older adults: a systematic review. J Nutr Health Aging 2011;15(10):933–8.

47. Huang IC, Brinkman TM, Kenzik K, et al. Association between the prevalence of symptoms and health-related quality of life in adult survivors of childhood cancer: a report from the St Jude Lifetime Cohort study. J Clin Oncol 2013;31(33):4242–51.

48. Alesi ER, del Fabbro E. Opportunities for targeting the fatigue-anorexia-cachexia symptom cluster. Cancer J 2014;20(5):325–9.

49. Del Fabbro E. More is better: a multimodality approach to cancer cachexia. Oncologist 2010;15(2):119–21.

50. Savard J, Morin CM. Insomnia in the context of cancer: a review of a neglected problem. J Clin Oncol 2001;19(3):895–908.

51. Giacalone A, Quitadamo D, Zanet E, et al. Cancer-related fatigue in the elderly. Support Care Cancer 2013;21(10):2899–911.

52. Irwin MR. Depression and insomnia in cancer: prevalence, risk factors, and effects on cancer outcomes. Curr Psychiatry Rep 2013;15(11):404.

53. Irwin MR, Olmstead RE, Ganz PA, et al. Sleep disturbance, inflammation and depression risk in cancer survivors. Brain Behav Immun 2013;30(Suppl):S58–67.

54. Yang P, Cheville AL, Wampfler JA, et al. Quality of life and symptom burden among long-term lung cancer survivors. J Thorac Oncol 2012;7(1):64–70.

55. Janz NK, Mujahid M, Chung LK, et al. Symptom experience and quality of life of women following breast cancer treatment. J women's Health 2007;16(9):1348–61.

56. Kent EE, Mitchell SA, Oakley-Girvan I, et al. The importance of symptom surveillance during follow-up care of leukemia, bladder, and colorectal cancer survivors. Support Care Cancer 2014;22(1):163–72.

57. Adams E, Boulton MG, Horne A, et al. The effects of pelvic radiotherapy on cancer survivors: symptom profile, psychological morbidity and quality of life. Clin Oncol 2014;26(1):10–7.

58. Wilmore JH. Exercise prescription: role of the physiatrist and allied health professional. Arch Phys Med Rehabil 1976;57(1):315–9.

59. Heit JA, O'Fallon WM, Petterson TM, et al. Relative impact of risk factors for deep vein thrombosis and pulmonary embolism: a population-based study. Arch Intern Med 2002;162(11):1245–8.

60. Knight K, Wade S, Balducci L. Prevalence and outcomes of anemia in cancer: a systematic review of the literature. Am J Med 2004;116(Suppl 7A):11S–26S.

61. Strasser F, Palmer JL, Schover LR, et al. The impact of hypogonadism and autonomic dysfunction on fatigue, emotional function, and sexual desire in male patients with advanced cancer: a pilot study. Cancer 2006;107(12):2949–57.

62. Stone CA, Kenny RA, Nolan B, et al. Autonomic dysfunction in patients with advanced cancer; prevalence, clinical correlates and challenges in assessment. BMC Palliat Care 2012;11:3.

Palliative Care and Physiatry in the Oncology Care Spectrum

An Opportunity for Distinct and Collaborative Approaches

Vishwa S. Raj, MD[a,b,]*, Julie K. Silver, MD[c],
Terrence M. Pugh, MD[b], Jack B. Fu, MD[d]

KEYWORDS

- Cancer rehabilitation • Function • Palliative care • Quality of life
- Supportive oncology • Survivorship • Symptom management

KEY POINTS

- Cancer survivorship can vary from living cancer free for the remainder of life to living with cancer continuously without a disease-free period.
- Palliative care and rehabilitation can impact overall quality of life and will increase in acceptance and prominence as valuable resources for the cancer patient.
- Although physiatry and palliative care remain distinct subspecialties, they share several common traits that complement care for the oncology survivor.
- Impairments such as deconditioning, neurologic deficits, and muscle weakness may adversely affect function; however, cancer symptoms also impact function.
- Opportunities for collaboration between the fields exist to more effectively improve patient outcomes.

Disclosure Statement: The authors have nothing to disclose (V.S. Raj, T.M. Pugh and J.B. Fu). J.K. Silver discloses that she founded Oncology Rehab Partners that developed the STAR Program certification.
[a] Division of Rehabilitation Medicine, Levine Cancer Institute, 1021 Morehead Medical Drive, Charlotte, NC 28204, USA; [b] Department of Physical Medicine and Rehabilitation, Carolinas Rehabilitation, 1100 Blythe Boulevard, Charlotte, NC 28203, USA; [c] Department of Physical Medicine and Rehabilitation, Spaulding Rehabilitation Hospital, Harvard Medical School, 300 First Avenue, Charlestown, MA 02129, USA; [d] Department of Palliative, Rehabilitation, and Integrative Medicine, MD Anderson Cancer Center, University of Texas, 1515 Holcombe Boulevard, Unit 1414, Houston, TX 77030, USA
* Corresponding author. Division of Rehabilitation Medicine, Levine Cancer Institute, 1021 Morehead Medical Drive, Charlotte, NC 28204.
E-mail address: vishwa.raj@carolinashealthcare.org

Phys Med Rehabil Clin N Am 28 (2017) 35–47
http://dx.doi.org/10.1016/j.pmr.2016.08.006

INTRODUCTION

As cancer evolves from a terminal illness to a chronic medical condition, so too does the need for clinical services beyond medical, surgical, and radiation oncology that principally focus on disease modification. The concept of survivorship for individuals with cancer is broad in scope. Although a cancer survivor is anyone who lives with cancer, from the time of diagnosis throughout the balance of life, the context can vary from living cancer free for the remainder of life to living with cancer continuously without a disease-free period. With more than 15 million individuals living who have a history of cancer, and a projection of almost 19 million by 2024, comprehensive approaches to care will be necessary to address the ongoing clinical needs of survivors. Two areas that warrant specific emphasis include impairment-driven cancer rehabilitation and palliative care.[1]

According to the Institute of Medicine, barriers to the delivery of high-quality cancer care exist secondary to rapidly increasing incidence, disease and treatment complexity, and costs, as well as a shrinking workforce. Given that aging is considered one of the greatest risk factors for cancer, several characteristics of the aging population may affect prognoses and care plans, such as altered physiology, premorbid functional and cognitive impairments, multimorbidity, increased side effects of treatment, distinct goals of care, and an increased need for social support.[2] Understanding the importance of function and symptomatology, and their integration into the continuum of cancer care is critical for successful care delivery in the future.

THE IMPORTANCE OF CANCER REHABILITATION AND PALLIATIVE CARE

According to The Surveillance, Epidemiology, and End Results Program, the total estimated new cancer cases in the United States for 2015 is approximately 1.6 million, occurring at a rate of 457.2 per 100,000, for both males and females.[3] The long-term mortality trend analysis, however, shows that the overall cancer death rate in the United States has declined by an average of 1.5% per year (between 2003 and 2012).[4] Although the number of cancer survivors continues to increase, deficits exist in addressing their long-term clinical needs. For example, according to a recent survey, physical problems were the most frequently unmet need among cancer survivors (**Table 1**), in addition to provision of information regarding their future care, and mental health.[5] Understanding that both physical and psychological impairments can contribute to decreased health-related quality of life (QOL),[6] and that treatment of physical, psychosocial, and spiritual needs can improve quality of care,[7] both rehabilitation and palliative care can play critical roles in the oncology care continuum. Realizing the importance of these services, the Commission on Cancer has incorporated standards regarding rehabilitation and palliative care as core components for program accreditation (**Table 2**).[8]

Barriers to the integration of palliative care and rehabilitation into comprehensive cancer care relate to limited understanding of the definitions of both specialties and how they may be applied throughout the continuum. The World Health Organization defines palliative care as:

[A]n approach that improves the quality of life of patients and their families facing the problem associated with life-threatening illness, through the prevention and relief of suffering by means of early identification and impeccable assessment and treatment of pain and other problems, physical, psychosocial and spiritual.

Aspects of clinical palliative care may include alleviation of pain and other distressing symptoms, attention to psychological and spiritual aspects of care, and

Table 1
Current themes for unmet needs

Unmet Need Domain	n	%	Codebook Description
Physical	578	38.2	Needs and issues experienced in or affecting the body, including pain, symptoms, sexual dysfunction, and care of body (such as diet, exercise, and rest).
Financial	307	20.3	Needs related to money, insurance, and the affordability of needed services and products.
Education/ information	295	19.5	Needs related to unanswered questions and the lack of knowledge regarding what to expect as a cancer survivor, follow-up care, self-care, cancer and health research, and cancer risks, causes, and prevention.
Personal control	249	16.4	Needs related to an individual's ability to maintain autonomy in terms of the physical self (sexual function, evacuation, and ambulation) and the social self (disclosure about cancer and ability to make plans and socialize). Also includes wishes to return to "normal" and finding a "new normal."
System of care	235	15.5	Needs related to the health care system, including constraints and flaws that affect early detection, diagnosis, treatment, follow-up care, continuity of care, and inadequate response from health care providers.
Resources	209	13.8	Needs related to availability and access to supplies, equipment, therapies and medications (including alternative and complementary), and transportation services.
Emotions/ mental health	207	13.7	Needs related to psychological issues, including fear (recurrence, new cancers, death, and dying), depression, anxiety, and negative feelings (mistrust toward body, anger, and guilt).
Social support	193	12.7	Needs related to psychosocial and interpersonal issues, including intimacy, access to support groups, opportunities to use one's own experiences to help others, and participation in social situations.
Societal	151	10.0	Needs revealed from respondents' commentary about conditions and issues related to society's response to cancer, including social norms, discrimination, misinformation, policies, and resource allocation (insurance coverage).
Communication	129	8.5	Needs related to discourse (talking) and information exchange (explaining) about cancer and cancer experience with others (including survivor and doctor and survivor and family/friends/employers) and among medical providers.
Provider relationship	124	8.5	Needs related to trust in health care providers, including decision making, follow-through, follow-up, and support.
Cure	53	3.5	Needs related to a wish for a cure for cancer and hopes of effective treatments for self and others.

(continued on next page)

Table 1 (continued)			
Unmet Need Domain	**n**	**%**	**Codebook Description**
Body image	53	3.5	Needs related to negative perception of body, including feeling unattractive and/or ashamed and loss of trust in body.
Survivor identity	47	3.1	Pertains to the respondent either explicitly identifying or not identifying as a cancer survivor because the respondent does not like the term "survivor" or feels that he or she has not reached a specific milestone to be called a survivor (eg, not still in treatment or living a specific number of years since the diagnosis).
Employment	35	2.3	Needs pertaining to maintaining or obtaining a source of income that is appropriate given the cancer experience.
Existential	9	0.6	Needs pertaining to attaining peace in life and spirituality and making sense or meaning of the cancer experience.

From Burg MA, Adorno G, Lopez ED, et al. Current unmet needs of cancer survivors: analysis of open-ended responses to the American Cancer Society Study of Cancer Survivors II. Cancer 2015;121(4):626; with permission.

enhancement of QOL to positively influence the course of illness. A team approach is used to address the needs of patients and their families. If appropriate, palliative care should be integrated early in the course of illness, in association with other therapies meant to prolong life, to comprehensively detect and address clinical complications.[9]

Similarly, oncology rehabilitation incorporates both a comprehensive and interdisciplinary approach that addresses the scope of clinical care. Specifically, cancer rehabilitation is defined as

> [M]edical care that should be integrated throughout the oncology care continuum and delivered by trained rehabilitation professionals who have it within their scope of practice to diagnose and treat patients' physical, psychological, and cognitive impairments in an effort to maintain or restore function, reduce symptom burden, maximize independence and improve quality of life in this medically complex population.[10]

The application of rehabilitation principles may benefit patients across all phases of cancer care, including the preventative, restorative, supportive, or palliative aspects of

Table 2 Eligibility requirements and standards for Commission on Cancer program accreditation	
Standard	**Description**
Eligibility Requirement 11: Rehabilitation Services	Policies and procedures are in place to ensure patient access to rehabilitation services either on site or by referral.
Standard 2.4: Palliative Care Services	Palliative care services are available to patients either on site or by referral.

From American College of Surgeons. Cancer program standards: ensuring patient-centered care. Chicago: American College of Surgeons; 2016.

care.[11] However, the ability to provide these services throughout the spectrum of oncology care is critical to ensure patients maintain appropriate access to care.

As cancer care continues to advance, the role for comprehensive oncological care has become a priority for the survivor. However, recent trends have shifted the care of cancer patients from tertiary centers to community-based models, potentially limiting their access to specialty services such as rehabilitation.[12] Access to care must remain a critical issue as it relates to palliative and rehabilitation services. With improved efficacy of treatment and decreased comorbidities, survival rates will continue to improve regardless of the setting, and survivors' needs will undoubtedly include symptom control and functional optimization before, during, and after acute oncological measures. Given that palliative care and rehabilitation can both exert major potential positive impacts on overall QOL, and diverse health outcomes, and that patients are becoming more engaged and involved in their care, the roles of these specialties are likely to increase in acceptance and prominence.

GAPS IN DELIVERING HIGH-QUALITY CANCER CARE

Cancer rehabilitation and palliative care are both critical components of high-quality oncology services. A recent report by Silver and colleagues[10] highlighted the important similarities and differences and focused on how these services could be better integrated in cancer care. This report emphasized that rehabilitation and palliative care practitioners are important referral sources for each other. Working collaboratively they can enhance survivors' ability to function and improve QOL.

Indeed, gaps in cancer rehabilitation training and care delivery have been well-documented in the literature.[6] Although cancer rehabilitation has been highlighted as an important area for targeted education across stakeholder groups, the quality and quantity of patient experiences remains a target for improvement.[13] For example, in a cohort of women with advanced stage breast cancer, Cheville and colleagues[14] found that approximately 92% had impairments and less than 2% of those were addressed proactively in an ambulatory setting. It was noted that systematic disability screening may be required to reliably detect functional decline and address a decades-long pattern of underuse of rehabilitation services among people with advanced cancer.[15] Pergolotti and colleagues[16] studied 529 older adults with cancer and found that 341 (65%) had potentially modifiable functional deficits with the potential to benefit from physical and/or occupational therapy, but only 9% received these services.

Similarly, gaps exist in the delivery of palliative care. Students and residents feel unprepared to provide, and faculty and residents feel unprepared to teach, end-of-life care.[17] Despite empirical evidence for spiritual care as part of palliative care, religion and spirituality remain insufficiently addressed by the medical system.[18] Access to palliative care services remains limited, with an acute shortage of hospice and palliative medicine physicians (potentially 6000–18,000 practitioners). Furthermore, evidence suggests decreased use of palliative care with increasing regional Medicare expenditure ($1387 difference per beneficiary between the first and fourth quartiles of palliative care use), and attention is still needed to address access barriers in underserved regions.[19] Some access-related issues may stem from patients' and clinicians' perceptions of palliative services. After completion of semistructured interviews with providers in Pennsylvania, palliative care was perceived as end-of-life or hospice, and often underrecognized as a resource for managing symptoms and addressing the psychosocial needs of patients with chronic illnesses.[20]

REDEFINING CANCER REHABILITATION AND PALLIATIVE CARE IN AN EVOLVING ONCOLOGY CONTINUUM

As both palliative care and rehabilitation services become more integrated into the oncology continuum, it is useful to understand their similarities and differences. Although physiatry and palliative care remain distinct subspecialties, they share several common traits that complement the disease-direct care delivered to patients with cancer. Disability frequently develops secondary to bed rest, deconditioning, and neurologic and musculoskeletal complications. Disability may also develop consequent to function-degrading symptoms such as pain and fatigue.[21] Although they share common targets—namely, QOL and optimal functioning—palliative care and rehabilitation have different emphases, with the former focusing disproportionately on symptoms and the latter on physical impairments.

Physiatry coordinates the functional remediation of acute injuries and chronic conditions, with emphasis on long-term improvement and prevention of future disablement. Physiatry also emphasizes patient empowerment, which promotes autonomy and reduces dependence on external support.[22] Physiatrists have a distinct skill set that may make them uniquely qualified to diagnose and treat various impairments in oncology populations, particularly those that are related to neurologic or musculoskeletal sequelae.[23] When caring for the cancer patient, however, the approach must be adapted to consider diagnoses, short-term goal planning, and oncological treatments to optimally address function, cognition, and QOL. Conversely, palliative care mitigates distress and enhances QOL through symptom control; alleviation of existential, spiritual, and psychological suffering; advanced care planning; and caregiver support, among other approaches. Ideally both palliative care and rehabilitation should be considered from the time of diagnosis throughout survivorship and end of life. When integrated into the care continuum, these services have been shown to positively impact important outcomes such as QOL, mood, health care use, patient satisfaction, and survival.[7]

Similarities between both areas become more evident when understanding their clinical philosophies. Overarching themes for both specialties include improving cancer-related symptoms and treatment-related side effects, lessening caregiver burden, and valuing patient-centered care and shared decision making. Both use interdisciplinary models to provide comprehensive, holistic care. With this interdisciplinary approach, both attempt to improve health care efficiencies by reducing hospital lengths of stay, unanticipated readmissions and other use parameters. Psychooncology and behavioral health are greatly valued and integrated by both rehabilitation and palliative care. Furthermore, both address cognitive dysfunction through pharmacologic and psychological approaches. Using a patient-centered approach, rehabilitation and palliative care can improve QOL and functional outcomes.[10]

COLLABORATION FOR SYMPTOMATIC MANAGEMENT

Although impairments such as deconditioning, neurologic deficits, and muscle weakness adversely affect function, adverse symptoms also impact function.[24] Both physiatrists and palliative care specialists may participate in symptom management. Improving cancer symptoms may result in functional improvements even before a therapist has worked with the patient. Because uncontrolled symptoms may undermine therapy participation and hinder therapy progress, minimizing symptom burden is an important dimension of cancer rehabilitation. It has also been shown that cancer patient symptom burden improves during inpatient rehabilitation facility admissions.

For inpatient rehabilitation facilities, symptom improvement is attributed, in part, to the use of medications and increased physical activity.[25,26] Cancer fatigue has been associated with reduced function.[27] Addressing symptoms that exacerbate fatigue such as insomnia and cachexia may also improve function.[28] Physical activity itself reduces cancer fatigue.[29] For individuals with "chemo-brain," cognitive rehabilitation programs may help patients to achieve higher level functional goals. Neurostimulants and compensatory strategies may be useful,[30] as well as antipsychotics and sedatives for delirium and agitation.[31]

Pain Management

Pain affects more than 70% of cancer patients, and is often undertreated.[32] Using a combination of physical therapy, home exercises, modalities, medications, and injections, physical medicine and rehabilitation (PM&R) and palliative care specialists can collaborate to develop effective, individualized treatment regimens.

Pain is often a prominent symptom at the end of life. In cancer patients, pain is often generated by malignant invasion of adjacent structures. Also survivors may suffer from common nononcologic causes of pain, including musculoskeletal sources such as osteoarthritis, bursitis, and tendonitis. Injections may be used for noncancer pain at the end of life.[33,34] Radiation treatment can lead to radiation fibrosis syndrome, trismus, and postmastectomy reconstruction syndrome with painful spastic muscles within or adjacent to the radiation field. Trigger point and botulinum toxin injections have been shown to be effective in these patients, although a lack of controlled trials is a problematic deficit in the current evidence base.[35] Cancer patients may be at increased risk for musculoskeletal pain compared with the general population owing to muscle weakness and imbalances from neuropathy, myopathy, deconditioning, and cachexia, although this remains conjectural.

Neuropathic discomfort is common in cancer patients either owing to chemotherapy, tumor invasion of nerves, surgeries, or radiation therapy. Antidepressant and antiepileptic medications are commonly used. However, nerve blocks and botulinum toxin injections may be trialed as well. Desensitization may also be effective.[36] If pain is more somatic or visceral in nature, medication administration may follow the World Health Organization's 3-step ladder as a guide for pain management (**Fig. 1**), which starts with nonopioid and adjuvant medications with initial signs of pain, and progresses to opioid mediations as pain severity increases.[37] Common opioid medications used for treatment may include tramadol, hydrocodone, and oxycodone, with progression for more severe pain to fentanyl and methadone.

Nausea and Bowel Irregularity

Nausea can often lead to reduced appetite and oral intake, as well as cachexia. Vomiting can lead to dehydration and electrolyte abnormalities. Acute chemotherapy-induced nausea is common among cancer patients. Serotonin receptor antagonists (eg, ondansetron) can be available in oral tablet, intravenous, and sublingual disintegrating tablet. Other oral antiemetics, such a chlorpromazine, promethazine, and cannaboids, can be sedating and thus affect function and therapy performance.

When approaching nausea from a palliative care perspective, common causes include gastric stasis, biochemical causes, increased intracranial pressure, vestibular issues, and bowel obstruction.[38] However, nausea may also be related to bowel hypomotility secondary to opioid use, which can then lead to constipation and anorexia. Questions regarding bowel movement frequency should be taken into consideration for patients using chronic opiate medications, especially if they are already receiving

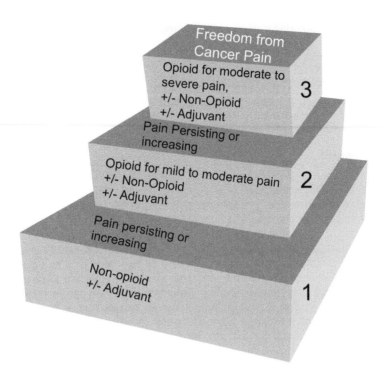

Fig. 1. World Health Organization pain relief ladder. (*From* World Health Organization. WHO's cancer pain ladder for adults. Available at: http://www.who.int/cancer/palliative/painladder/en/. Accessed April 17, 2016; with permission.)

antiemetic therapy without relief. Daily oral laxatives and stool softeners may help to maintain regular bowel movements. Promotility agents such as metoclopramide may also help, but clinicians should be aware of their side effects.

Cancer patients can also suffer from neurogenic bowel owing to central and peripheral nervous system cancer invasion, surgical resections, and radiation therapies; this may be an additional cause of nausea and vomiting. Many cancer patients present with spastic neurogenic bowel from upper motor neuron disease; however, damage to the sacral nerves and plexus owing to sacral tumors (eg, chondrosarcomas) and radiation are not uncommon and may lead to flaccidity with a lower motor neuron presentation. Patients with a flaccid neurogenic bowel, in particular, can retain large amounts of stool leading to ileus or obstruction. In this case, bowel programs are typically designed to reduce stool production. Programs may be needed more than once a day.[39] Monitoring bowel movement frequency and maintaining regular bowel movements are critical.

The principles of rehabilitation neurogenic bowel management can be applied to many constipated cancer patients with and without a neurologic cause. A daily bowel program including a large meal with hot liquid coffee or tea and use of a rectal suppository stimulant may be beneficial. Severe thrombocytopenia and leukopenia, common issues in cancer patients, may prohibit the use of a rectal suppository and rectal digital stimulation. During times of severe pancytopenia, an oral bowel program, which excludes the rectal portions of the program, can be used. Oral bowel programs may not produce as consistent results, but can still benefit some patients.[40]

CONSIDERATIONS FOR THE FUTURE COLLABORATION

It has previously been stated that cancer rehabilitation and palliative care are key components of high-quality oncology services.[10] Both specialties use interdisciplinary teams to regularly assess patients' medical, physical, cognitive, and functional status. More intentional collaboration between the fields may further improve patient outcomes. Gagnon and colleagues[41] showed that patient physical endurance, psychological health, and disease-related weight loss improved with an interdisciplinary nutrition rehabilitation program for patients with advanced stage cancers. A similar model that integrates physicians specializing in PM&R and palliative care along with physical, occupational, and speech therapies, nursing, clinical nutrition, psychology, and social work may be effective at other points along the cancer trajectory. Although there is some integration of PM&R and palliative care in oncology units, this is not a routine practice.[42] Physiatrists' knowledge and skill in identifying and treating physical and cognitive impairments complements the palliative care specialists' expertise in symptom management and relief of suffering. The potentially synergistic benefits of systematically integrating these approaches are obvious, but more research is needed to empirically validate models of care.

PM&R and palliative care departments are well-equipped to develop patient-centered care protocols. These protocols could ensure that patient goals remain relevant and inform medical, surgical, and radiation oncology treatment plans. The ability to treat disease while minimizing symptoms and maintaining functionality and QOL has clear benefits for all stakeholders and preliminary reports suggest that it may be cost saving. Although Round and colleagues[43] did not show significant cost reduction with the incorporation of rehabilitation interventions in a hospice day program, it has been shown that physical activity improves mental and physical well-being in diverse cancer populations.[44]

Cancer rehabilitation physicians are trained to care for patients with many different oncologic diagnoses and a broad range of symptoms. Although there are similarities between various cancers, each diagnosis presents impairments and symptoms unique to its specific pathology and treatment. This underscores the challenge of accurately and patient-centrically weighing treatment burden, prognosis, individual goals, and QOL as a disease progresses. In this both rehabilitation and palliative care physicians play a vital role. Osborne and colleagues[45] attempted to identify important QOL factors for patients with multiple myeloma, but found that existing QOL questionnaires did not capture all relevant factors adequately. This led to the development of a new QOL measure specific to patients with multiple myeloma, thus highlighting the tension between generic QOL measures that allow cross-population comparisons and disease-specific measures that are less generalizable, but may more accurately and comprehensively capture issues unique to a particular disease state.[46] Palliative care and rehabilitation specialists may contribute to current efforts to develop broadly applicable measures that assess constructs valued by patients and their caregivers, for example, symptom control and function.

Physiatrists and palliative care physicians may play an important role in developing universal measures of performance status to promote cross-disciplinary, function-related communication. Oncologists routinely use the Eastern Cooperative Oncology Group (**Table 3**) or Karnofsky (**Table 4**) scores to measure performance status whereas rehabilitation physicians use the Functional Independence Measure (**Table 5**). The Eastern Cooperative Oncology Group and/or the Karnofsky score

Table 3
ECOG Performance Status scale

Grade	ECOG Performance Status
0	Fully active, able to carry on all predisease performance without restriction
1	Restricted in physically strenuous activity but ambulatory and able to carry out work of a light or sedentary nature, for example, light house work, office work
2	Ambulatory and capable of all self-care but unable to carry out any work activities; up and about more than 50% of waking hours
3	Capable of only limited self-care; confined to bed or chair more than 50% of waking hours
4	Completely disabled; cannot carry on any self-care; totally confined to bed or chair
5	Dead

Abbreviation: ECOG, Eastern Cooperative Oncology Group.
From Oken MM, Creech RH, Tormey DC, et al. Toxicity and response criteria of the Eastern Cooperative Oncology Group. Am J Clin Oncol 1982;5(6):654; with permission.

contributes to determinations of whether a patient can receive cancer treatment. Rehabilitation physicians use Functional Independence Measure scoring to determine levels of functional independence. There are limitations to both scoring systems. The Eastern Cooperative Oncology Group and Karnofsky scores and the Functional Independence Measure score are clinician rated and therefore subject to issues of inter-rater reliability. Kelly and Shahrokni proposed a new method for monitoring performance status in cancer patients.[47] The different measures and the current lack of a cross walk make it difficult for clinicians, therapists and nurses to communicate accurately about patients' functional status, which may undermine clinical decision making.

Table 4
Karnofsky Performance Status scale

	Karnofsky Performance Status
100	Normal, no complaints; no evidence of disease
90	Able to carry on normal activity; minor signs or symptoms of disease
80	Normal activity with effort, some signs or symptoms of disease
70	Cares for self, but unable to carry on normal activity or to do active work
60	Requires occasional assistance but is able to care for most of personal needs
50	Requires considerable assistance and frequent medical care
40	Disabled; requires special care and assistance
30	Severely disabled; hospitalization is indicated although death not imminent
20	Very ill; hospitalization and active supportive care necessary
10	Moribund
0	Dead

From Karnofsky D, Burchenal J. The clinical evaluation of chemotherapeutic agents in cancer. In: MacLeod C, editor. Evaluation of chemotherapeutic agents. New York: Columbia University Press; 1949. p. 196.

Table 5
FIM

FIM Instrument Scoring Criteria	
Score	Description
No helper required	
7	Complete independence
6	Modified independence (patient requires use of a device, but no physical assistance)
Helper (modified dependence)	
5	Supervision or setup
4	Minimal contact assistance (patient can perform $\geq$75% of task)
3	Moderate assistance (patient can perform 50%–74% of task)
Helper (complete dependence)	
2	Maximal assistance (patient can perform 25%–49% of tasks)
1	Total assistance (patient can perform <25% of the task or requires >1 person to assist)

Abbreviation: FIM, Functional Independence Measure.
From Rehabilitation Measures Database. FIM® instrument (FIM); FIM® is a trademark of the Uniform Data System for Medical Rehabilitation. Available at: http://www.rehabmeasures.org/lists/rehabmeasures/dispform.aspx?id=889. Accessed April 20, 2016.

SUMMARY

Although palliative care and physiatry remain distinct subspecialties, both provide unique skills sets to address common issues related to disablement and symptomatology. With the growing need for patient-centered care that optimizes function and QOL, collaboration will be essential to maximize efficiencies while achieving the highest quality cancer care. This synergistic approach is expected to advance standardized, effective, and cost-sensitive care for cancer populations.

REFERENCES

1. American Cancer Society. Cancer treatment and survivorship facts & figures 2014-2015. Atlanta (GA): American Cancer Society; 2014.
2. IOM (Institute of Medicine). Delivering high-quality cancer care: charting a new course for a system in crisis. Washington, DC: The National Academies Press; 2013.
3. Cancer trends progress report. Bethesda (MD): National Cancer Institute, NIH, DHHS; 2015. Available at: http://www.who.int/cancer/palliative/definition/en/.
4. Ryerson AB, Eheman CR, Altekruse SF, et al. Annual report to the nation on the status of cancer, 1975–2012, featuring the increasing incidence of liver cancer. Cancer 2016;122(9):1312–37.
5. Burg MA, Adorno G, Lopez ED, et al. Current unmet needs of cancer survivors: analysis of open-ended responses to the American Cancer Society Study of Cancer Survivors II. Cancer 2015;121(4):623–30.
6. Silver JK, Baima J, Mayer RS. Impairment-driven cancer rehabilitation: an essential component of quality care and survivorship. CA Cancer J Clin 2013;63(5):295–317.
7. Ramchandran K, Tribett E, Dietrich B, et al. Integrating palliative care into oncology: a way forward. Cancer Control 2015;22(4):386–95.
8. American College of Surgeons. Cancer program standards: ensuring patient-centered care. Chicago: American College of Surgeons; 2016.

9. World Health Organization (WHO). WHO definition of palliative care. Available at: http://www.who.int/cancer/palliative/definition/en/. Accessed April 2, 2016.
10. Silver JK, Raj VS, Fu JB, et al. Cancer rehabilitation and palliative care: critical components in the delivery of high-quality oncology services. Support Care Cancer 2015;23(12):3633–43.
11. Dietz JH Jr. Rehabilitation oncology. New York: John Wiley & Sons Inc; 1981.
12. Alfano CM, Ganz PA, Rowland JH, et al. Cancer survivorship and cancer rehabilitation: revitalizing the link. J Clin Oncol 2012;30(9):904–6.
13. Raj VS, Balouch J, Norton JH. Cancer rehabilitation education during physical medicine and rehabilitation residency: preliminary data regarding the quality and quantity of experiences. Am J Phys Med Rehabil 2014;93(5):445–52.
14. Cheville AL, Troxel AB, Basford JR, et al. Prevalence and treatment patterns of physical impairments in patients with metastatic breast cancer. J Clin Oncol 2008;26(16):2621–9.
15. Cheville AL, Kornblith AB, Basford JR. An examination of the causes for the underutilization of rehabilitation services among people with advanced cancer. Am J Phys Med Rehabil 2011;90(5 Suppl 1):S27–37.
16. Pergolotti M, Deal AM, Lavery J, et al. The prevalence of potentially modifiable functional deficits and the subsequent use of occupational and physical therapy by older adults with cancer. J Geriatr Oncol 2015;6(3):194–201.
17. Sullivan AM, Lakoma MD, Block SD. The status of medical education in end-of-life care: a national report. J Gen Intern Med 2003;18(9):685–95.
18. El Nawawi NM, Balboni MJ, Balboni TA. Palliative care and spiritual care: the crucial role of spiritual care in the care of patients with advanced illness. Curr Opin Support Palliat Care 2012;6(2):269–74.
19. Roeland EJ, Triplett DP, Matsuno RK, et al. Patterns of palliative care consultation among elderly patients with cancer. J Natl Compr Canc Netw 2016;14(4):439–45.
20. Rodriguez KL, Barnato AE, Arnold RM. Perceptions and utilization of palliative care services in acute care hospitals. J Palliat Med 2007;10(1):99–110.
21. Santiago-Palma J, Payne R. Palliative care and rehabilitation. Cancer 2001;92(4 Suppl):1049–52.
22. Mukai A. The future of physiatry: with challenges come opportunities. PM R 2011;3(3):189–92.
23. Smith SR, Reish AG, Andrews C. Cancer survivorship: a growing role for physiatric care. PM R 2015;7(5):527–31.
24. Lin S, Chen Y, Yang L, et al. Pain, fatigue, disturbed sleep and distress comprised a symptom cluster that related to quality of life and functional status of lung cancer surgery patients. J Clin Nurs 2013;22(9–10):1281–90.
25. Guo Y, Persyn L, Palmer JL, et al. Incidence of and risk factors for transferring cancer patients from rehabilitation to acute care units. Am J Phys Med Rehabil 2008;87(8):647–53.
26. Fu JB, Lee J, Tran KB, et al. Gains in a cancer rehabilitation unit. Int J Ther Rehabil 2015;22(11):517–23.
27. Hung R, Krebs P, Coups EJ, et al. Fatigue and functional impairment in early-stage non-small cell lung cancer survivors. J Pain Symptom Manage 2011;41(2):426–35.
28. Asher A, Fu JB, Bailey C, et al. Fatigue among patients with brain tumors. CNS Oncol 2016;5(2):91–100.
29. LaVoy EC, Fagundes CP, Dantzer R. Exercise, inflammation, and fatigue in cancer survivors. Exerc Immunol Rev 2016;22:82–93.

30. Asher A. Cognitive dysfunction among cancer survivors. Am J Phys Med Rehabil 2011;90(5 Suppl 1):S16–26.
31. Breitbart W, Alici Y. Agitation and delirium at the end of life: "We couldn't manage him". JAMA 2008;300(24):2898–910.
32. Perron V, Schonwetter RS. Assessment and management of pain in palliative care patients. Cancer Control 2001;8(1):15–24.
33. Fu JB, Dhah SS, Bruera E. Corticosteroid injections for knee pain at the end of life. J Palliat Med 2015;18(7):570–1.
34. Fu J, Ngo A, Shin K, et al. Botulinum toxin injection and phenol nerve block for reduction of end-of-life pain. J Palliat Med 2013;16(12):1637–40.
35. Stubblefield MD, Levine A, Custodio CM, et al. The role of botulinum toxin type A in the radiation fibrosis syndrome: a preliminary report. Arch Phys Med Rehabil 2008;89(3):417–21.
36. Stubblefield MD. Radiation fibrosis syndrome: trismus, trigeminal neuralgia, and cervical dystonia. In: Cooper G, editor. Therapeutic uses of botulinum toxin. Totowa (NJ): Humana Press; 2007. p. 31–2.
37. World Health Organization (WHO). WHO's cancer pain ladder for adults. Available at: http://www.who.int/cancer/palliative/painladder/en/. Accessed April 17, 2016.
38. Glare P, Miller J, Nikolova T, et al. Treating nausea and vomiting in palliative care: a review. Clin Interv Aging 2011;6:243–59.
39. Yim SY, Yoon SH, Lee IY, et al. A comparison of bowel care patterns in patients with spinal cord injury: upper motor neuron bowel vs lower motor neuron bowel. Spinal Cord 2001;39(4):204–7.
40. Raj VS, Lofton L. Rehabilitation and treatment of spinal cord tumors. J Spinal Cord Med 2013;36(1):4–11.
41. Gagnon B, Murphy J, Eades M, et al. A prospective evaluation of an interdisciplinary nutrition-rehabilitation program for patients with advanced cancer. Curr Oncol 2013;20(6):310–8.
42. Palacio A, Calmels P, Genty M, et al. Oncology and physical medicine and rehabilitation. Ann Phys Rehabil Med 2009;52(7–8):568–78.
43. Round J, Leurent B, Jones L. A cost-utility analysis of a rehabilitation service for people living with and beyond cancer. BMC Health Serv Res 2014;14:558.
44. Dieli-Conwright CM, Orozco BZ. Exercise after breast cancer treatment: current perspectives. Breast Cancer (Dove Med Press) 2015;7:353–62.
45. Osborne TR, Ramsenthaler C, de Wolf-Linder S, et al. Understanding what matters most to people with multiple myeloma: a qualitative study of views on quality of life. BMC Cancer 2014;14:496.
46. Osborne TR, Ramsenthaler C, Schey SA, et al. Improving the assessment of quality of life in the clinical care of myeloma patients: the development and validation of the Myeloma Patient Outcome Scale (MyPOS). BMC Cancer 2015;15:280.
47. Kelly CM, Shahrokni A. Moving beyond Karnofsky and ECOG Performance Status Assessments with New Technologies. J Oncol 2016;2016:6186543.

Surgical Prehabilitation in Patients with Cancer

State-of-the-Science and Recommendations for Future Research from a Panel of Subject Matter Experts

Francesco Carli, MD, MPhil[a,1,]*, Julie K. Silver, MD[b,1],
Liane S. Feldman, MD[c], Andrea McKee, MD[d], Sean Gilman, MD[e],
Chelsia Gillis, MSc, RD[a], Celena Scheede-Bergdahl, PhD[f],
Ann Gamsa, PhD[a], Nicole Stout, DPT, CLT-LANA[g],
Bradford Hirsch, MD[h]

KEYWORDS

- Cancer • Surgery • Exercise • Nutrition • Prehabilitation • Anxiety • Outcome

KEY POINTS

- Surgical prehabilitation is the process on the continuum of care that occurs between cancer diagnosis and surgical treatment.
- Physiologic principles support the implementation of either unimodal or multimodal preoperative interventions in patients diagnosed with cancer and requiring surgical intervention.

Continued

This work was supported by the Peri-Operative Program, a Nonprofit Charitable Foundation, Montreal, Quebec, Canada.

Disclosure: The opinions expressed in this publication are not an official policy or position of the National Institutes of Health, the Department of Health and Human Services, or the U.S. Government.

[a] Department of Anesthesia, McGill University Health Centre, Montreal, Quebec, Canada; [b] Department of Physical Medicine and Rehabilitation, Spaulding Rehabilitation Hospital, Harvard Medical School, Boston, MA, USA; [c] Department of Surgery, McGill University Health Centre, Montreal, Quebec, Canada; [d] Department of Radiation Oncology, Lahey Hospital and Medical Center, Burlington, MA, USA; [e] Department of Medicine, McGill University Health Centre, Montreal, Quebec, Canada; [f] Department of Kinesiology and Physical Education, McGill University, Montreal, Quebec, Canada; [g] Rehabilitation Medicine Department, National Institutes of Health, Clinical Center, Bethesda, MD, USA; [h] Flatiron Health, New York, NY, USA
[1] Contributed equally to the publication of this article.
* Corresponding author. Department of Anesthesia, Montreal General Hospital, McGill University Health Centre, 1950 Cedar Avenue, Room D10.144, Montreal, Quebec H3G 1A4, Canada.
E-mail address: franco.carli@mcgill.ca

Phys Med Rehabil Clin N Am 28 (2017) 49–64
http://dx.doi.org/10.1016/j.pmr.2016.09.002
1047-9651/17/© 2016 Elsevier Inc. All rights reserved.

Continued

- Recommendations are proposed to advance research in surgical prehabilitation by identifying the role of exercise, nutritional optimization, and psychological stress reduction in order to increase physiologic reserves in anticipation of surgery.
- There is a need to determine the impact of prehabilitation on length of stay, unanticipated readmissions and emergency department visits, perioperative complications, short-term impairments, long-term impairments, late effects, and associated disability and delays to planned postsurgical oncologic treatment.

INTRODUCTION

Surgery remains a cornerstone of oncology treatment, and minimally invasive approaches, enhanced recovery pathways (ERPs), and other interventions have improved safety and patient outcomes.[1] However, despite these advances, major cancer resections of the bladder, pancreas, lung, or esophagus have mortalities of 4% to 9%[2] and high morbidities persist even for lower-risk procedures like colorectal resection, ranging from 25% to 50%.[3] Postoperative complications prolong hospital lengths of stay, increase readmissions and elevate costs, impact patient functioning and quality of life, and may have long-term implications on mortality.[4] Tissue trauma, reduced physical activity, quasi-starvation, and psychological distress associated with major surgery result in a rapid decline in functional capacity, followed by slow recovery.[5] At-risk populations, including the elderly, are more susceptible to the negative effects of surgical stress, and some never regain their baseline functioning. Poor preoperative fitness and physical status are risk factors for serious postoperative complications and prolonged disability.[6] Neoadjuvant oncologic therapies may be associated with additional degradations of physical fitness before surgery.[7]

The preoperative period may provide an opportunity to increase the physiologic reserve in the anticipation of neoadjuvant therapies and surgery with the intention to improve outcomes and accelerate recovery (**Fig. 1**).[8] Much as someone might train for any upcoming physical challenge, prehabilitation is a compelling strategy to address modifiable risk factors that impact cancer treatment outcomes.

Cancer prehabilitation is "A process on the cancer continuum of care that occurs between the time of cancer diagnosis and the beginning of acute treatment and

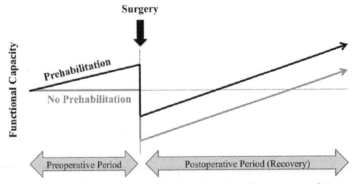

Fig. 1. Theoretic model of surgical prehabilitation based on the concept of increasing functional capacity before surgery. (*Adapted from* Carli F, Zavorsky GS. Optimizing functional exercise capacity in the elderly surgical population. Curr Opin Clin Nutr Metab Care 2005;8(1):25; with permission.)

includes physical and psychological assessments that establish a baseline functional level, identify impairments, and provide interventions that promote physical and psychological health to reduce the incidence and/or severity of future impairments" (**Fig. 2**).[9] Of note, prehabilitation is not a "one size fits all" program before surgery, but rather involves specific individualized assessments and interventions that are likely to improve outcomes for each patient. Much of the early cancer prehabilitation literature focused on exercise as a single modality intervention[9]; however, recent reports have investigated other modalities such as nutritional[10] and psychological[11] interventions either alone or in combination with exercise.[12,13] This expanding scope of prehabilitation is likely due to the acknowledgment that non–exercise interventions may be beneficial as well as that prescribing exercise as a single modality shortly before surgery may actually be detrimental to some patients who lack physiologic reserves. For example, frail elderly patients known to be at high risk for postoperative complications often present with decreased muscle mass and low protein reserves, and they may not tolerate an increase in exercise before surgery without protein supplementation. Although there is encouraging evidence in support of surgical prehabilitation in abdominal surgery,[14,15] much remains to be studied.

Beginning in early 2015, a 10-member panel of Canadian and US prehabilitation subject matter experts was invited to work collaboratively in an effort to describe the current state-of-the-science in oncology surgical prehabilitation. The panel then convened in November 2015 for 2 days at the McGill University Health Centre in Montreal, Quebec, Canada, to discuss their findings and reach consensus on recommendations for future research directions. This report summarizes the current state-of-the-science and recommends directions for future research.

THE ROLE OF EXERCISE IN SURGICAL PREHABILITATION
Exercise in the Cancer Trajectory

Regular exercise has long been recognized as an effective means of preventing disease.[16] Cardiac and other types of rehabilitation have also incorporated exercise into comprehensive disease management. Studies of subjects confined to bed rest highlight the rapid loss of physical function[17] and insulin sensitivity[18] that occur with sedentary behavior.

Robust evidence supports the role of structured exercise as a means of enhancing diverse outcomes during and following the active phase of cancer treatment.[19] Of late, exercise is also gaining acceptance for its potential in the preintervention period.[13] As it becomes increasingly clear that exercise plays an important role in both cancer

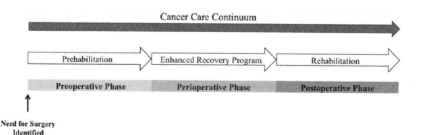

Fig. 2. Assessment and interventions designed to improve outcomes and reduce health care costs are possible across the care continuum beginning with the preoperative phase (prehabilitation) and transitioning to the perioperative phase (enhanced recovery programs) and postoperative phase (rehabilitation).

prevention and treatment, tailoring validated exercise programs can be challenging in this patient population.

Precisely defining exercise is challenging because there are many definitions in the literature. For the purposes of this report, exercise encompasses regular physical activity that is incorporated into a planned and structured program. This planned program contrasts with generic recommendations to increase physical activity preoperatively.[14] Furthermore, exercise designed to improve overall cardiovascular or muscular fitness is distinct from exercise that is, "targeted" and focuses on the training or retraining of specific muscles to facilitate disease-specific outcomes such as improving swallowing in head and neck cancer survivors,[20] urinary continence in patients with prostate cancer,[21] and reducing arm, shoulder, and upper quadrant pain and disability in patients with breast cancer.[22]

This discussion is focused on the overall cardiovascular and strength training components of exercise with specified intensity, frequency, and modality,[13] as more prehabilitation research currently supports this than "targeted" exercise. However, future studies may demonstrate the benefit of targeted exercises in optimizing patient outcomes.

Prescribing Exercise in the Prehabilitation Period

At the present time, there are no guidelines specific for general cardiovascular or resistance exercise in the prehabilitation period. However, the American Cancer Society has published broad exercise guidelines that recommend[23] at least 150 minutes of moderate or 75 minutes of vigorous intensity (or combination of) exercise per week and include 2 to 3 sessions of resistance training, involving major muscle groups. An individual's baseline health and fitness, as well as cancer diagnosis, treatment sequelae, and comorbid conditions, should inform exercise prescribing for the patient with cancer.[24] A growing body of evidence highlights the need to consider the type and amount of activity that is performed during non-exercise time.[25] Adequate recovery/rest time (both between sets and sessions) should be included in the prescription, especially if the individual is unaccustomed to the prescribed activity.[26] When considering exercise as a prehabilitation intervention, "one size does not fit all." Exercise prescriptions are ideally tailored to baseline levels of fitness (determined by formal assessment), current health status, and the planned surgical procedure. In some individuals, exercise is contraindicated altogether or should be modified based on their health status, and safety in the cancer population is an important consideration.

There is a need in patients with cancer to compare the cost-effectiveness, health benefits, and adherence rates of different modes of exercise delivery (eg, supervised personal training, supervised group training, home-based training).[27] It is also important to establish who should be supervising these exercise programs and what qualifications they should have in order to ensure the safety and address the specific needs of a patient. Sensor technology has only recently allowed for the generation of objective data to inform the discussion of fatigue and health-related quality of life (HRQOL), as well as to inform care delivery. In oncology, the main focus of sensor-based analyses has been in the survivor population. Trials using sensor technologies have shown a relationship between moderate to vigorous physical activity (MVPA), sedentary time (SED), and health-related quality of life (HRQOL). Examples include a study of 199 breast cancer survivors showing that levels of pain, fatigue, and dysphoria are related to the amount of MVPA and SED experienced,[28] and a study showing that participants who achieved 150 minutes of MVPA per week had 18% higher HRQOL relative to those who reported no MVPA.[29] Even more nascent, yet equally important, is the use of sensors in the analysis of sleep among oncology patients. The rate of sleep disturbance among patients with cancer ranges from 25%

to 59%,[30,31] and the quality of sleep may impact quality of life. The increasing use of sensors in the community and acceptance by the public have paved the way to integrating them into research studies and clinical care.

THE ROLE OF NUTRITION IN SURGICAL PREHABILITATION
Malnutrition and Nutritional Risk

Malnutrition arises from inadequate intake and/or metabolic and inflammatory alterations that alter nutrient requirements or absorption, which, ultimately, leads to wasting and diminished physical function. The cause of malnutrition is generally multifactorial and includes gastrointestinal (GI) abnormalities (eg, nausea, diarrhea), tumor-related mechanisms (eg, obstruction), and tumor-induced metabolic abnormalities (eg, insulin resistance, catabolism), as well as anticancer therapies that provoke anorexia and GI derangements.[32] Data on the prevalence of malnutrition vary based on tumor type, site, and advancement of disease as well as anticancer treatment; however, the prevalence of malnutrition associated with body wasting among patients with cancer with either early or late disease has been estimated to range between 28% and 57%.[33] Perioperative treatment of disease-related malnutrition with oral nutrition supplements or enteral nutrition might reduce rates of mortality and morbidity.[34] Moreover, recent North American surgical consensus recommendations suggest moving beyond treating malnutrition to proactive preoperative nutritional therapy in all "at-risk" patients to potentially mitigate complication rates and severity.[35] As a result, early determination of malnutrition risk, for the purpose of eliciting a comprehensive dietary consult, throughout the continuum of care for oncologic and surgical patients, is increasingly recognized as a significant component of quality care.[36]

A systematic approach to identifying and treating patients at nutritional risk should be established. Several nutrition screening tools, such as the Nutrition Risk Screening 2002 and Subjective Global Assessment, have been used and validated in surgical populations.[37,38]

Nutritional Care Goals

The primary goal of oncologic and perioperative nutritional care is to decrease the incidence and severity of nausea and vomiting, improve appetite recovery, enhance immunity, support normoglycemia, and provide sufficient protein intake to achieve anabolism and enough energy to maintain body weight. It is becoming increasingly evident that these interventions should begin *preoperatively*. The use of appropriate assessments, such as that to detect malnutrition, before surgery permits patient-specific treatments that can improve metabolic status. The goals would include improved postoperative outcomes as well as less nutritional support needed after surgery.

Optimal Nutrition Care: A Combination of Oral Nutrition Supplements and Dietary Counseling

A *Cochrane Review* did not find a reduction of complications or length of hospital stay with the use of standard preoperative oral nutritional supplements in patients undergoing GI surgery.[36] Although some benefits were found with immune-enhancing nutrients, these results cannot yet be generalized to the ERP population. A combination of both individualized nutrition counseling and oral nutritional supplements has been proven to be effective in building functional capacity in prehabilitation trials.[39]

Integrating Nutrition with Exercise

Observational evidence suggests that patients with higher preoperative lean body mass (ie, reserve) are better able to cope with surgical stress as determined by reduced complications and earlier discharge.[40] In order to generate a positive net protein balance in favor of lean body mass accretion, exogenous amino acids must be administered to produce a state in which protein synthesis exceeds that of protein breakdown. Twenty grams of protein (in liquid form) taken immediately after resistance exercise is regarded as sufficient to maximally stimulate muscle protein synthesis in healthy individuals.[41] The optimal after-exercise diet to support lean body mass accretion in patients with cancer should be investigated. Although most of the literature has focused on assessing malnutrition and providing interventions to those with documented problems, a recent study suggests that even patients with cancer with no clinical signs of malnutrition may have better outcomes with dietary intervention.[10] Finally, omega-3 fatty acids, particularly eicosapentaenoic acid and docosahexaenoic acid, which are found naturally in fish oils, have been identified in several randomized controlled trials to reduce oxidative stress and inflammation in cancer and surgical patients,[42] which may translate into minimized loss of lean body tissue.[43] Adequate dietary intake of these nutrients should thus be a consideration in dietary planning.

THE ROLE OF PSYCHOLOGICAL STRESS REDUCTION IN SURGICAL PREHABILITATION
Emotional Stress and Its Impact on Perioperative Outcome

A recently published systematic review on psychological surgical prehabilitation suggests a positive role.[11] A large body of published literature suggests associations of patients' preoperative psychological state with their postoperative recovery, including wound healing, infection, function, and length of hospital stay.[44] For instance, anxiety and depression can predict surgical outcome, even after known physiologic factors are accounted for.[45] Presence of depression increases the length of hospitalization for patients undergoing thoracic surgery for cancer[46] and is associated with poor compliance to medical treatment.[47]

Preoperative anxiety and its concomitant stress response are the most frequently cited psychological factors to affect wound healing, hospital stay, return to function, and satisfaction with surgery.[48] Trait and state anxiety have been shown to have significant effect on postoperative complications and impaired wound healing.[49] The diagnosis of cancer and the addition of neoadjuvant chemoradiation therapy enhance even further the emotional stress in anticipation of surgery.

Preoperative Strategies to Attenuate Anxiety

Evidence-based perioperative psychological interventions effectively reduce anxiety in surgical patients.[49] Reduced anxiety has been empirically linked to improvements in patients' immunologic function, as well as self-reported psychological outcomes, quality of life, and somatic symptoms. However, these strategies did not affect traditional surgical outcomes, including length of hospital stay, complications, analgesic use, or mortality. A wide variety of anxiety-reducing approaches have been used, including relaxation training and education, deep breathing exercises, visualization, yoga, and music in the perioperative setting.[11] Music therapy can reduce postoperative anxiety, pain, and analgesia requirements as well as improve patient satisfaction, by reducing sympathetic arousal.[50]

THE ROLE OF SMOKING CESSATION IN SURGICAL PREHABILITATION

The literature shows that patients with cancer who successfully abstain from smoking before surgery have reduced risk of postoperative complications and improved performance status and quality-of-life measures.[51] In contrast, patients with cancer who continue to smoke face an increased risk of postoperative complications, impaired wound healing, delays to adjuvant chemotherapy, increased recurrence and second primaries, and increased mortality.[52,53]

Although smoking cessation has not been well studied as a prehabilitation intervention, this panel of subject matter experts recommends addressing nicotine dependence at the time of cancer diagnosis, initiating smoking cessation therapy, and using the eventual hospitalization to reinforce abstinence. Best practices in smoking cessation suggest counseling along with either combination nicotine replacement therapy (cNRT) or Varenicline.[54] cNRT is a recommended first-line treatment especially in those more motivated to quit. Prescriptions consist of appropriately dosed transdermal nicotine (patch) and a short-acting nicotine to be used as needed for cravings. If there are no contraindications, Varenicline is an equally good choice[54] and may be a preferred treatment in the ambivalent smoker due to its flexible target quit date of 8 to 35 days.[55] Nicotine replacement can be combined with Varenicline to help additional cravings.[56] Either NRT or Varenicline monotherapy may also be used in those patients who are not ready to quit but are willing to reduce tobacco consumption (**Table 1**).[57,58]

PREHABILITATION AS PART OF AN ENHANCED RECOVERY STRATEGY TO ATTENUATE SURGICAL STRESS AND IMPROVE RECOVERY

Major surgery triggers a range of endocrinologic, immunologic, and hematologic changes as a result of inflammatory mediators released in response to tissue injury as well as afferent impulses from the injury site. A central feature of the metabolic

Table 1
Therapeutic strategies of smoking cessation

	Combination NRT	Varenicline ± Short-Acting NRT	NRT Monotherapy
Motivated to quit	Appropriately dosed TD nicotine patch in combination with short acting NRT used PRN for cravings	Acceptable regimen	Not recommended as first line
Ambivalent smoker	Acceptable regimen	Encourage continued smoking until target quit date chosen by patient, usually day 8–35	Not recommended as first line
Unwilling to make a quit attempt	Acceptable regimen	Acceptable regimen in patient willing to make a quit attempt within 3 mo	Long-term TD nicotine patch to significantly reduce the number of cigarettes smoked

Appropriately dosed patch depends on daily smoking. Typical starting dose is 21 mg daily. For smokers of 25 to 30 cigarettes per day, start TD nicotine at 28 mg daily. For smokers of 30 to 40 cigarettes per day, start TD nicotine at 35 mg.

Short-acting NRT includes nicotine gum, lozenge, spray, or inhaler, used hourly as needed for cravings.

Varenicline may be prescribed as long as there are no identified contraindications. Usual prescription is the Starter Pack followed by 1 mg BID.

Abbreviations: NRT, nicotine replacement therapy; TD, transdermal.

response to injury is the development of a state of acute insulin resistance,[59] which is greatest on the day of surgery but may persist for weeks and is associated with increased morbidity. Clinically, the stress response is manifested as hyperglycemia, pain, tachycardia, hypoxia, cognitive disturbance, anxiety, acidosis, ileus, hypercoagulability, and loss of muscle mass.[59] As mentioned earlier, ERPs are care pathways that integrate multiple evidence-based perioperative interventions into a cohesive plan with the aim to attenuate the stress response. A large body of evidence supports the use of ERPs to organize perioperative care.[60] One meta-analysis of 38 randomized trials concluded that ERPs reduced the risk of complications by about 30% and was associated with reduced hospital stay by about 1 day overall and no increase in readmissions.[61]

Prehabilitation and ERPs should both be part of an integrated surgical care continuum (see **Fig. 2**). A single modality may not be powerful enough to change outcomes, but combined with other modalities, the effect may be more significant. This effect is often called the "sum of small gains," whereby multiple interventions, each of which may have a small benefit on its own, have a synergistic effect when combined.[1] Although prehabilitation is distinct from other preoperative preparation, there is some overlap, and it is important that prehabilitation be part of a continuum of care in which changes made preoperatively are supported throughout the perioperative period, as in an ERP.

SPECIFIC EXAMPLES OF SURGICAL PREHABILITATION

Although surgical prehabilitation programs are not routinely part of current clinical practice, specialties such as thoracic, colorectal, and breast surgery have introduced some interventions to mitigate the surgical stress and facilitate recovery. In this section, examples of surgical prehabilitation are presented for each of the 3 specialties with particular attention to the characteristics of the specific patient population.

Surgical Prehabilitation for Lung Cancer

Lung cancer is the leading cause of cancer-related mortality in both men and women in the United States.[62] The 2 most important risk factors for the development of lung cancer are tobacco use and advanced age.[63] Computed tomographic lung screening is being widely implemented in the United States for high-risk patients, because it has been shown to be an effective secondary prevention intervention, which has the potential to improve the 5-year overall survival of patients with lung cancer—currently at 17.4%.[64] The anticipated growth in the population of early stage patients with lung cancer identified through screening will result in a significant increase in the number of patients with potentially resectable disease but who are aging and often sedentary patients with lung cancer with multiple comorbidities. Therefore, prehabilitation may provide a unique opportunity to facilitate better surgical outcomes.

Most of the literature on rehabilitation in patients undergoing thoracic surgery has addressed the role of respiratory therapy either before or after surgery with moderate impact on postoperative outcome.[65] A recent systematic review on the effect of preoperative exercise therapy based on moderate to intense exercise in patients scheduled for lung surgery showed beneficial effects on aerobic capacity, physical fitness, and quality of life.[66] The rationale of assessing lung reserve by cardiopulmonary exercise testing (CPET) in this population is to increase aerobic reserve in anticipation of the removal of part of the lung. Although most of the studies looked at the role of exercise alone, it is important to also consider multimodal interventions (**Box 1**).

Box 1
Surgical prehabilitation for lung cancer

What is known:

- Several publications on standard pulmonary rehabilitation (physical therapy, smoking cessation) started before surgery confirm some improvement in dyspnea scores and in functional exercise capacity (6-minute walk distance), and reduction on postoperative morbidity, with fewer days of chest tube in place. Little effect if pulmonary rehabilitation is performed after surgery.

- Preoperative moderate or intense exercise improves aerobic capacity, physical fitness, and quality of life.

- High level of depression impacts negatively on duration of hospital stay and mortality.

Gaps in research:

- Determine the impact of introducing a lung surgery–specific standardized ERPs on postoperative outcome.

- Develop structured, patient-tailored, exercise programs based on objective assessment of cardiopulmonary function (anaerobic threshold, Vo_2 peak, 6 MWT), physical strength, flexibility and pulmonary function tests.

- Define timing, intensity, duration of training methods to be used also in presence of chronic obstructive pulmonary disease.

- Develop nutritional assessment and determine which nutritional intake (proteins and energy) is appropriate to overcome respiratory muscle weakness.

- Introduce group therapy to mitigate the impact of anxiety and depression on postoperative outcome.

- Determine, by using appropriate metrics, the impact of multimodal interventions on postoperative complications, length of stay (LOS), readmission rate, progression of the disease.

Surgical Prehabilitation for Colorectal Cancer

The incidence of colorectal cancer continues to increase, and although the mortality has decreased over the years, the burden of the disease is still high. Modifiable risk factors for colorectal cancer include sedentary lifestyle as well as high-fat and low-fiber diets, heavy alcohol consumption, and cigarette smoking. These risk factors also have an impact on cardiorespiratory and metabolic systems, thus leading to high comorbidity rate in this population.[67] In view of the great number of postoperative complications and a 30% to 40% reduction in functional walking capacity,[68] this type of surgery may be amenable to outcome enhancement through prehabilitation. ERPs for colorectal surgery have been in place for more than a decade demonstrating the positive impact of evidence-based multidisciplinary interventions on postoperative outcomes.[69] Although the initial introduction of prehabilitation programs using intense exercise showed poor compliance and modest changes in postoperative functional capacity,[70] multimodal structured prehabilitation protocols, which included aerobic and resistance exercises together with protein supplementation and relaxation strategies, showed a positive impact on preoperative physiologic reserve with sustained levels of functional capacity after surgery.[12] More than 80% of patients who received the multimodal prehabilitation program returned to baseline values of functional walking capacity by 8 weeks. In contrast, only 40% of patients who did not receive prehabilitation returned to baseline values.[12] Recently, a consensus among an expert group of colorectal surgeons highlighted the potential benefits of preoperative exercise in patients undergoing tumor resections.[71] The ongoing CHALLENGE (Colon Health and Life Health and Life-Long Exercise Change) trial will determine the impact of supervised exercise on survival.[72]

Although the early evidence that prehabilitation may support better outcomes in the colorectal cancer surgery populations is encouraging, it remains to be seen if preoperative interventions will reduce complications and unplanned health care utilization (**Box 2**).

Surgical Prehabilitation for Breast Cancer

Breast cancer is the most commonly diagnosed cancer among women and has one of the highest survival rates of all cancer diagnoses.[73] Morbidity and disability rates are reported in up to 60% of breast cancer survivors.[74] Despite recent evidence supporting pretreatment and prospective screening and assessment for early identification and treatment of breast cancer treatment-related impairments,[75,76] there have been very few reports on breast cancer prehabilitation and its effect on improving outcomes. One recent study reported positive results on upper extremity prehabilitation to improve shoulder pain and abduction range of motion after breast cancer surgery.[77] Further research in this population is needed because there is merit to considering systemic prehabilitation as a value added intervention (**Box 3**).

Box 2
Surgical prehabilitation for colorectal cancer

What is known:

- ERPs in colorectal surgery are well documented with positive impact on LOS, but not significant reduction in on postoperative morbidity.

- Consensus among an expert group of colorectal surgeons on potential benefits of preoperative exercise.

- Only 2 randomized controlled trials (RCTs) using exercise preoperatively, one with moderate exercise and positive impact on postoperative complications, and the other using an intensive exercise program and no effect on postoperative functional capacity.

- One pilot and one RCT comparing 4-week multimodal (exercise, nutritional supplements, relaxation) prehabilitation versus rehabilitation. Significant postoperative improvement in functional capacity in the prehabilitation group.

- Modest increase in functional capacity if nutritional supplementation alone.

- Supervised intense exercise after neoadjuvant chemoradiotherapy improved significantly cardiopulmonary function.

Gaps in research:

- Standardize assessment of exercise capacity (CPET, walk test, physical activity) to plan the tailored exercise (aerobic, resistance) and measures of detecting improvement.

- Determine whether the intensity, duration, and supervision of endurance exercise before surgery, by increasing levels of activity before and after surgery, impact positively on postoperative LOS, unanticipated readmission or emergency department visits, and complications.

- Identify if vulnerable patients, such as frail, elderly, with many comorbidities, would benefit from multimodal prehabilitation.

- Verify whether multimodal prehabilitation may improve diagnosis by reducing the time frame from surgery to the start of chemotherapy or other treatment.

Box 3
Surgical prehabilitation for breast cancer

What is known:

- Many studies report the beneficial effect of postoperative therapeutic exercises to minimize the disability burden associated with breast surgery.

- No structured systemic prehabilitation program to prevent breast cancer treatment–related morbidity and disability has been addressed.

Gaps in research:

- Identify valid and reliable patient-reported outcomes measures that are most sensitive to assess the premorbid condition of the patient.

- Identify clinical measurement tools with sensitivity and specificity sufficient to contribute to accurate screening for morbidity before and during cancer treatment.

- Identify an evidence-based, upper quadrant therapeutic exercise program and study its impact on functional recovery when taught and incorporated into a prehabilitation plan of care.

- Study the impact of pretreatment education for health-promoting skills and behaviors, including exercise, nutrition, and cognitive function.

- Determine if prehabilitation intervention for a cohort of patients with pre-existing shoulder and arm morbidity impacts overall functional recovery after treatment.

- Investigate patient perceptions and perspectives on the benefits of prehabilitation and identify if cancer treatment outcomes and adherence to treatment recommendations are different among patients undergoing a prehabilitation plan of care.

SUMMARY

Prehabilitation in patients with cancer may offer an opportunity to preserve or enhance physiologic integrity and optimize surgical recovery. This panel of subject matter experts reached consensus on the following recommendations for future research on surgical prehabilitation.

RESEARCH RECOMMENDATIONS

1. Determine the impact of prehabilitation on physical and psychological health in patients with cancer
   a. which patients are most likely to benefit
   b. whether prehabilitation can increase surgical candidacy in high-risk patients
2. Determine the impact of prehabilitation on
   a. health care utilization
   b. perioperative complications
   c. the metabolic response to surgery
   d. physical functioning
   e. timing of recommended oncologic treatment
   f. adherence to recommended oncologic treatment
3. Characterize the performance of measures to assess baseline status and evaluate effectiveness of prehabilitation.
4. Identify procedure-specific prehabilitation assessments and interventions for specific patient populations.

ACKNOWLEDGMENTS

The authors would like to thank the Peri-Operative Program Team, Mary Guay, and the McGill University Health Centre, Montreal General Hospital site, for their assistance with the Surgical Prehabilitation Subject Matter Experts meeting held at the Montreal General Hospital, Montreal, Quebec, Canada on November 6 to 7, 2015.

REFERENCES

1. Lassen K, Soop M, Nygren J, et al. Consensus review of optimal perioperative care in colorectal surgery: enhanced recovery after surgery (ERAS) group recommendations. Arch Surg 2009;144(10):961–9.
2. Finks JF, Osborne NH, Birkmeyer JD. Trends in hospital volume and operative mortality for high-risk surgery. N Engl J Med 2011;364(22):2128–37.
3. Lucas DJ, Pawlik TM. Quality improvement in gastrointestinal surgical oncology with American College of Surgeons National Surgical Quality Improvement Program. Surgery 2014;155(4):593–601.
4. Khuri SF, Henderson WG, DePalma RG, et al. Determinants of long-term survival after major surgery and the adverse effect of postoperative complications. Ann Surg 2005;242(3):326–41 [discussion: 41–3].
5. Christensen T, Bendix T, Kehlet H. Fatigue and cardiorespiratory function following abdominal surgery. Br J Surg 1982;69(7):417–9.
6. Wilson RJ, Davies S, Yates D, et al. Impaired functional capacity is associated with all-cause mortality after major elective intra-abdominal surgery. Br J Anaesth 2010;105(3):297–303.
7. West MA, Loughney L, Lythgoe D, et al. Effect of prehabilitation on objectively measured physical fitness after neoadjuvant treatment in preoperative rectal cancer patients: a blinded interventional pilot study. Br J Anaesth 2015;114(2): 244–51.
8. Carli F, Zavorsky GS. Optimizing functional exercise capacity in the elderly surgical population. Curr Opin Clin Nutr Metab Care 2005;8(1):23–32.
9. Silver JK, Baima J. Cancer prehabilitation: an opportunity to decrease treatment-related morbidity, increase cancer treatment options, and improve physical and psychological health outcomes. Am J Phys Med Rehabil 2013;92(8):715–27.
10. Kabata P, Jastrzebski T, Kakol M, et al. Preoperative nutritional support in cancer patients with no clinical signs of malnutrition–prospective randomized controlled trial. Support Care Cancer 2015;23(2):365–70.
11. Tsimopoulou I, Pasquali S, Howard R, et al. Psychological prehabilitation before cancer surgery: a systematic review. Ann Surg Oncol 2015;22(13):4117–23.
12. Gillis C, Li C, Lee L, et al. Prehabilitation versus rehabilitation: a randomized control trial in patients undergoing colorectal resection for cancer. Anesthesiology 2014;121(5):937–47.
13. Carli F, Scheede-Bergdahl C. Prehabilitation to enhance perioperative care. Anesthesiol Clin 2015;33(1):17–33.
14. Englesbe MJ, Lussiez AD, Friedman JF, et al. Starting a surgical home. Ann Surg 2015;262(6):901–3.
15. Dunne DF, Jack S, Jones RP, et al. Randomized clinical trial of prehabilitation before planned liver resection. Br J Surg 2016;103(5):504–12.
16. Buffart LM, Galvao DA, Brug J, et al. Evidence-based physical activity guidelines for cancer survivors: current guidelines, knowledge gaps and future research directions. Cancer Treat Rev 2014;40(2):327–40.

17. Coker RH, Hays NP, Williams RH, et al. Bed rest promotes reductions in walking speed, functional parameters, and aerobic fitness in older, healthy adults. J Gerontol A Biol Sci Med Sci 2015;70(1):91–6.
18. Alibegovic AC, Sonne MP, Hojbjerre L, et al. Insulin resistance induced by physical inactivity is associated with multiple transcriptional changes in skeletal muscle in young men. Am J Physiol Endocrinol Metab 2010;299(5):E752–63.
19. Courneya KS, Friedenreich CM. Physical activity and cancer: an introduction. Recent Results Cancer Res 2011;186:1–10.
20. Kraaijenga SA, van der Molen L, Jacobi I, et al. Prospective clinical study on long-term swallowing function and voice quality in advanced head and neck cancer patients treated with concurrent chemoradiotherapy and preventive swallowing exercises. Eur Arch Otorhinolaryngol 2015;272(11):3521–31.
21. Wang W, Huang QM, Liu FP, et al. Effectiveness of preoperative pelvic floor muscle. BMC Urol 2014;14:99.
22. Springer BA, Levy E, McGarvey C, et al. Pre-operative assessment enables early diagnosis and recovery of shoulder function in patients with breast cancer. Breast Cancer Res Treat 2010;120(1):135–47.
23. Kushi LH, Doyle C, McCullough M, et al. American Cancer Society guidelines on nutrition and physical activity for cancer prevention: reducing the risk of cancer with healthy food choices and physical activity. CA Cancer J Clin 2012;62(1):30–67.
24. Denlinger CS, Engstrom PF. Colorectal cancer survivorship: movement matters. Cancer Prev Res (Phila) 2011;4(4):502–11.
25. Lemanne D, Cassileth B, Gubili J. The role of physical activity in cancer prevention, treatment, recovery, and survivorship. Oncology (Williston Park) 2013;27(6):580–5.
26. Sasso JP, Eves ND, Christensen JF, et al. A framework for prescription in exercise-oncology research. J Cachexia Sarcopenia Muscle 2015;6(2):115–24.
27. Alibhai SM, Santa Mina D, Ritvo P, et al. A phase II RCT and economic analysis of three exercise delivery methods in men with prostate cancer on androgen deprivation therapy. BMC Cancer 2015;15:312.
28. Sabiston CM, Brunet J, Vallance JK, et al. Prospective examination of objectively assessed physical activity and sedentary time after breast cancer treatment: sitting on the crest of the teachable moment. Cancer Epidemiol Biomarkers Prev 2014;23(7):1324–30.
29. Lynch BM, Cerin E, Owen N, et al. Prospective relationships of physical activity with quality of life among colorectal cancer survivors. J Clin Oncol 2008;26(27):4480–7.
30. Savard J, Villa J, Ivers H, et al. Prevalence, natural course, and risk factors of insomnia comorbid with cancer over a 2-month period. J Clin Oncol 2009;27(31):5233–9.
31. Palesh OG, Roscoe JA, Mustian KM, et al. Prevalence, demographics, and psychological associations of sleep disruption in patients with cancer: University of Rochester Cancer Center-Community Clinical Oncology Program. J Clin Oncol 2010;28(2):292–8.
32. Nicolini A, Ferrari P, Masoni MC, et al. Malnutrition, anorexia and cachexia in cancer patients: a mini-review on pathogenesis and treatment. Biomed Pharmacother 2013;67(8):807–17.
33. von Haehling S, Anker SD. Cachexia as major underestimated unmet medical need: facts and numbers. Int J Cardiol 2012;161(3):121–3.

34. Jie B, Jiang ZM, Nolan MT, et al. Impact of preoperative nutritional support on clinical outcome in abdominal surgical patients at nutritional risk. Nutrition 2012;28(10):1022–7.

35. McClave SA, Kozar R, Martindale RG, et al. Summary points and consensus recommendations from the North American Surgical Nutrition Summit. JPEN J Parenter Enteral Nutr 2013;37(5 Suppl):99s–105s.

36. Burden S, Todd C, Hill J, et al. Pre-operative nutrition support in patients undergoing gastrointestinal surgery. Cochrane Database Syst Rev 2012;(11):CD008879.

37. Bauer J, Capra S, Ferguson M. Use of the scored Patient-Generated Subjective Global Assessment (PG-SGA) as a nutrition assessment tool in patients with cancer. Eur J Clin Nutr 2002;56(8):779–85.

38. Kondrup J, Rasmussen HH, Hamberg O, et al. Nutritional risk screening (NRS 2002): a new method based on an analysis of controlled clinical trials. Clin Nutr 2003;22(3):321–36.

39. Gillis C, Loiselle SE, Fiore JF Jr, et al. Prehabilitation with whey protein supplementation on perioperative functional exercise capacity in patients undergoing colorectal resection for cancer: a pilot double-blinded randomized controlled trial. J Acad Nutr Diet 2016;116(5):802–12.

40. Pichard C, Kyle UG, Morabia A, et al. Nutritional assessment: lean body mass depletion at hospital admission is associated with an increased length of stay. Am J Clin Nutr 2004;79(4):613–8.

41. Burke LM, Hawley JA, Ross ML, et al. Preexercise aminoacidemia and muscle protein synthesis after resistance exercise. Med Sci Sports Exerc 2012;44(10):1968–77.

42. Chen B, Zhou Y, Yang P, et al. Safety and efficacy of fish oil-enriched parenteral nutrition regimen on postoperative patients undergoing major abdominal surgery: a meta-analysis of randomized controlled trials. JPEN J Parenter Enteral Nutr 2010;34(4):387–94.

43. Ryan AM, Reynolds JV, Healy L, et al. Enteral nutrition enriched with eicosapentaenoic acid (EPA) preserves lean body mass following esophageal cancer surgery: results of a double-blinded randomized controlled trial. Ann Surg 2009;249(3):355–63.

44. Mavros MN, Athanasiou S, Gkegkes ID, et al. Do psychological variables affect early surgical recovery? PLoS One 2011;6(5):e20306.

45. Rosenberger PH, Jokl P, Ickovics J. Psychosocial factors and surgical outcomes: an evidence-based literature review. J Am Acad Orthop Surg 2006;14(7):397–405.

46. Kitagawa R, Yasui-Furukori N, Tsushima T, et al. Depression increases the length of hospitalization for patients undergoing thoracic surgery: a preliminary study. Psychosomatics 2011;52(5):428–32.

47. DiMatteo MR, Lepper HS, Croghan TW. Depression is a risk factor for noncompliance with medical treatment: meta-analysis of the effects of anxiety and depression on patient adherence. Arch Intern Med 2000;160(14):2101–7.

48. Webster Marketon JI, Glaser R. Stress hormones and immune function. Cell Immunol 2008;252(1–2):16–26.

49. Bailey L. Strategies for decreasing patient anxiety in the perioperative setting. AORN J 2010;92(4):445–57 [quiz: 58–60].

50. Bradt J, Dileo C, Shim M. Music interventions for preoperative anxiety. Cochrane Database Syst Rev 2013;(6):CD006908.

51. Sorensen LT. Wound healing and infection in surgery: the pathophysiological impact of smoking, smoking cessation, and nicotine replacement therapy: a systematic review. Ann Surg 2012;255(6):1069–79.

52. Schnoll RA, Martinez E, Langer C, et al. Predictors of smoking cessation among cancer patients enrolled in a smoking cessation program. Acta Oncol 2011;50(5): 678–84.

53. Kim SW, Kong KA, Kim DY, et al. Multiple primary cancers involving lung cancer at a single tertiary hospital: clinical features and prognosis. Thorac Cancer 2015; 6(2):159–65.

54. Cahill K, Stevens S, Perera R, et al. Pharmacological interventions for smoking cessation: an overview and network meta-analysis. Cochrane Database Syst Rev 2013;(5):CD009329.

55. Rennard S, Hughes J, Cinciripini PM, et al. A randomized placebo-controlled trial of varenicline for smoking cessation allowing flexible quit dates. Nicotine Tob Res 2012;14(3):343–50.

56. Koegelenberg CF, Noor F, Bateman ED, et al. Efficacy of varenicline combined with nicotine replacement therapy vs varenicline alone for smoking cessation: a randomized clinical trial. JAMA 2014;312(2):155–61.

57. Ebbert JO, Hughes JR, West RJ, et al. Effect of varenicline on smoking cessation through smoking reduction: a randomized clinical trial. JAMA 2015;313(7): 687–94.

58. Moore DR, Tang JE, Burd NA, et al. Differential stimulation of myofibrillar and sarcoplasmic protein synthesis with protein ingestion at rest and after resistance exercise. J Physiol 2009;587(Pt 4):897–904.

59. Carli F. Physiologic considerations of enhanced recovery after surgery (ERAS) programs: implications of the stress response. Can J Anaesth 2015;62(2):110–9.

60. Spanjersberg WR, Reurings J, Keus F, et al. Fast track surgery versus conventional recovery strategies for colorectal surgery. Cochrane Database Syst Rev 2011;(2):CD007635.

61. Nicholson A, Lowe MC, Parker J, et al. Systematic review and meta-analysis of enhanced recovery programmes in surgical patients. Br J Surg 2014;101(3): 172–88.

62. Surveillance epidemiology and end results stat fact sheets: Lung and bronchus cancer. 2014. Available at: http://seer.cancer.gov/statfacts/html/lungb.html. Accessed October 5, 2016.

63. NCCN Lung Cancer Screening Guidelines. 2014. Available at: http://www.rrmginc.com/docs/NCCN_GuidelinesLungCancerScreening.pdf. Accessed October 5, 2016.

64. Aberle DR, Adams AM, Berg CD, et al. Reduced lung-cancer mortality with low-dose computed tomographic screening. N Engl J Med 2011;365(5):395–409.

65. Rodriguez-Larrad A, Lascurain-Aguirrebena I, Abecia-Inchaurregui LC, et al. Perioperative physiotherapy in patients undergoing lung cancer resection. Interact Cardiovasc Thorac Surg 2014;19(2):269–81.

66. Pouwels S, Fiddelaers J, Teijink JA, et al. Preoperative exercise therapy in lung surgery patients: a systematic review. Respir Med 2015;109(12):1495–504.

67. Edwards BK, Noone AM, Mariotto AB, et al. Annual Report to the Nation on the status of cancer, 1975-2010, featuring prevalence of comorbidity and impact on survival among persons with lung, colorectal, breast, or prostate cancer. Cancer 2014;120(9):1290–314.

68. Lawson EH, Wang X, Cohen ME, et al. Morbidity and mortality after colorectal procedures: comparison of data from the American College of Surgeons case log system and the ACS NSQIP. J Am Coll Surg 2011;212(6):1077–85.

69. Zhuang CL, Ye XZ, Zhang XD, et al. Enhanced recovery after surgery programs versus traditional care for colorectal surgery: a meta-analysis of randomized controlled trials. Dis Colon Rectum 2013;56(5):667–78.

70. Carli F, Charlebois P, Stein B, et al. Randomized clinical trial of prehabilitation in colorectal surgery. Br J Surg 2010;97(8):1187–97.

71. Boereboom CL, Williams JP, Leighton P, et al. Forming a consensus opinion on exercise prehabilitation in elderly colorectal cancer patients: a Delphi study. Tech Coloproctol 2015;19(6):347–54.

72. Courneya KS, Booth CM, Gill S, et al. The colon health and life-long exercise change trial: a randomized trial of the National Cancer Institute of Canada Clinical Trials Group. Curr Oncol 2008;15(6):279–85.

73. Siegel RL, Fedewa SA, Miller KD, et al. Cancer statistics for Hispanics/Latinos, 2015. CA Cancer J Clin 2015;65(6):457–80.

74. Schmitz KH, Speck RM, Rye SA, et al. Prevalence of breast cancer treatment sequelae over 6 years of follow-up: the Pulling Through Study. Cancer 2012; 118(8 Suppl):2217–25.

75. Stout NL, Binkley JM, Schmitz KH, et al. A prospective surveillance model for rehabilitation for women with breast cancer. Cancer 2012;118(8 Suppl): 2191–200.

76. Brunelle C, Skolny M, Ferguson C, et al. Establishing and sustaining a prospective screening program for breast cancer-related lymphedema at the massachusetts general hospital: lessons learned. J Pers Med 2015;5(2):153–64.

77. Baima J, Reynolds SG, Edmiston K, et al. Teaching of independent exercises for prehabilitation in breast cancer. J Cancer Educ 2015. [Epub ahead of print].

Cancer-Related Fatigue
Persistent, Pervasive, and Problematic

Lynn H. Gerber, MD[a,b,*]

KEYWORDS

- Cancer • Rehabilitation • Fatigue exercise • Cognitive behavioral therapy

KEY POINTS

- Cancer-related fatigue (CRF) is common, persistent, and difficult to treat.
- Causes for CRF are not known, but associations with anemia, high body mass index, diabetes with some tumor types (breast, colon, liver), inflammatory cytokines, insomnia, and cortisol dysregulation are reported.
- One of the most effective treatments for CRF is exercise. Aerobic and resistance exercise are both effective.
- Cognitive and behavioral therapy mitigate symptoms, as does modafinil.

BACKGROUND

Cancer and its treatments have been reported to be associated with fatigue in a significant number of patients. Fatigue has been a finding during all phases of treatment, from pretreatment through treatment completion and survivorship.[1–3] Additionally, it was noted to be associated with significant patient distress.[4–6] These early reports helped establish an awareness that fatigue was common in patients with cancer diagnoses. What also resulted from these descriptive studies was the belief, later substantiated, that this fatigue was pathologic; that is, persistent and not easily resolved with the usual antidote to fatigue, rest. The early reports proposed that this fatigue was unusual and possibly specific to cancer, in part because its onset was often related to the diagnosis and became almost universal during treatment. Consensus was reached about identifying this as cancer-related fatigue (CRF).[1,2]

The National Comprehensive Cancer Network (NCCN), a network of practitioners from many disciplines who treat and study patients with cancer, has helped spearhead an effort to bring the needs of patients with cancer into a forum that can help

Conflicts of Interest/Grant Support: Grant support received from PNC Foundation: 2010 (221577/PNC), 2014 to 2016 (GMU:115085, COEUS00004226).
[a] Center for the Study of Chronic Illness and Disability, George Mason University, 4400 University Drive, MS 2G7, Fairfax, VA 22030, USA; [b] Department of Medicine, Inova Fairfax Medical Campus, 3300 Gallows Road Falls Church, VA 22042, USA
* Center for the Study of Chronic Illness and Disability, George Mason University, 4400 University Drive, MS 2G7, Fairfax, VA 22030.
E-mail address: ngerber1@gmu.edu

improve and possibly prolong their lives. CRF is one area that NCCN has provided a forum for discussion to raise awareness, and provide data and written guidelines and other tools for management.[7]

NCCN has defined CRF as "an unusual, persistent, subjective sense of tiredness related to cancer or cancer treatment that interferes with usual functioning."[8] Others have suggested that possibly a better approach might be to use a case definition to describe CRF. This approach suggests 4 criteria to establish the diagnosis: (1) a period of 2 weeks or longer within the preceding month during which significant CRF or diminished energy was experienced each day or almost every day along with additional CRF-related symptoms; (2) the experience of CRF results in significant distress or impairment of function; (3) the presence of clinical evidence suggesting that CRF is a consequence of cancer or cancer therapy; and (4) CRF is not primarily a consequence of a concurrent psychiatric condition, such as major depression. Many agree that CRF is associated with significant distress; interferes with usual activity; is not the result of a psychiatric condition; is likely to be the result of multiple causes, as a result of the disease itself or its treatments; and is difficult to treat.[9,10]

Because of its prevalence, consensus about the criteria for diagnosis and its impact of function and well-being, CRF has been accepted as a diagnosis in the *International Classification of Diseases, 10th Revision* (World Health Organization. International Statistical Classification of Diseases and Related Health Problems, 10th Revision. Version for 2003: http://www.who.int/classifications/icf/en/). Many have stated that fatigue is nearly a universal symptom in patients with cancer, mainly during treatment. However, nearly 30% of cancer survivors with no existing disease still have significant fatigue symptoms.[11–14] Cella and colleagues[12] demonstrated that patients with cancer with anemia, even after successful anemia therapy, and patients with cancer without anemia were significantly more fatigued than controls without either.

In general, CRF is a descriptive term widely accepted by practitioners and patients. The criteria for establishing the diagnosis and its importance as a symptom that needs be followed over time and treated are not questioned. Nonetheless, diagnosis is dependent on a mix of clinical observations and patient self-reports. As of this writing, no metric establishes the diagnosis of CRF and its etiology is not known.

Is CRF a unique form of fatigue? Does it differ from other pathologic fatigue conditions associated with chronic illness? Does it share similar clinical and physiologic findings with chronic fatigue syndrome? In part, the answers to these questions depend on the way fatigue is measured. Improvements in understanding have resulted through the use of operationalized criteria, but classification methods and the validity of diagnostic criteria also are important. Some common findings from other diseases and syndromes may help answer these questions and are discussed in the sections pertaining to clinical presentations and possible biological associations or mechanisms of fatigue.

CLINICAL PRESENTATIONS

One of the most frequently heard comments from my patients over the decades of treating them is "Why am I so tired? I am exhausted all the time and I am terribly frustrated by this." My approach has been to enable them to describe their experiences in their own words and hopefully enable me to sort out the contributors to their symptom. I often begin with a thorough evaluation of their medical status and try to identify comorbidities that are treatable, conditions resulting from the cancer and its treatments that might resolve with time, and an overall assessment of the impact fatigue has had on the individual's life activities. Specifically, it is helpful to ask about the duration, frequency, onset, pattern, and intensity.

Another important, often difficult to quantify issue is the sense of hopefulness and resourcefulness about their disease and its impact. Some have suggested that a patient's resilience, which correlates well with coping skills, may mitigate treatment-related fatigue. At least one study questions this assumption.[15] In that study, resilience turned out to be a predictor of patients' fatigue early in the course of receiving radiation therapy. This result is similar to findings from other studies, showing resilience to be a predictor of quality of life and coping in patients with cancer, but it seems to have little influence on treatment-related fatigue for patients receiving radiation therapy.

A list of medical conditions and their association with fatigue is presented in **Table 1**, and a list of other conditions associated with fatigue is presented in **Box 1**.

CRF differs from fatigue that is "ordinarily" associated with muscle exertion, delayed-onset muscle soreness, overuse, the flu, or overly exuberant celebration, because it is not relieved by rest or sleep, and does not spontaneously resolve, as following a viral illness.[16] It is, however, entirely consistent that people with CRF may also present with other self-limited fatiguing conditions, such as muscle fatigue or postviral fatigue increasing the intensity in a time-limited way.

CRF has both subjective and objective components and may involve dysfunction in physical performance (physical weakness or tiredness), mood (depression, anxiety), motivation (lack of initiative), cognition (slowing of thought processes, distraction, memory deficits), and social functions (reduced ability to sustain social relationships). All components should be evaluated using proper instruments.

One useful approach to sorting through the presentation of symptoms is to assess whether the individual associates the fatigue with activity or notices that activity exacerbates fatigue to a point thought to be out of proportion to the level of effort. If the latter is an accurate characterization of the fatigue, it is likely to be peripheral fatigue. Peripheral fatigue is usually the result of neuromuscular fatigue and may be the result of depletion of glycogen, sarcolemmal excitability, or the impact of cardiorespiratory limitations. This is thought to be independent of the central nervous system (**Table 2**).

If the symptom is present independent of physical activity and is present most if not all of the time, the fatigue is more likely to be related to central fatigue. Central fatigue is a term used to describe a decrement in performance that is not due to a failure in the capacity of muscle to perform. In other words, the muscle has not fatigued to a point where it can no longer contract, suggesting that a mechanism other than local, muscular fatigue is influencing the performance. The explanation is attributed to a central mechanism. One way of measuring this is using a measure of perceived exertion. The most commonly used is the Borg scale.[17]

Central fatigue is the failure to initiate or sustain tasks and activities requiring motivation.[18] The nature of the symptoms associated with central fatigue is difficult to attribute to a specific activity. This type of fatigue has affective components and is

Table 1		
Comorbid conditions associated with fatigue		
Common	**Less Common**	**Rare**
Anemia	Renal failure	Adrenal insufficiency
Hyper/hypothyroidism	Liver disease	Lyme disease
Atrial fibrillation	Chronic obstructive pulmonary	Fibromyalgia
Infection	disease/multiple sclerosis	
Medications (eg, hypnotics,	Hypercalcemia	
opioids)	Arthritis	
Depression/anxiety	Autoimmune disease	
	Vitamin D deficiency	

Box 1
Conditions contributing to fatigue

Deconditioning

Inactivity

Insomnia

Stress (physical and emotional)

Dehydration

Nutritional deficiencies

---

frequently experienced by individuals as having no energy, motivation, overall/general fatigue, or changes in mood.[19] This type of fatigue is sometimes equated with not being able to think "clearly" or as rapidly as usual. The term "chemobrain" has been used to link the receipt of anticancer treatment with "fuzzy" thinking. Additionally, people notice memory and recall deficiencies that are often disturbing. It may or may not be associated with depressive symptoms.

Although the distinction between central and peripheral fatigue is a useful framework in which to work, sometimes it is difficult to reliably separate the 2 into distinct entities. One explanation is that individuals select words to describe their feelings and experiences associated with the symptom. Not everyone uses the same words for these. Second, there are more objective measures for physical fatigue determination, and although these provide validity, they do not prove causality. The distinction between peripheral and central fatigue is not universally accepted. Nonetheless, researchers in the field have supported the view that the symptoms can be accurately measured[20] and can distinguish between physical and central fatigue. With the recent interest in brain imaging, and its application to imaging patients with fatigue, pilot data are emerging that suggest there may be abnormal neural network communication in people with persistent fatigue.[21]

There are additional important aspects of fatigue that should be ascertained through patient interviews. These include asking whether the fatigue antedated the diagnosis, or whether it was contemporaneous with treatment (surgery, radiation, chemotherapy, and/or adjuvant). The group whose fatigue is contemporaneous with treatment is less likely to suffer persistent CRF. Data also suggest that migraine, analgesic use,

---

Table 2
Associations used to help distinguish between physical and central fatigue

Symptoms	Physical Fatigue	Central Fatigue
Decreased ability to perform activity, decreased exercise tolerance	+++	+/−
Dyspnea on exertion	+++	+
Muscle fatigue/weakness	+++	−
Mood/behavioral change	+	+++
Change in reaction time and attention to task	+/−	+
Decline in cognitive performance	+/−	+++
Lack of motivation	+/−	+++

+++, most likely associated with type of fatigue; ++, less likely associated with type of fatigue; +, least likely associated with type of fatigue; +/−, occasionally associated with type of fatigue; − not associated with type of fatigue.

peripheral arterial obstructive disease, and arthritis also are associated with long-term fatigue. Patients who are obese and primarily sedentary have a high risk for CRF. Predictors of long-term CRF are likely to include premorbid depression and fatigue, lack of physical activity, and elevated body mass index (BMI).[22] Other studies have shown similar findings and have included pain as a predictor.[23,24]

FATIGUE MEASUREMENT

Fatigue management has been targeted as a critical need for cancer survivors that warrants continuous evaluation and treatment. NCCN has issued guidelines for practice with respect to this symptom in patients with cancer (http://www.nccn.org/professionals/physician_gls/pdf/fatigue.pdf). Among them are that all patients should be screened for fatigue initially and on subsequent visits, treated promptly, and patients and families should be informed that management of fatigue is integral to care for patients with cancer.

This recommendation has been made in part because of the accumulation of significant evidence about the high prevalence of fatigue in patients being treated for and surviving cancer and its adverse impact on life, function, and on patients' sense of well-being.[5,6,25,26] It is prevalent among all types of cancer, but breast, lung, and pancreatic are among the most frequently associated with persistent fatigue. Some of this may be because patients with breast cancer are among the most frequently studied. Breast and lung are highly prevalent, and breast cancer research has been among the top 3 diagnoses that have received research funds, making it among the most studied cancers, which may partially explain the findings.[27]

Patients and clinicians acknowledge that fatigue is a formidable foe. This is, in part, because there are many possible contributors. Even though we have accepted criteria for diagnosing CRF, not everyone agrees on its cause(s), how to measure it, or how to best mitigate the symptom.

Measuring fatigue has been problematic for researchers studying CRF. One explanation is that most fatigue measures are self-reports, which may not have the precision of objective measures. Nonetheless, significant effort has been mounted to ensure the reliability and validity of these instruments. In fact, seminal work done by a variety of professionals, including nurses, psychometricians, and others has helped develop measurement tools that have placed measurement of patient-reported outcomes (PROs) on a strong methodological footing, demonstrating strong psychometric properties.[28]

Others have reviewed fatigue metrics and recommended a variety of instruments useful for CRF.[29–31] A recent review of 40 fatigue assessments used to evaluate patients with advanced cancer has found many instruments to be burdensome and therefore favored those that are less complex and with fewer questions. They recommend the Brief Fatigue Inventory and 3 fatigue items of the European Organization for Research and Treatment Quality of Life Questionnaire Fatigue Scale (EORTC QLQ-C30) for assessing patients with advanced cancer.[32] A systematic review of the use and psychometric properties of the multidimensional fatigue symptom inventory short form suggests this instrument has good psychometric properties, clinical utility, and is valid.[33]

In particular, fatigue metrics need discriminant properties to help distinguish between central and peripheral fatigue. Fatigue needs to be distinguished from depression and sleepiness. In reviewing published research for CRF, instruments frequently used are presented in **Table 2**. The instruments also need to be sensitive to change so that treatment response can be monitored accurately and the items presented to patients for selection have to align with the kinds of phrases/words likely to be recognized as associated with the fatigue that individuals experience.

Item response theory-based advances in the fatigue measurement have enabled researchers to specifically select questions from an item bank and tailor these to the patient population being studied. Advances in thinking about PROs have led to applying newer technological approaches that use item response theory, including computer adaptive testing.[34] The first steps were to develop a domain framework that focused efforts to organize item pools. The domains are 3 broad areas for self-reports: physical, mental, and social health.

The Patient-Reported Outcomes Measurement Information System (PROMIS) effort has provided options for fatigue and other symptom measurement.[35] One way to use PROMIS is to adopt short forms that have questions preselected based on their link to the constructs being studied. Alternatively, one can select an item bank of one's own choosing from a larger pool (95 items in the fatigue bank for adults and 23 for children). A recently reported study indicates that PROMIS fatigue measures are responsive to change in 6 different chronic conditions, including cancer.[36]

Another important consideration for measuring fatigue is to be able to identify the ability of the instrument to assess clinically significant findings. Investigators are committed to presenting statistically significant findings, but these should be seen within the context of meaningful differences and clinical relevance. In general, there is consensus about what is meant by clinically meaningful fatigue.[37] Several measures have been evaluated for clinical significance. The SF-36 vitality subscale score of greater than 45 has been shown to be clinically significant fatigue and the Fatigue Severity Index of ≥ 3.[38,39]

The other difficulty with respect to fatigue and its measurement is a conceptual one. The word fatigue has many different meanings (connotations and denotations). Using grounded theory, some investigators have been able to identify themes that classify fatigue into physical, affective, and cognitive components. For example, using the Fatigue Assessment Questionnaire, investigators were able to discriminate between fatigue experienced by patients with cancer and controls without cancer diagnoses. A tentative steplike theoretic explanation for the production, perception, and expression of fatigue proposed at the end of one study was supported by factor analysis suggesting that the themes do load separately and can be considered different factors.[40] Other studies have performed factor analysis on a variety of symptoms. One examined symptoms reported by 208 patients with postviral fatigue, and found 4 factors emerged: emotional distress, fatigue, somatic symptoms, and cognitive difficulty.[41] Another analyzed fatigue-related symptoms reported by 780 respondents of persons with chronic fatigue. They found 4 factors: lack of energy, physical exertion, cognitive problems, and fatigue and rest.[42] There remains confusion about these distinctions, and how to determine the different contributors to fatigue. Nonetheless, investigators agree that fatigue is a multidimensional construct.[30]

Measuring physical activity also has been a critical part of the clinical investigation of fatigue for decades. This has been particularly important since the increase in the prevalence of obesity and its apparent connection with sedentary behavior at work and during leisure time. To date, when one speaks of objective measures of fatigue they usually include performance-based measures, such as strength, local muscle endurance, and cardio/respiratory measures of exercise tolerance, such as Vo_2 maximum. However, several self-reports of activity have been shown to correlate with these measures. The Human Activity Profile, a self-report of 94 graded questions records what one is able to do, what one can no longer do, and what one never did. The first question asks about one's ability to arise from a chair (2 metabolic equivalents [mets] of energy) and the 94th asks whether you run 3 miles in 30 minutes (10 mets of work). This questionnaire provides a reliable measure of level of activity and correlates well with aerobic capacity, as does the International Physical Activity Questionnaire.[43,44] A recent review of the correlations between findings from the self-reported physical activity measures and objective measures, including accelerometers, energy expenditure, and aerobic measures suggest they measure different factors and points out that the basis for the linkage between obesity and lack of physical activity was established using self-reports. Further, that the context of activity, not only its frequency and intensity is important to determine when assessing the activities in which people engage.[45]

Effective management and treatment of CRF symptoms is enhanced when the symptom is well described using qualitative and quantitative measures. The more precisely patients can describe their fatigue and the more accurately it can be measured, the greater the likelihood it can be managed effectively. Meeting these conditions poses a problem because, as described previously, individuals often describe the same symptom differently from each other, and use the same wording to describe different symptoms. Comorbidities (arthritis, diabetes, cardiovascular disease) and clustering of other symptoms (depression, pain, and insomnia) may influence the experience and/or the severity of fatigue, hence these often need to be concurrently evaluated with the fatigue.[46,47]

One important approach is to provide patients with a careful review of systems and history of prior illness and a comprehensive review of medications. Good control of comorbidities and reduction in medication that may contribute to fatigue should be considered. Medications for control of the primary cancer also are known to cause secondary conditions (eg, arthritis/arthralgia) that associate with fatigue, such as aromatase inhibitors.[48,49] Once a careful review of systems, determination of comorbidities, and ascertainment of medications are learned, the evaluation should result in a better understanding of the nature of the fatigue, its functional impact, and its possible likely contributors. This will help select targeted, specific treatment.

There has been interest in this concept of clustering of symptoms and efforts to link these in terms of gene expression and proteomics (cytokine profiles). As of now, this has not been shown to be the case. Nonetheless, a unifying theory about mechanism or relationships among these frequently paired symptoms remains an active area for research.

A brief summary of commonly used fatigue scales is presented in **Table 3**.

Table 3
Fatigue scales commonly used to evaluate cancer-related fatigue

	Name of Instrument	Dimensions of Measurement	CSF Score	Reference
1	Fatigue Inventory Scale	Physical, cognitive, and psychosocial fatigue	≥ 3	Fisk
2	Fatigue Severity Scale	9 questions, no clear dimensional separate	≥ 40	Krupp
3	Visual Analog Scale	One dimension	4	
4	Medical Outcome Study Short Form-36	Vitality subscale	>45	Ware
5	FACIT-F	Multidimensional		Yellen
6	EORTC	Physical and mental fatigue		Knobel
7	PROMIS	Multidimensional, custom questions from item banks		

Abbreviations: CSF, clinically significant fatigue; EORTC, European Organization for Research and Treatment; FACIT-F, Functional Assessment of Chronic Illness Therapy-F; PROMIS, Patient-Reported Outcomes Measurement Information System.

MECHANISMS AND CONTRIBUTORS TO FATIGUE
Inflammation

Cytokines are a group of proteins that communicate between cells. Their effects are protean in that they mediate inflammatory reactions and can stimulate the stress reaction via the hypothalamic-pituitary axis. They either stimulate inflammation (are proinflammatory) or suppress inflammation (are anti-inflammatory). The proinflammatory cytokines, such as interleukins, interferon, and tumor necrosis factors activate corticotropin-releasing hormone. Cytokines and interferon, also used for treatment of melanoma and hepatitis C, have been observed to engender cognitive impairments, mood, and affective changes.[50,51] Symptoms associated with these treatments also include somatic symptoms, such as headache and fatigue. In part, based on these observations, researchers have sought to investigate the potential role of inflammatory markers in the CRF.

Researchers now need to help explain CRF from the perspective of multiple systems (neuroimmunoregulatory, cardiorespiratory, and musculoskeletal) by creating a biological profile that can connect these systems. Much effort has been spent on assessing associations between inflammatory cytokines as correlates and predictors of fatigue. Studies have documented associations among interleukins, tumor necrosis factors, chemokines, and C-reactive protein in most tumor types.[52–59] Data support some possible correlations, including the significant rise in plasma interleukin-1 receptor antagonist (IL-1ra) in breast cancer survivors .[53] Elevated levels of IL-1ra, soluble tumor necrosis factor receptor type II (sTNF-RII), neopterin, and soluble IL-6 receptor, have been correlated with fatigue in breast cancer survivors at 5 years after diagnosis.[54,56] Sleep disruption is associated with CRF, which in turn can be affected by IL-1, IL-6, and TNF-a.[60,61]

Several longitudinal studies have noted high levels of IL-1ra, and IL-6 during radiation in patients with early-stage breast cancer, as well as elevated IL-1β and IL-6 with stressing stimuli in patients with CRF.[62] The findings are not consistent and when controlled for other variables, age, gender, BMI, and ethnicity, they lose statistical significance. Nonetheless, associations have been reported and have been shown during pretreatment, treatment, and posttreatment phases. This suggests that although the biological insults may differ (tumor, treatment, posttreatment), biological events in patients with cancer diagnoses are likely to have correlations among cytokines and fatigue symptoms.

Several difficulties remain in addition to those mentioned previously. One is that most of these studies are performed in women with breast cancer. Other tumor types are beginning to be reported and share some of the observations about associations with IL-6 and TNF-a, but we await confirmation of the generalizability of the findings. Many of the studies tend to be reported by the same investigative groups and lack confirmatory evidence. Finally, none of the studies has demonstrated a causal relationship between the cytokines and symptom severity or types of fatigue.

Cellular Considerations

Changes in levels of neutrophils and lymphocytes,[63] in particular CD3+, CD4+, and natural killer (NK) cells have been measured in patients with cancer.[64] Similar to the studies in which cytokines and other inflammatory products have been measured, the cross-sectional and longitudinal assessments provide somewhat inconsistent findings. This may be due to the administration of different fatigue metrics, thereby providing a large variance in the severity of fatigue and the lack of control for biological variations, such as BMI.[62] There have been reports of cellular changes following

radiation,[64] and indications that the cellular changes persist.[65] Immune dysregulation has been associated with cancer treatment, with a demonstrated decrease in NK cell activity (NKCA).[66] NK cells defend against tumor metastasis, tumor initiation, and tumor growth, and may be of particular importance in epithelial tumors, such as breast cancer.[67] During the early phase after completion of adjuvant radiation therapy, NK cell–mediated antitumor defense becomes particularly important.

Hormonal Factors

The hypothalamic-pituitary-adrenal axis controls the releasing factors that influence thyroid, parathyroid, and adrenal glands and provides cortisol regulation.[68] Cortisol regulation is an important contributor to alterations in glucocorticoid production (including dysregulated circadian profiles) and decreased receptivity of its receptor to hormone attachment. Cortisol is an important regulator of inflammation, both in stimulating demargination of white blood cells and through its anti-inflammatory effects. The role of cortisol has been actively researched as a potential link to the biology of CRF. In other words, it plays an important role in regulating inflammation and in energy production; both phenomena have been identified as correlated with fatigue,[69] suggesting to researchers that there may be a link to metabolic abnormalities, such as seen during the treatment phase of breast cancer, most notably. Reported findings include data suggesting fatigued breast cancer survivors have a significantly more blunted cortisol response to a stressor when compared with those who are not fatigued, even when the frequency of depression is controlled.

Others have found that the phenomenon of blunting the diurnal variation of cortisol occurs only in those who experience physical fatigue. In those patients, the evening cortisol level remains high and the total cortisol secretion is higher than those who do not experience fatigue. Patients with cognitive fatigue do not demonstrate cortisol blunting.[70]

Also reported, and of some interest, is that androgen depletion treatment for men with prostate cancer has accelerated fatigue symptoms during the first year of treatment. This apparently resolves a year into treatment and suggests that significant shifts in circulating levels of androgen may be another contributor to CRF.[71]

Fig. 1 presents a schematic of the neurohormonal interactions thought to be integral to CRF.

Genetic Factors

During the past decade, investigators have been studying the relationships between gene polymorphisms and symptoms in patients with cancer. This may have begun as an interest in identifying specific tumor signatures so as to target tumor characteristics to maximize therapeutic kill. As gene technological capabilities have progressed, attention has expanded to include unique patient characteristics, to try to maximize the understanding of the host response. This has led to explorations between genetic profiles and cancer-related symptoms.

Most approaches used by these investigators have been to determine whether there are genetic associations between fatigue and various genotypes. The investigators usually select genotypes associated with cytokines that have been shown to be associated with proinflammatory cytokines. Saligan and Kim[62] cite 7 cross-sectional studies in which a variety of genetic findings associated with patterns of fatigue.[72–74] These included common, homozygous (AA) alleles of IL-6 associating with higher levels of evening and morning fatigue symptoms; higher morning fatigue, but not evening fatigue was with homozygous (GG) alleles of the TNF-α gene; and single nucleotide polymorphisms (SNPs) associated with various cytokines.

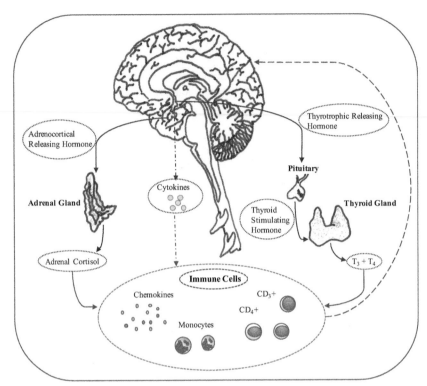

Fig. 1. Schematic for neuro-immune regulation.

SNPs of several cytokines, including IL-1β (rs1143633, rs2853550), IL-1RN (rs397211, rs4252041), and IL-10 (rs1878672, rs3021094) showed significant associations with fatigue levels in lung cancer survivors. The G/G genotype of IL-6-174 and TNF-308; specific catechol-O-methyltransferase (COMT) genotypes (Valine [Val]/ Methionine [Met] and Met/Met) were significantly correlated with higher fatigue scores compared with survivors with the Val/Val genotype.[75]

Other descriptive studies report that the presence of specific genetic factors need to be assessed within the context of social and biological milieu, possibly because epigenetic changes may occur. Such factors include that younger, female, unmarried, and black people had more comorbidities, a lower functional status, and were more likely to be in the low morning energy class. Two polymorphisms (IL2 rs1479923 and NFKB1 rs4648110) were associated with this energy descriptive group. Two groups with distinct evening energy trajectories were identified. One is described as younger and male and who had more comorbidities, decreased body weight, and a lower functional status, and were more likely to be in the moderate evening energy class. This group was associated with 5 different polymorphisms (IL1R2 rs4141134, IL6 rs4719714, IL17A rs8193036, NFKB2 rs1056890, and TNFA rs1800683) and had an evening energy pattern.[76] This work points out a very important aspect of fatigue studies that, unfortunately, are not usually addressed. Attending to descriptors of fatigue that differentiate the times of day likely to be "low energy" or more fatigue may be very important to the understanding of fatigue biology. The variable of "when," not only "how much," fatigue is one experiencing is not easily measured using standard fatigue instruments. Objective measures of activity are inadequate to determine the details about the symptom.

One issue frequently discussed in the literature reporting genetic associations with cancer-related symptoms is how to sort out the relative contributions of treatment toxicity and tumor effects. In fact, some of the genetic data are questioned with respect to its relevance because of the influence of toxicity.[62] This is a complicated topic and is well reviewed by Vichaya and colleagues.[77]

Based on the number of publications attempting to elucidate relationships between symptoms and genetic profiles of patients, gene expression data, and possible mechanisms for symptom manifestation and control, there is clearly interest in linking biological findings to causal relationships. In my opinion, as of this time, the genetic data provide interesting statistical correlations between symptoms and SNPs, and the biological and demographic information suggest fatigue is a complex symptom and is likely to be influenced by multiple factors and are best considered correlates.[62,76-78]

Metabolic Factors

Patients with diabetes are at a higher risk of developing breast cancer than those without either type 1 or 2 diabetes mellitus.[79] Moreover, diabetes is one of the most common comorbidities of breast cancer, at 18%. In one breast cancer survivor study, diabetic patients also obtained higher scores in symptom dimensions, including fatigue, nausea and vomiting, pain, dyspnea, insomnia, constipation, and diarrhea measured by the EORTC QLQ-C30.[80]

Long-term cancer survivors have been reported to have a high prevalence of metabolic syndrome, which poses a significant threat to longevity unless treated. Often the dyslipidemia and glucose intolerance are accompanied by fatigue. Additionally, the survivors most affected are likely to be sedentary. This combination of findings is a significant challenge because it depends on engaging the patients in a long-term commitment to lifestyle changes.[81-83]

Other Factors

Very robust discussions have appeared in the literature regarding the key features of CRF, in which the similarities and differences lie in comparison with other types of fatigue. These discussions have stimulated research and resulted in statements about the need for continued effort to clarify etiology. Physical fatigue in cancer survivors is frequently associated with inactivity, deconditioning, cardiorespiratory dysfunction secondary to chemotherapy, radiation and/or surgery, and various endocrine and hematological abnormalities. Possible explanations for this have led to explorations about energy production and mitochondrial function at the muscle level.[84] The contributions of local mechanisms, such as contractile properties of muscle, how these contribute to exhaustion, and the central mechanisms of fatigue in the cancer population are currently being actively investigated.[85] Investigators have argued that in the patient with cancer, energy production may have undergone a shift toward the glycolytic pathway, resulting in a greater buildup of lactate and less efficiency of muscle contraction.[86,87] These abnormalities could possibly link mechanisms of central and peripheral fatigue. Fatigue during prolonged exercise clearly is influenced by a complex interaction between peripheral and central factors. One theory has been that this is a result of central serotonin levels because of its effects on sleep, lethargy and drowsiness, and loss of motivation.[88]

As of the current time, no unifying hypothesis has been convincingly developed to define the mechanism of CRF, despite the considerable literature exploring the chronic fatigue syndrome and its relationship to viral illnesses and neuroinflammation and its relationship to sickness behaviors.[20,42]

TREATMENT AND MANAGEMENT OF CANCER-RELATED FATIGUE EDUCATION AND COUNSELING

In my view, treatment and management of CRF must start with education. Cancer rehabilitation is a collaboration among patients, their caregivers, and families, as well as other medical specialists likely to be participating in care. Education of health care professionals is an important part of the process. The oncology specialists (medical, surgical, and radiation), frequently consider primary cancer treatment as acute care. The treatments must provide best possible evaluation, staging, and selection of definitive interventions and are designed to eliminate tumor. Once the primary treatment is concluded, ongoing care may be shared among oncology specialists and primary care physicians and/or rehabilitation professionals. Cancer survivorship has steadily increased as treatment has become more effective and early screening and detection have become routine practice. Management of the survivorship phase is just beginning to undergo effectiveness trials from which guidelines are being developed and tested.

The results of some studies have reported efforts to educate primary care physicians so as to improve functional outcomes among cancer survivors.[89] The goals of the study cited were to determine if an educational intervention was successful in engaging general practitioners (GPs) in cancer rehabilitation. The level of proactivity was no different in the intervention group compared with the controls. That is, the GPs receiving the educational intervention were no more proactive about patients being involved in rehabilitation, nor were the patients of GPs who had received the intervention more participatory in rehabilitation. However, there was a significant association between the GPs' proactivity and patient participation in rehabilitation. The investigators concluded that a GP who was more proactive in obtaining rehabilitation for patients was likely to facilitate patient participation in rehabilitation activities.

Data also suggest that the psychoeducational approach may be beneficial for a variety of patients with different cancer diagnoses. Whether this is because of the amount of time spent discussing symptoms with health professionals or the result of specific interventions is unclear. This type of patient interaction may enable patients to problem solve and use information about energy conservation, coping, and symptom control so as to assist in improving function. Several systematic reviews have been published showing generally good results for this type of intervention.[90–92]

Education may be a powerful tool and may be useful for patients with CRF. One scoping review reported results of 447 trials and 37 systematic reviews in a mixed cancer diagnosis cohort. The most frequent interventions reported for the treatment of CRF included exercise and pharmacologic, psychoeducation, and mind-body interventions. Fatigue was identified as a primary outcome measure (OM) in 58% of studies, with 58 different fatigue measures reported. Emerging evidence exists for the effectiveness of fatigue interventions for some cancer types. More research on interventions with participants with the same cancer type and illness phase is needed. Measurement of severity and impact of CRF using fewer, robust OMs will permit comparisons across studies.[93] A systematic review resulted in identifying 10 randomized controlled trials involving 1534 adults for whom a variety of educational interventions were provided. The effects of the interventions on CRF were inconsistent. The reviewers concluded that there is limited support for the clinical use of patient education programs to reduce CRF. There were some outcomes that seemed to be associated with the educational intervention about benefits of exercise, sleep hygiene, nutrition, and relaxation.[94]

Counseling and therapy are designed to promote symptom reduction often through use of individual or group therapy. These sessions use educational interventions, coping strategies and problem solving, emotional support, and psychotherapy. Although these approaches have been successful in reducing overall cancer-related symptoms, they have not been definitively shown to be effective in treating CRF.

In a landmark study by Goodwin and colleagues,[95] women with metastatic breast cancer were randomized to receive either supportive-expressive group therapy or standard of care. The primary outcome was survival, and there was no survival benefit to those receiving the intervention. However, there was improvement in levels of distress, pain, and mood.

PHARMACOLOGIC INTERVENTIONS

There have been numerous trials of pharmacologic interventions performed to assess their effectiveness in reducing the symptom and its impact. I have divided them into 3 general classes of interventions. Of necessity, these include interventions that are aimed at a particular underlying physiologic abnormality, such as thyroid dysfunction when diagnostic tests are abnormal, or targeting symptom management, such as psychostimulants aimed at improving cognitive fatigue. Some trials use medications for CRF when the diagnostic tests are "borderline" or within the normal range. The 3 categories include hematopoietic stimulants designed to raise hemoglobin concentration, hormones including corticosteroids/anabolic steroids, and psychostimulants and antidepressants.

Recent reviews of CRF have included pharmacologic interventions and are recommended for your attention.[96,97] The new (2016) NCCN guidelines are available for review. One precaution is that the references for the pharmacological interventions are nearly 10 years since publication and more recent data are available (https://www.nccn.org/professionals/physician_gls/pdf/fatigue.pdf).

Hematopoietic Stimulants

Many trials have been conducted attempting to determine the effectiveness of erythropoietic stimulation on fatigue in patients with CRF. In general, these have shown effectiveness in treating anemia in patients with cancer and with increase in hemoglobin, patients report improvement in CRF. However, improvement in CRF did not reach a clinically significant level, and although reducing need for transfusions, increased thromboembolic events were part of the overall risk profile.[98] An additional report of long-term survivors who had prophylactically received erythropoietic stimulation for cancer-induced anemia, who participated in a randomized trial of stimulant versus placebo that was prematurely discontinued in 2007, remained under biological surveillance. A total of 630 subjects were evaluated over the ensuing decade. There was a significant increase in median hemoglobin levels in patients with mixed tumor types and who were receiving chemotherapy for advanced cancer. This was particularly true for the subset of patients with nonmetastatic disease (2-sided $P<.01$) There was also a significant difference in fatigue levels for those receiving the treatment (all tumor grades: $P<.001$, grades 3–4: $P = .055$). These investigators noted a higher rate of all thrombosis-related events in the treated group (all tumor grades: $P = .043$, grades 3–4: $P = .099$).[99] Another recent study reported slightly different findings. In patients with cancer receiving chemotherapy, erythropoietic stimulation provided a small but clinically important improvement in anemia-related symptoms (Functional Assessment of Cancer Therapy–Anemia [FACT-An]) but for general fatigue-related symptoms, it did not reach clinically meaningful improvement.[100]

Hormones

There have been only a few studies reporting the use of corticosteroids for treatment of fatigue in CRF as a primary outcome. A Cochrane review reported no research on corticosteroids with fatigue as the primary outcome in 2010[101]; however, a multicenter physician survey sent to palliative care physicians reported that there were "high response rates when treating appetite loss, nausea, fatigue or poor wellbeing."[102] In 2013, Yennurajalingam and colleagues[103] published a randomized placebo-controlled trial of corticosteroids with fatigue as the primary end point. Participants were outpatients with advanced cancer. The study demonstrated a significant improvement in fatigue using the Functional Assessment of Chronic Illness Therapy–Fatigue (FACIT-F) subscale with a mean improvement of 5.9 points, which is a clinically significant improvement for the group receiving dexamethasone.[103] Since then, several studies, whose primary outcome has been pain, have reported significant and clinically meaningful improvement for both fatigue and appetite, as well as patient satisfaction in the treated groups as compared with those receiving placebo, although it had no significant effect on pain or analgesic consumption.[104] Additional studies confirm the benefit of corticosteroids in advanced cancer. In some, there is a suggestion that patients with prostate cancer are more likely to respond than those with lung cancer, response is likely to be within the first week of treatment, and has only been confirmed for short-term treatment regimens.[105,106]

One preliminary placebo-controlled trial of dexamethasone attempted to assess the effects of treatment on symptom clusters.[107] There were only 114 participants in the study and 3 clusters selected: fatigue/anorexia-cachexia/depression (FAD), sleep/anxiety/drowsiness, and pain/dyspnea. Only the FAD cluster significantly improved. This study was also a short-term intervention, and outcomes were assessed at day 8 and day 15. This is a small sample size, and the clustering was determined by the predominance of symptoms. Nonetheless, the evidence is accumulating in support of corticosteroids that have a potential role in controlling fatigue in patients with advanced cancer in the short term.

Various other hormones (progestational agents, thyrotropin-releasing hormone) have not shown significant effect sizes, consistent convincing benefit.[108]

Psychostimulants and Antidepressants

Methylphenidate is probably the most studied pharmacologic agent for the treatment of CRF. Minton and colleagues,[109] in a meta-analysis of 2 studies (n = 264 patients), indicated that methylphenidate was superior to placebo (standardized mean difference [SMD] in change in fatigue score = -0.30, 95% confidence interval [CI] = -0.54 to -0.05; $P = .02$) for treating CRF. In a subsequent meta-analysis,[110] with 426 participants, there was an overall SMD of -0.28 (95% CI -0.48 to -0.09; $P = .005$). In this analysis, several trials failed to find any benefit over placebo. This subsequent analysis supported the earlier finding of fatigue reduction with methylphenidate. There were no adverse effects reported.

Modafinil has been evaluated in several settings. It has been studied in outpatient, inpatient, and palliative care settings. A comprehensive systematic review and meta-analysis selected randomized controlled trials of pharmacologic treatments compared with placebo, another medication, or a nonpharmacological intervention. The primary outcome was fatigue, not temporally related to primary cancer treatments. Forty-five met the inclusion criteria. In total, they analyzed data from 18 drugs and 4696 participants; however, there were significant problems with this review. They included patients with fatigue with a diagnoses of multiple sclerosis. There was a very high degree of statistical and clinical heterogeneity, difficulties with blinding, and some difficulty with definitions of fatigue. Nonetheless, despite the methodological faults with many of the studies and the small sample sizes, a meta-analysis showed a positive effect for methylphenidate in CRF (SMD 0.49, 95% CI 0.15–0.83).[111]

To date, donepezil, an acetylcholinesterase inhibitor, has not been shown to be effective in CRF. Paroxetine and sertraline also have been shown to have no increased benefit for reducing symptoms of CRF when compared with placebo.[110,112] Finally, despite significant numbers of testimonials and some trials, the data in support of herbals and dietary supplements for treatment of CRF do not reach a level of evidence to support a generalized statement for their effectiveness.

NONPHARMACOLOGICAL INTERVENTIONS
Exercise and Rehabilitation Modalities

The goals of rehabilitation are to prevent functional decline and improve or restore functional outcome. As a specialty, rehabilitation is interdisciplinary and evaluates multiple domains of function so as to meet individual patients' functional needs and wishes to lead their lives. It is patient centered and the goals of treatment are established by patients, their caregivers, and the health professionals involved in their care.

Rehabilitation interventions include physical and biopsychosocial treatments to improve impairments, promote function, and assist with participation and integration into societal aspects of life.

Exercise has been a cornerstone of rehabilitation intervention for the patient with cancer and has been one of the most researched areas. It is 30 years since MacVicar and Winningham[113] published their seminal observation about the positive effect of exercise for women with breast cancer.[114] It was a small study, with a quasi-experimental design using bicycle ergometry and patients were not randomized; however, it did have a small control group. OMs included symptom-limited exercise testing for oxygen consumption and the Profile of Mood States to evaluate mood and fatigue. The study results demonstrated that patients and controls had improved symptoms (mood and fatigue) and that functional aerobic capacity improved after the 10-week intervention. These findings changed thinking about cancer treatment. The study demonstrated safety of the intervention for patients with cancer, a physiologic response to treatment, and improvement in symptoms. The study opened the way for many investigators to further pursue the possible benefits of exercise, to refine the nature of the intervention, and to try to learn what to do, how to do it, and where it could/should be done for maximal benefit while ensuring patient safety.

Within a short period, many well-designed and some bold efforts were undertaken to test a variety of factors pertaining to exercise for CRF. These included determining (1) the effect size for exercise studies, (2) when during the course of an individual's life with cancer (eg, during active treatment, posttreatment, during survivorship, end of life) treatment should be prescribed, (3) the venues in which exercise can be delivered (eg, home, community, hospital, with/without supervision), and (4) the approaches needed to maximize adherence (eg, groups, individual supervision, automated activity monitors, Web-based programs).

Multiple systematic reviews of the level of evidence in support of exercise as an effective treatment for CRF have been reported, with an increasing number being published over the past 5 years.[96,97,113,115–121] In general, positive effects of exercise interventions are more pronounced with moderate-intensity or vigorous-intensity versus mild-intensity exercise programs. The reports all support its efficacy.

Specific reports identify that aerobic exercise has been shown to be effective for patients with prostate cancer.[117,122] Resistance exercise is an effective and safe intervention to improve muscular strength and performance, fatigue, and quality of life.[123,124] Patients with colorectal cancer,[125] lung cancer,[126] and stem cell transplantation[127] have results similar to patients with breast cancer.

Other studies have shown that multimodal interventions in which exercise is combined with other interventions, such as supervised exercise, comprising high-intensity cardiovascular and heavy resistance training, relaxation, and body awareness training and massage had a 3-point reduction in fatigue score[128]; or relaxation, body awareness, and massage reduced fatigue and improved vitality, aerobic capacity, muscular strength, and physical and functional activity, and emotional well-being.[129]

In summary, the strongest evidence for effectiveness in treating CRF is exercise. Aerobic, resistance, and multimodal with higher-intensity exercise is more likely to reduce CRF. The venue for treatment does not seem to be a critical factor. The studies support exercise for inpatients, outpatients, at home,[130] and community based.[131] Improvements were significant in blood pressure, upper and lower body strength, the 6-minute walk test, and fatigue ($P < .001$). The timing of the exercise, although not entirely determined, has shown safety and effectiveness during treatment, posttreatment, and survivorship. Although the specifics of exercise prescriptions have been explored, the general principles are intensity (60%–85% of maximal heart rate) for at least 3 times per week in accordance with the American College of Sports Medicine Guidelines.[132]

Cognitive Behavioral Therapy

Although the data from exercise studies have been strong and reasonably well accepted, other rehabilitation interventions have been used to treat CRF. In particular, treatments that have included cognitive behavioral therapies (CBTs). This type of therapy explores the relationships among thoughts, feelings, and relationships. "The core principles of CBT are identifying negative or false beliefs and testing or restructuring them" (http://www.nami.org/Learn-More/Treatment/Psychotherapy#sthash. Hqu2Tyrh.dpuf).

There is strong evidence that this type of intervention is effective in reducing fatigue, and after CBT, the number of those experiencing clinical insomnia and clinical fatigue decreased. Baseline data from 113 participants with insomnia were explored to establish rates of and associations among clinical levels of fatigue, anxiety, and depression across the sample.[133,134] CBT, especially designed for postcancer fatigue, is successful in reducing fatigue and functional impairment in cancer survivors. Moreover, these positive effects were maintained at approximately 2 years after finishing CBT.[135] Additionally, Web-based and teleconferencing can be used effectively to provide treatment.[136,137] Another study reported that the CBT intervention worked equally well whether additional physical activity was part of the study treatment regimen.[138]

Many facilities offer a combination of treatments under the overall heading of rehabilitation interventions. It is the belief of some practitioners that the addition of meditation, yoga, mindfulness, hypnosis, relaxation training, energy conservation, and stress management provide support for other interventions designed to promote fatigue mitigation. The evidence from controlled intervention trials does not reach the level of evidence to support the effectiveness of these interventions and hence recommendation for treatment.

A recent monograph has been published addressing the role of integrative therapies for cancer symptoms. The investigators suggest that the level of evidence supporting recommendation of massage and stress management for mood improvement and energy conservation in the context of treatment-associated fatigue is modest and in need of further trials and study.[139]

SUMMARY OF EVIDENCE SUPPORTING TREATMENT OF CANCER-RELATED FATIGUE

The most persuasive evidence for effective management of CRF is exercise: aerobic, resistance, and multimodal therapies all work well.

The use of corticosteroids for patients with advanced cancer, for short periods of time, has been effective in reducing CRF.

The literature does support the effectiveness in reducing CRF for CBTs when they include improved understanding of the nature of fatigue and techniques to recognize and manage it.

Many studies report outcomes for the use of methylphenidate and there has been a recent review and meta-analysis. The trial designs, the number of patients studied, and the heterogeneity of the sample have thwarted the ability to endorse its use based on a high level of evidence.

The use of erythropoietic therapy is effective in treating anemia but not effective for reduction of CRF.

REFERENCES

1. Haylock PJ, Hart LK. Fatigue in patients receiving localized radiation. Cancer Nurs 1979;2:461–7.
2. Cassileth BR, Lusk EJ, Bodenheimer BJ, et al. Chemotherapeutic toxicity–the relationship between patients' pretreatment expectations and post-treatment results. Am J Clin Oncol 1985;8:419–25.
3. Meyerowitz BE, Sparks FC, Spears IK. Adjuvant chemotherapy for breast carcinoma: psychosocial implications. Cancer 1979;43:1613–8.
4. Winningham ML, Nail LM, Burke MB, et al. Fatigue and the cancer experience: the state of the knowledge. Oncol Nurs Forum 1994;21:23–36.
5. Portenoy RK, Thaler HT, Kornblith AB, et al. Symptom prevalence, characteristics, and distress in a cancer population. Qual Life Res 1994;3:183–9.
6. Curt GA. Impact of fatigue on quality of life in oncology patients. Semin Hematol 2000;37:14–7.
7. National Comprehensive Cancer Network (NCCN). NCCN clinical practice guidelines in oncology: cancer-related fatigue. Fort Washington (PA): NCCN; 2011.
8. Mock V, Atkinson A, Barsevick A, et al. NCCN practice guidelines for cancer-related fatigue. Oncology (Williston Park) 2000;14:151–61.
9. Andrykowski MA, Schmidt JE, Salsman JM, et al. Use of a case definition approach to identify cancer related fatigue in women undergoing adjuvant therapy for breast cancer. J Clin Oncol 2005;23:6613–22.
10. Cella D, Peterman A, Passik S, et al. Progress toward guidelines for the management of fatigue. Oncology (Williston Park) 1998;12:369–77.
11. Servaes P, Verhagen S, Bleijenberg G. Determinants of chronic fatigue in disease-free breast cancer patients: a cross-sectional study. Ann Oncol 2002; 13(4):589–98.
12. Cella D, Lai JS, Chang CH, et al. Fatigue in cancer patients compared with fatigue in the general United States population. Cancer 2002;94:528–38.
13. Minton O, Stone P. How common is fatigue in disease-free breast cancer survivors? A systematic review of the literature. Breast Cancer Res Treat 2008;112: 5–13.

14. Glaus A. Fatigue in patients with cancer: analysis and assessment. Heidelberg (Germany): Springer-Verlag Berlin; 1998.

15. Strauss B, Brix C, Fischer B, et al. The influence of resilience on fatigue in cancer patients undergoing radiation therapy. J Cancer Res Clin Oncol 2007;133: 511–8.

16. Morrow GR. Cancer related fatigue: causes, consequences and management. Oncologist 2007;12(Suppl 1):1–3.

17. Borg G. Perceived exertion as an indicator of somatic stress. Scand J Rehabil Med 1970;2:92–8.

18. Meeusen R, Piacentini MF. Exercise, fatigue, neurotransmission and the influence of the neuroendocrine axis. Adv Exp Med Biol 2003;527:521–5.

19. Kirk J, Douglass R, Nelson E, et al. Chief complaint of fatigue: a prospective study. J Fam Pract 1990;30:33–9.

20. Wessely S, Powell R. Fatigue syndromes: a comparison of chronic "postviral" fatigue with neuromuscular and affective disorders. J Neurol Neurosurg Psychiatry 1989;52:940–8.

21. Askren MK, Jung M, Berman MG, et al. Neuromarkers of fatigue and cognitive complaints following chemotherapy for breast cancer: a prospective fMRI investigation. Breast Cancer Res Treat 2014;147:445–55.

22. Schmidt ME, Chang-Claude J, Seibold P, et al. Determinants of long-term fatigue in breast cancer survivors: results of a prospective patient cohort study. Psychooncology 2015;24:40–6.

23. Bower J, Ganz PA, Desmond KA, et al. Fatigue in long term breast carcinoma survivors: a longitudinal investigation. Cancer 2006;106:751–8.

24. Reinertsen KV, Cvancarova M, Loge JH, et al. Predictors and correlates of chronic fatigue in long-term breast cancer survivors. J Cancer Surviv 2010;4: 405–14.

25. Hofman M, Ryan JL, Figueroa-Moseley CD, et al. Cancer-related fatigue: the scale of the problem. Oncologist 2007;12(Suppl 1):4–10.

26. de Jong N, Candel MJ, Schouten HC, et al. Prevalence and course of fatigue in breast cancer patients receiving adjuvant chemotherapy. Ann Oncol 2004;15: 896–905.

27. Carter AJ, Nguyen CN. A comparison of cancer burden and research spending reveals discrepancies in the distribution of research funding. BMC Public Health 2012;12:526.

28. Yellen S, Cella DF, Webster L, et al. Measuring fatigue and other anemia-related symptoms with the Functional Assessment of Cancer Therapy (FACT) measurement system. J Pain Symptom Manage 1997;13:63–74.

29. Minton O, Stone P. A systematic review of the scales used for the measurement of cancer-related fatigue (CRF). Ann Oncol 2009;20:17–25.

30. Jacobsen PB. Assessment of fatigue in cancer patients. J Natl Cancer Inst Monogr 2004;32:93–7.

31. Whitehead L. The measurement of fatigue in chronic illness: a systematic review of unidimensional and multidimensional fatigue measures. J Pain Symptom Manage 2009;37:107–28.

32. Dilara Seyidova-Khoshknabi D, Davis MP, Walsh D. Review article: a systematic review of cancer-related fatigue measurement questionnaires. Am J Hosp Palliat Care 2011;28:119–29.

33. Donovan KA, Stein KD, Lee M, et al. Systematic review of the multidimensional fatigue symptom inventory-short form. Support Care Cancer 2015;23:191–212.

34. Cella D, Riley W, Stone A, et al. Initial adult health item banks and first wave testing of the Patient-Reported Outcomes Measurement Information System (PROMIS™) network: 2005–2008. J Clin Epidemiol 2010;63:1179–94.
35. Lai J, Cella D, Choi S, et al. How item banks and their application can influence measurement practice in rehabilitation medicine: a PROMIS fatigue item bank example. Arch Phys Med Rehabil 2011;92:S20–7.
36. Cella D, Lai JS, Jensen SE, et al. PROMIS fatigue item bank had clinical validity across diverse chronic conditions. J Clin Epidemiol 2016;73:128–34.
37. Cella D, Eton D, Lai J-S, et al. Combining anchor and distribution-based methods to derive minimal clinically important differences on the Functional Assessment of Cancer Therapy (FACT) anemia and fatigue scales. J Pain Symptom Manage 2002;24:547–61.
38. Dittner AJ, Wessely SC, Brown RG. The assessment of fatigue: a practical guide for clinicians and researchers. J Psychosom Res 2004;56:157–70.
39. Donovan KA, Jacobsen PB, Small BJ, et al. Identifying clinically meaningful fatigue with the fatigue symptom inventory. J Pain Symptom Manage 2006;36:480–7.
40. Beutel ME, Hinz A, Albani C, et al. Fatigue assessment questionnaire: standardization of a cancer-specific instrument based on the general population. Oncology 2006;70:351–7.
41. Weir RC, Cullen S, Phillips S. Illness perception and symptom components in chronic fatigue syndrome. J Psychosom Res 1992;36(3):243–56.
42. Jason LA, Taylor RR, Kennedy CL, et al. A factor analysis of chronic fatigue symptoms in a community-based sample. Soc Psychiatry Psychiatr Epidemiol 2002;37:183–9.
43. Daughton DM, Fix AJ, Kass I, et al. Maximum oxygen consumption and the ADAPT quality-of-life scale. Arch Phys Med Rehabil 1982;63:620–2.
44. Craig C, Marshall AL, Sjostrom M, et al. International Physical Activity Questionnaire: 12-country reliability and validity. Med Sci Sports Exerc 2003;35:1381–95.
45. Haskell WL. Physical activity by self-report: a brief history and future issues. J Phys Act Health 2012;9(Suppl 1):5–10.
46. Wright F, Hammer MJ, D'Eramo Melkus G. Associations between multiple chronic conditions and cancer-related fatigue: an integrative review. Oncol Nurs Forum 2014;41:399–410.
47. Alexander S, Minton O, Andrews P. Comparison of the characteristics of disease-free breast cancer survivors with or without cancer-related fatigue syndrome. Eur J Cancer 2009;45:384–92.
48. Bauml J, Chen L, Chen J, et al. Arthralgia among women taking aromatase inhibitors: is there a shared inflammatory mechanism with co-morbid fatigue and insomnia? Breast Cancer Res 2015;17:89.
49. Sprauten M, Haugnes HS, Brydøy M, et al. Chronic fatigue in 812 testicular cancer survivors during long-term follow-up: increasing prevalence and risk factors. Ann Oncol 2015;26:2133–40.
50. Cole BF, Gelber RD, Kirkwood JM, et al. Quality-of-life adjusted survival analysis of interferon alfa-2b adjuvant treatment for high-risk resected cutaneous melanoma: an Eastern Cooperative Oncology Group Study. J Clin Oncol 1996;14:2666–73.
51. Bonaccorso S, Marino V, Biondi M, et al. Depression induced by treatment with interferon-alpha in patients affected by hepatitis C virus. J Affect Disord 2002;72:237–41.
52. Coussens LM, Werb Z. Inflammation and cancer. Nature 2002;420:860–7.

53. Bower JE, Ganz PA, Aziz N, et al. Fatigue and proinflammatory cytokine activity in breast cancer survivors. Psychosom Med 2002;64:604–11.

54. Collado-Hidalgo A, Bower JE, Ganz PA, et al. Inflammatory biomarkers for persistent fatigue in breast cancer survivors. Clin Cancer Res 2006;12:2759–66.

55. Bower JE. Cancer-related fatigue: links with inflammation in cancer patients and survivors. Brain Behav Immun 2007;21:863–71.

56. Karayiannakis AJ, Syrigos KN, Polychronidis A, et al. Serum levels of tumor necrosis factor-alpha and nutritional status in pancreatic cancer patients. Anticancer Res 2001;21:1355–8.

57. Orre IJ, Murison R, Dahl AA, et al. Levels of circulating interleukin-1 receptor antagonist and C-reactive protein in long-term survivors of testicular cancer with chronic cancer-related fatigue. Brain Behav Immun 2009;23:868–74.

58. Orre IJ, Reinertsen KV, Aukrust P, et al. Higher levels of fatigue are associated with higher CRP levels in disease-free breast cancer survivors. J Psychosom Res 2011;71:136–41.

59. Schubert C, Hong S, Natarajan L, et al. The association between fatigue and inflammatory marker levels in cancer patients: a quantitative review. Brain Behav Immun 2007;21:413–27.

60. Vgontzas AN, Papanicolaou DA, Bixler EO, et al. Elevation of plasma cytokines in disorders of excessive daytime sleepiness: role of sleep disturbance and obesity. J Clin Endocrinol Metab 1997;82:1313–6.

61. Schultz SL, Dalton SO, Christensen J, et al. Factors correlated with fatigue in breast cancer survivors undergoing a rehabilitation course, Denmark, 2002–2005. Psychooncology 2011;20:352–60.

62. Saligan L, Kim HS. A systematic review of the association between immunogenic markers and cancer related fatigue. Brain Behav Immun 2012;21:830–48.

63. Gerber LH, Stout N, McGarvey C, et al. Factors predicting clinically significant fatigue in women following treatment for primary breast cancer. Support Care Cancer 2011;19:1581–91.

64. Rotstein S, Blomgren H, Petrini B, et al. Long term effects on the immune system following local radiation therapy for breast cancer. I. Cellular composition of the peripheral blood lymphocyte population. Int J Radiat Oncol Biol Phys 1985;11:921–5.

65. Bower JE, Ganz PA, Aziz N, et al. T-cell homeostasis in breast cancer survivors with persistent fatigue. J Natl Cancer Inst 2003;95:1165–8.

66. Witek-Janusek L, Albuquerque K, Chroniak KR, et al. Effect of mindfulness based stress reduction on immune function, quality of life and coping in women newly diagnosed with early stage breast cancer. Brain Behav Immun 2008;22:969–81.

67. Vivier E, Raulet DH, Moretta A, et al. Innate or adaptive immunity? The example of natural killer cells. Science 2011;331:44–9.

68. McEwen BS, Biron CA, Brunson KW, et al. The role of adrenocorticoids as modulators of immune function in health and disease: neural, endocrine and immune interactions. Brain Res Brain Res Rev 1997;23:79–133.

69. Bower J, Ganz PA, Aziz N. Altered cortisol response to psychologic stress in breast cancer survivors with persistent fatigue. Psychosom Med 2005;67:277–80.

70. Schmidt ME, Semik J, Habermann N, et al. Cancer-related fatigue shows a stable association with diurnal cortisol dysregulation in breast cancer patients. Brain Behav Immun 2016;52:98–105.

71. Nelson AM, Gonzalez BD, Jim HS, et al. Characteristics and predictors of fatigue among men receiving androgen deprivation therapy for prostate cancer: a controlled comparison. Support Care Cancer 2016;24:4159–66.
72. Aouizerat BE, Dhruva A, Paul SM, et al. Phenotypic and molecular evidence suggests that decrements in morning and evening energy are distinct but related symptoms. J Pain Symptom Manage 2015;50:599–614.
73. Miaskowski C, Dodd M, Lee K, et al. Preliminary evidence of an association between a functional interleukin-6 polymorphism and fatigue and sleep disturbance in oncology patients and their family caregivers. J Pain Symptom Manage 2010;40:531–44.
74. Ng T, Chan M, Khor CC, et al. The genetic variants underlying breast cancer treatment-induced chronic and late toxicities: a systematic review. Cancer Treat Rev 2014;40:1199–214.
75. Fernandez-de-las-Penas C, Fernandez-Lao C, Cantarero-Villanueva I, et al. Catechol-O-methyltransferase genotype (Val158met) modulates cancer-related fatigue and pain sensitivity in breast cancer survivors. Breast Cancer Res Treat 2011;133:405–12.
76. Barsevick A, Frost M, Zwinderman A, et al. GENEQOL Consortium. I'm so tired: biological and genetic mechanisms of cancer-related fatigue. Qual Life Res 2010;19:1419–27.
77. Vichaya EG, Chiu GS, Krukowski K, et al. Mechanisms of chemotherapy-induced behavioral toxicities. Front Neurosci 2015;9:131.
78. Reinertsen KV, Grenaker Alnæs GI, Landmark-Høyvik H, et al. Fatigued breast cancer survivors and gene polymorphisms in the inflammatory pathway. Brain Behav Immun 2011;25:1376–83.
79. Giovannucci E, Harlan DM, Archer MC, et al. Diabetes and cancer: a consensus report. Diabetes Care 2010;33:1674–85.
80. Tang Z, Wang J, Zhang H, et al. Associations between diabetes and quality of life among breast cancer survivors. PLoS One 2016;11(6):e0157791.
81. Nuver J, Smit AJ, Wolffenbuttel BH, et al. The metabolic syndrome and disturbances in hormone levels in long-term survivors of disseminated testicular cancer. J Clin Oncol 2005;23(16):3718–25.
82. Nuver J, Smit AJ, Postma A, et al. The metabolic syndrome in long-term cancer survivors, an important target for secondary preventive measures. Cancer Treat Rev 2002;28:195–214.
83. Hoffman KE, Derdak J, Bernstein D, et al. Metabolic syndrome traits in long-term survivors of pediatric sarcoma. Pediatr Blood Cancer 2008;50(2):341–6.
84. Fontes-Oliveira CC, Busquets S, Toledo M, et al. Mitochondrial and sarcoplasmic reticulum abnormalities in cancer cachexia: altered energetic efficiency? Biochim Biophys Acta 2013;1830:2770–8.
85. Kisiel-Sajewicz K, Davis MP, Siemionow V, et al. Lack of muscle contractile property changes at the time of perceived physical exhaustion suggests central mechanisms contributing to early motor task failure in patients with cancer-related fatigue. J Pain Symptom Manage 2012;44:351–61.
86. Gatenby RA, Gillies RJ. Why do cancers have high aerobic glycolysis? Nat Rev Cancer 2004;4:891–9.
87. Fantin VR, St-Pierre J, Leder P. Attenuation of LDH-A expression uncovers a link between glycolysis, mitochondrial physiology, and tumor maintenance. Cancer Cell 2006;9:425–34.
88. Meeusen R, Watson P, Hasegawa H, et al. Central fatigue: the serotonin hypothesis and beyond. Sports Med 2006;36:881–909.

89. Bergholdt SH, Søndergaard J, Larsen PV, et al. A randomised controlled trial to improve general practitioners' services in cancer rehabilitation: effects on general practitioners' proactivity and on patients' participation in rehabilitation activities. Acta Oncol 2013;52:400–9.

90. Goedendorp MM, Gielissen MF, Verhagen CA, et al. Psychosocial interventions for reducing fatigue during cancer treatment in adults [serial online]. Cochrane Database Syst Rev 2009;(91):CD006953.

91. Jacobsen P, Donovan KA, Vadaparampil S, et al. Systematic review and meta-analysis of psychological and activity based interventions for cancer-related fatigue. Health Psychol 2007;26:660–7.

92. Purcell A, Fleming J, Burmeister B, et al. Is education an effective management strategy for reducing cancer-related fatigue? Support Care Cancer 2011;19: 1429–39.

93. Pearson EJ, Morris ME, di Stefano M, et al. Interventions for cancer-related fatigue: a scoping review. Eur J Cancer Care (Engl) 2016. http://dx.doi.org/10. 1111/ecc.12516.

94. Du S, Hu L, Dong J, et al. Patient education programs for cancer-related fatigue: a systematic review. Patient Educ Couns 2015;98:1308–19.

95. Goodwin PJ, Leszcz M, Ennis M. The effect of group psychosocial support on survival in metastatic breast cancer. N Engl J Med 2001;345:1719–26.

96. Berger AM, Mitchell SA, Jacobsen PB. Screening, evaluation, and management of cancer-related fatigue: ready for implementation to practice? CA Cancer J Clin 2015;65:190–211.

97. Bower JE. Cancer-related fatigue: mechanisms, risk factors, and treatments. Nat Rev Clin Oncol 2014;11:597–609.

98. Grant MD, Piper M, Bohlius J, et al. Epoetin and darbepoetin for managing anemia in patients undergoing cancer treatment: comparative effectiveness update. Rockville (MD): Agency for Healthcare Research and Quality (US); 2013.

99. Mountzios G, Aravantinos G, Alexopoulou Z, et al. Lessons from the past: Long-term safety and survival outcomes of a prematurely terminated randomized controlled trial on prophylactic vs. hemoglobin-based administration of erythropoiesis-stimulating agents in patients with chemotherapy-induced anemia. Mol Clin Oncol 2016;4:211–20.

100. Bohlius J, Tonia T, Nüesch E, et al. Effects of erythropoiesis-stimulating agents on fatigue- and anaemia-related symptoms in cancer patients: systematic review and meta-analyses of published and unpublished data. Br J Cancer 2014;111(1):33–45.

101. Peuckmann V, Elsner F, Krumm N, et al. Pharmacological treatments for fatigue associated with palliative care. Cochrane Database Syst Rev 2010;(11):CD006788.

102. Lundström SH, Fürst CJ. The use of corticosteroids in Swedish palliative care. Acta Oncol 2006;45:430–7.

103. Yennurajalingam S, Frisbee-Hume S, Palmer JL, et al. Reduction of cancer-related fatigue with dexamethasone: a double-blind, randomized, placebo-controlled trial in patients with advanced cancer. J Clin Oncol 2013;31(25): 3076–82.

104. Paulsen O, Klepstad P, Rosland JH, et al. Efficacy of methylprednisolone on pain, fatigue, and appetite loss in patients with advanced cancer using opioids: a randomized, placebo-controlled, double-blind trial. J Clin Oncol 2014;10(32): 3221–8.

105. Haywood A, Good P, Khan S, et al. Corticosteroids for the management of cancer-related pain in adults. Cochrane Database Syst Rev 2015;(4):CD010756.
106. Begley S, Rose K, O'Connor M. The use of corticosteroids in reducing cancer-related fatigue: assessing the evidence for clinical practice. Int J Palliat Nurs 2016;22:5–9.
107. Yennurajalingam S, Williams JL, Chisholm G, et al. Effects of dexamethasone and placebo on symptom clusters in advanced cancer patients: a preliminary report. Oncologist 2016;21:384–90.
108. Kamath J. Cancer-related fatigue, inflammation and thyrotropin-releasing hormone. Curr Aging Sci 2012;5:195–202.
109. Minton O, Richardson A, Sharpe M, et al. A systematic review and meta-analysis of the pharmacological treatment of cancer-related fatigue. J Natl Cancer Inst 2008;100:1155–66.
110. Minton O, Richardson A, Sharpe M. Psychostimulants for the management of cancer-related fatigue: a systematic review and meta-analysis. J Pain Symptom Manage 2011;41:761–7.
111. Mücke M, Mochamat M, Cuhls H. Pharmacological treatments for fatigue associated with palliative care. Cochrane Database Syst Rev 2015;(5):CD006788.
112. Roscoe JA, Morrow GR, Hickok JT, et al. Effect of paroxetine hydrochloride (Paxil) on fatigue and depression in breast cancer patients receiving chemotherapy. Breast Cancer Res Treat 2005;89:243–9.
113. MacVicar MG, Winningham ML. Promoting the functional capacity of cancer patients. Cancer Bull 1986;38:235–9.
114. Mock V. Evidence-based treatment for cancer-related fatigue. J Natl Cancer Inst Monogr 2004;32:112–8.
115. Dimeo FC, Tilmann MH, Bertz H, et al. Aerobic exercise in the rehabilitation of cancer patients after high dose chemotherapy and autologous peripheral stem cell transplantation. Cancer 1997;79:1717–22.
116. Tomlinson D, Diorio C, Beyene J, et al. Effect of exercise on cancer-related fatigue: a meta analysis. Am J Phys Med Rehabil 2014;93:675–86.
117. Cramp F, Byron-Daniel J. Exercise for the management of cancer related fatigue in adults. Cochrane Database Syst Rev 2012;(11):CD006145.
118. Eickmeyer SM, Gamble GL, Shahpar S, et al. The role and efficacy of exercise in persons with cancer. PM R 2012;4:874–81.
119. Puetz TW, Herring MP. Differential effects of exercise on cancer-related fatigue during and following treatment: a meta-analysis. Am J Prev Med 2012;43:e1–24.
120. Mishra SI, Scherer RW, Snyder C, et al. Exercise interventions on health-related quality of life for people with cancer during active treatment. Cochrane Database Syst Rev 2012;(8):CD008465.
121. Velthuis MJ, Agasi-Idenburg SC, Aufdemkampe G, et al. The effect of physical exercise on cancer-related fatigue during cancer treatment: a meta-analysis of randomised controlled trials. Clin Oncol (R Coll Radiol) 2010;22(3):208–21.
122. Larkin D, Lopez V, Aromataris E. Managing cancer-related fatigue in men with prostate cancer: a systematic review of non-pharmacological interventions. Int J Nurs Pract 2013;20:549–60.
123. Segal RJ, Reid RD, Courneya KS, et al. Resistance exercise in men receiving androgen deprivation therapy for prostate cancer. J Clin Oncol 2003;21:1653–9.
124. Hasenoehrl T, Keilani M, Sedghi Komanadj T, et al. The effects of resistance exercise on physical performance and health-related quality of life in prostate cancer patients: a systematic review. Support Care Cancer 2015;23:2479–97.

125. Cramer H, Lauche R, Klose P, et al. A systematic review and meta-analysis of exercise interventions for colorectal cancer patients. Eur J Cancer Care (Engl) 2014;23:3–14.
126. Paramanandam VS, Dunn V. Exercise for the management of cancer-related fatigue in lung cancer: a systematic review. Eur J Cancer Care (Engl) 2014;24: 4–14.
127. van Haren IE, Timmerman H, Potting CM. Physical exercise for patients undergoing hematopoietic stem cell transplantation: systematic review and meta-analyses of randomized controlled trials. Phys Ther 2013;93:514–28.
128. Andersen C, Rorth M, Ejlertsen B, et al. The effects of a six-week supervised multimodal exercise intervention during chemotherapy on cancer-related fatigue. Eur J Oncol Nurs 2013;17:331–9.
129. Adamsen L, Quist M, Andersen C, et al. Effect of a multimodal high intensity exercise intervention in cancer patients undergoing chemotherapy: randomised controlled trial. BMJ 2009;339:b3410.
130. Gracey JH, Watson M, Payne C, et al. Translation research: 'Back on Track', a multiprofessional rehabilitation service for cancer-related fatigue. BMJ Support Palliat Care 2016;6:94–6.
131. Rajotte EJ, Yi JC, Baker KS, et al. Community-based exercise program effectiveness and safety for cancer survivors. J Cancer Surviv 2012;6:219–28.
132. Pescatello LS, Arena R, Riebe D, et al. ACSM guide lines for exercise testing and prescription. 9th edition. Philadelphia: Wolters Kluwer/Lippincott Williams and Wilkens; 2014.
133. Fleming L, Randell K, Harvey CJ, et al. Does cognitive behaviour therapy for insomnia reduce clinical levels of fatigue, anxiety and depression in cancer patients? Psychooncology 2014;23:679–84.
134. Kwekkeboom KL, Abbott-Anderson K, Cherwin C, et al. Pilot randomized controlled trial of a patient-controlled cognitive-behavioral intervention for the pain, fatigue, and sleep disturbance symptom cluster in cancer. J Pain Symptom Manage 2012;44:810–22.
135. Gielissen MF, Verhagen CA, Bleijenberg G. Cognitive behaviour therapy for fatigued cancer survivors: long-term follow-up. Br J Cancer 2007;97:612–8.
136. Abrahams HJ, Gielissen MF, Goedendorp MM, et al. A randomized controlled trial of web-based cognitive behavioral therapy for severely fatigued breast cancer survivors (CHANGE-study): study protocol. BMC Cancer 2015;15:765.
137. Ferguson RJ, Sigmon ST, Pritchard AJ, et al. A randomized trial of videoconference-delivered cognitive behavioral therapy for survivors of breast cancer with self-reported cognitive dysfunction. Cancer 2016;122:1782–91.
138. van Weert E, May AM, Korstjens I, et al. Cancer-related fatigue and rehabilitation: a randomized controlled multicenter trial comparing physical training combined with cognitive-behavioral therapy with physical training only and with no intervention. Phys Ther 2010;90:1413–25.
139. Greenlee H, Balneaves LG, Carlson LE, et al. Clinical practice guidelines on the use of integrative therapies as supportive care in patients treated for breast cancer. J Natl Cancer Inst Monogr 2014;50:346–58.

Clinical Evaluation and Management of Radiation Fibrosis Syndrome

Michael D. Stubblefield, MD

KEYWORDS

- Cancer • Rehabilitation • Radiation fibrosis syndrome • Late effects
- Hodgkin lymphoma • Head and neck cancer • Neuromuscular • Musculoskeletal

KEY POINTS

- Radiation fibrosis syndrome (RFS) describes the multiple neuromuscular, musculoskeletal, visceral, and other late effects that result from radiation-induced fibrosis.
- Radiation can damage the spinal cord, nerve roots, plexus, local peripheral nerves, and muscles within the radiation field. This phenomenon is known as a "myelo-radiculo-plexo-neuro-myopathy" and results in multiple clinical manifestations.
- There is no cure for RFS, but supportive treatment of its clinical sequelae can potentially result in improved function and quality of life.

INTRODUCTION

The American Cancer Society estimates that there are approximately 14.5 million cancer survivors in the United States as of 2015.[1] Approximately one-half of patients treated for cancer will have required radiation therapy (RT) at some time during the course of their illness.[2] Despite the therapeutic goals of RT as either potentially curative (ie, head and neck cancer [HNC]), or palliative (ie, bone metastases), toxicity is commonly seen.[3] Such toxicity can manifest with treatment and remain (a long-term effect) or develop and progress weeks, months, or decades later (late effect).[4] This article describes the common neuromusculoskeletal late effects likely to be seen as a result of RT and the rehabilitation principles key to evaluating and managing these complex disorders.

RADIATION THERAPY DELIVERY

Understanding radiation injury requires a basic knowledge of what radiation is and how it is, and has historically been, delivered. The basic unit currently used in radiation

Disclosures: The author has no disclosures.
Kessler Institute for Rehabilitation, Department of Physical Medicine and Rehabilitation, 1199 Pleasant Valley Way, West Orange, NJ 07052, USA
E-mail address: mstubblefield@selectmedical.com

Phys Med Rehabil Clin N Am 28 (2017) 89–100
http://dx.doi.org/10.1016/j.pmr.2016.08.003
1047-9651/17/© 2016 Elsevier Inc. All rights reserved.

oncology is the gray (Gy). One gray is defined as the absorption of 1 J of radiation per 1 kg of matter. Radiation dosing was previously expressed in absorbed radiation dose or rads (1 rad = 0.1 J/kg = 0.01 Gy = 1 cGy). Therefore, a total dose of radiation of 5000 rad is equivalent to 5000 cGy or 50 Gy.

In general, as total dose increases, so too does the risk of radiation injury. **Table 1** lists the tolerances of select tissues to therapeutic radiation. The total dose of radiation delivered is not, however, the sole determinant of radiation injury. In addition to total dose, the size of each radiation fraction, the type of tissue radiated, the time from radiation treatment, individual patient tolerance, and concomitant oncologic treatments impact the development of RFS.[5]

The practice of RT has evolved significantly over past decades in an effort to minimize toxicity. Before the 1980s, radiation was generally delivered in an anterior-posterior (AP) and posterior-anterior (PA) fashion. Radiographic imaging was used for treatment planning, patient positioning, and tumor identification. Simple blocks were used to shape the radiation beam. Because large amounts of normal tissue were included in the radiation field, the radiation dose could not safely exceed what was tolerated by the most sensitive structure (ie, the lung or bowel) in the field. In addition to considerable amounts of normal tissue being affected, surface hotspots, and inability to maximize radiation dose to the tumor limited the effectiveness of conventional RT for some tumors. Despite these limitations, conventional AP/PA RT is still used today, as it is relatively uncomplicated and inexpensive compared with newer techniques.

To circumvent the many barriers of conventional AP/PA RT, conformal radiation techniques were developed and continue to evolve in concert with imaging and computer technology.[6] Three-dimensional (3D) conformal techniques use 3D imaging, such as computed tomography (CT) and MRI, to identify tumor and normal tissues.[7] As opposed to conventional 2D techniques, which direct radiation beams from only 2 directions, 3D conformal techniques use multiple beams of radiation from varied directions to sculpt the radiation to the tumor while minimizing exposure to normal tissue. In addition to delivering radiation from multiple directions, it is possible to modulate the intensity of radiation coming from each direction for enhanced control. This technique is known as intensity-modulated radiotherapy (IMRT). IMRT is a frequently used radiotherapy technique. It is often used where tumor is adjacent to critical structures. For example, in nasopharyngeal cancer, IMRT has been demonstrated to improve local recurrence-free survival while minimizing the incidence of complications, such as xerostomia.[8] **Fig. 1** compares a 3D and IMRT treatment plan in a patient with HNC.

The ability to sculpt and modulate radiation with exacting tolerances has allowed the development of stereotactic radiosurgical (RS) techniques. RS is similar to IMRT in that radiation is delivered from numerous angles and focused precisely on the tumor with relative sparing of surrounding normal tissue. The primary difference is that stereotactic RS is delivered in fewer fractions; that is, 1 to 5 of higher dose.[9] For instance, spine metastases that are considered radioresistant to conventional radiotherapy (30 Gy in 10 fractions) may be better controlled with stereotactic RS (24 Gy in 1 fraction).[9] **Fig. 2** depicts the isodose curve for radiosurgery of metastatic disease to L4 and L5.

PATHOPHYSIOLOGY OF RADIATION INJURY
Radiation Fibrosis

Radiation fibrosis (RF) is the term used to describe the insidious, progressive, and immortalized process that occurs in tissues as a result of RT. Although the

Table 1
Tissue tolerance to therapeutic radiation

Site	TD 5/5 (Gy)[a] Portion of Organ Irradiated			TD 50/5 (Gy)[b] Portion of Organ Irradiated			Complication/End Point (s)
	1/3	2/3	3/3	1/3	2/3	3/3	
Neuromusculoskeletal:							
Brachial plexus	62	61	60	77	76	75	Clinical nerve damage
Brain	60	50	45	75	65	60	Necrosis, infarct
Brainstem	60	53	50	—	—	65	Necrosis, infarct
Cauda equina	No volume effect		60	No volume effect		75	Clinical nerve damage
Optic nerve	No partial volume		50	No partial volume		65	Blindness
Spinal cord	50 (5 cm)	50 (10 cm)	47 (20 cm)	70 (5 cm)	70 (10 cm)	—	Myelitis, necrosis
Temporomandibular joint	65	60	60	77	72	72	Marked limitation in joint function
Femoral head	—	—	52	—	—	65	Necrosis
Visceral:							
Bladder	N/A	80	65	N/A	85	80	Contracture, volume loss
Colon	55	—	45	65	—	55	Obstruction, perforation, fistula, ulceration
Esophagus	60	58	55	72	70	68	Stricture, perforation
Heart	60	45	40	70	55	50	Pericarditis
Kidney	50	30	23	—	40	28	Nephritis
Liver	50	35	30	55	45	40	Liver failure
Lung	45	30	17.5	65	40	24.5	Radiation pneumonitis
Rectum	—	—	60	—	—	80	Severe proctitis, necrosis, fistula
Small intestine	50	—	40	60	—	55	Obstruction, perforation, fistula
Stomach	60	55	50	70	67	65	Ulceration, perforation

[a] TD 5/5 is the average dose that results in a 5% complication risk within 5 years.
[b] TD 50/5 is the average dose that results in a 50% complication risk within 5 years.
Adapted from Emami B, Lyman J, Brown A, et al. Tolerance of normal tissue to therapeutic irradiation. Int J Radiat Oncol Biol Phys 1991;21:109–22.

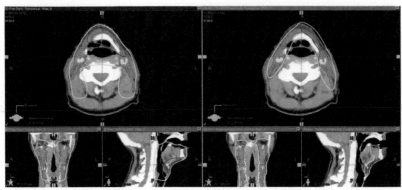

Fig. 1. Patient with HNC treated with 3D technique (*left*) or IMRT technique (*right*). Illustrative axial, coronal, and midsagittal slices are shown. A primary tumor from the floor of the mouth and a positive left anterior neck lymph node with focal extracapsular extension has been surgically resected. RT is given adjuvantly to areas at risk in the bilateral neck (*shaded magenta*) with a dose of 5130 cGy (*cyan outline*), and also to the area of higher risk in the operative bed (*shaded red*) with a dose of 6000 cGy (*red outline*). The IMRT plan on the right is significantly more conformal, with dose levels carefully shaped to the respective targets. Both plans spare the spinal canal, but epiglottis at the level of the vallecula is mostly spared the 5130-cGy dose level in the IMRT plan. A much more focused dose is possible for the area at higher risk. Acute and long-term side effects are dramatically improved with IMRT technique.

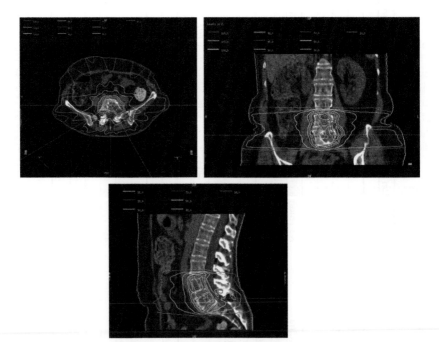

Fig. 2. The axial, coronal, and sagital isodose curves from a radiosurgical treatment plan for a patient with metastases to L4 and L5 is depicted. The radiation dose is 2400 cGy delivered in 1 fraction. Note the tight conformity to the tumor within the vertebral bodies with marked sparing of the spinal cord and surrounding tissues.

pathophysiology of RF has not been definitively elucidated, microvascular injury seems to be an important component in nerve injury.[10] Injury to the nervous system, and other tissues, progresses indefinitely. RF can be characterized by 3 distinct histopathological phases[11]:

1. Prefibrotic phase: This usually asymptomatic phase is characterized by endothelial cell dysfunction. Radiation injury is evidenced by signs of chronic nonspecific local inflammation with increased vascular permeability and edema. Endothelial cell dysfunction and vascular thrombosis can result in necrosis of the microvasculature and subsequent local ischemia.
2. Constitutive organized phase: Symptoms often develop during this stage. The radiated tissue contains patchy areas of activated fibroblasts (myofibroblasts) in a disorganized extracellular matrix that is found adjacent to senescent fibroblasts (fibrocytes) in a densely sclerotic (fibrotic) matrix. Immortalized damage to the endothelial and connective tissue cells, coupled with the action of cytokines, maintains and perpetuates the fibrosis.
3. Late fibroatrophic phase: In this phase, the radiated tissue becomes progressively dense as a result of successive remodeling of the extracellular matrix. The few fibroblasts that survive are encased by a dense extracellular matrix. This stage may develop and progress years or decades following RT. The result is tissue that is poorly vascularized, friable, and fragile.

Radiation Fibrosis Syndrome

Radiation fibrosis syndrome (RFS) defines the clinical manifestations of RF.[3] RF can affect any segment of the neuromuscular system as well as any visceral organ. The sequelae of RF are determined by the specific tissues affected. Clinical manifestations of RFS can develop months, years, or even decades after treatment. Functional decline is often insidious but can be punctuated by periods of rapid deterioration.

The literature is mixed with regard to the specific pathophysiology responsible for radiation-induced neuromuscular disease. Some investigators suggest that it is a result of selective injury to the lower motor neurons in the cord.[12–15] Others argue that the nerve roots or peripheral nerves are the primary site of injury.[16–18] Still others tout ischemic nerve injury and disruption of motor axon conduction based on cases of delayed post-RT plexopathy responding to anticoagulation.[19–21] It is more likely that radiation injury is multifactorial and that multiple levels of the neuromuscular axis are damaged.

CLINICAL EVALUATION AND TREATMENT OF RADIATION FIBROSIS SYNDROME

Hodgkin lymphoma (HL) survivors are frequently affected by RFS and can manifest an extraordinary variety of neuromusculoskeletal and visceral late effects due to radiation. Understanding the late effects in this complicated group of cancer survivors will facilitate accurate identification, informed evaluation, and effective rehabilitation of RFS in other groups, such as HNC survivors.

HL has been potentially curable with RT since the middle of the twentieth century.[22] This susceptibility to treatment is, in part, what separates HL from non-HL and other cancers. In 1902, Pusey[23] reported that enlarged lymph nodes in patients with Hodgkin disease could be treated by x-ray exposure. In 1950, Vera Peters[24] published a landmark publication on the treatment of histologically proven HL with RT and demonstrated a doubling of 5-year survival and a more than threefold increase in 10-year survival. The concept of using multiple chemotherapeutic agents (mechlorethamine, vincristine, procarbazine, and prednisone [MOPP]) to treat HL was introduced in 1964.[25,26] Combined-modality treatment with MOPP and RT was introduced in the mid-1970s.[27] Vera Peters developed the first clinical classification (staging system) for patients with HL.[22] Before the early 1980s, HL staging required laparotomy, which became unnecessary with the advent of CT and the expanded use of combined-modality therapy.[26]

Historically, the treatment of HL involved radiation techniques that are no longer in use today. The radiation fields treated depend on the specific lymph nodes involved by disease. **Fig. 3** depicts the common radiation classically used to treat HL. HL confined to lymph nodes above the diaphragm was treated with mantle field (MF) radiation. MF radiation included all lymph nodes in the neck, chest (mediastinum), and axilla. The lungs (and sometimes part of the heart and shoulders) were shielded. Patients would often report loosing hair on the back of their head to the level of the occipital inion. If disease was found below the diaphragm, then additional fields, including the peri-aortic, splenic, and ilioinguinal were added. A combination of MF and peri-aortic radiation was referred to as "subtotal" radiation. Radiation of the peri-aortic and ilioin-guinal fields was referred to as "inverted-Y" radiation. If all fields were radiated, the pa-tient was said to have received "total nodal" radiation.

The total dose of radiation used to treat HL varied but could be as high as 46 Gy. Because of the extensive nature of the radiation fields to use HL, considerable normal

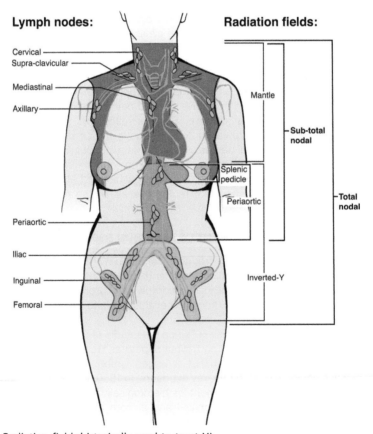

Fig. 3. Radiation fields historically used to treat HL.

tissue was involved. RT for HL has become progressively more sophisticated and now uses involved-field RT, which offers lower dosing to normal tissue as well as decreased secondary cancer risk.[28]

The clinical evaluation of HL survivor's radiation-induced neuromusculoskeletal late effects is greatly facilitated by understanding the specifics of their radiation treatment. Only structures that are in or traverse the radiation field are affected. Depending on the field used in treatment, the spinal cord, nerve roots, plexus, peripheral nerves, and muscles can all be affected. This pattern of neuromuscular damage has been termed a "myelo-radiculo-plexo-neuro-myopathy."[3] **Fig. 4** depicts the neuromusculoskeletal late effects in a typical HL survivor.

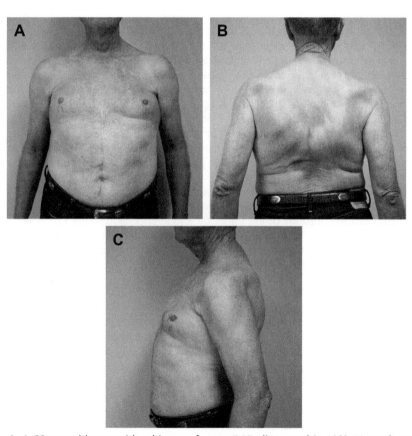

Fig. 4. A 66-year-old man with a history of stage II HL diagnosed in 1983. He underwent staging laparotomy with splenectomy but no disease was found below the diaphragm. He received MF radiation (dose unknown) and is currently without evidence of disease. He has multiple medical late effects of cancer treatment, including hypothyroidism, small bowel obstruction, pericarditis, cerebrovascular accident, and multiple basal and squamous cell carcinomas. Note the marked atrophy of the cervical, thoracic, and rotator cuff muscles. The pectoral muscles were shielded from radiation to protect the lungs and are relatively preserved. There is a left anterior shoulder biopsy scar and the staging laparotomy scar.(*A*) His humeral heads, scapulae, and neck are protracted.(*C*) Hyperlordosis of the lumbar spine is used to position the neck so that the head can be more easily supported.(*B,C*)

Myelopathy is a well-known complication of radiation injury that can be "early-delayed," which is usually reversible, or "late-delayed," which is almost always progressive and permanent.[29] Subacute myelopathy has been described as affecting up to 15% of HL survivors.[5] In the author's experience, this figure may be much higher. Subacute spinal cord injury in HL survivors can be evidenced clinically by typical symptoms of myelopathy, such as gait dysfunction, fatigue, detrusor-sphincter dyssynergia, and spasticity.[3] Frank paraplegia and quadriplegia are uncommon. Physical examination often reveals increased reflexes and clonus. For instance, HL survivors treated with MF radiation typically demonstrate a pattern of depressed reflexes in the biceps and potentially brachioradialis often associated with brisk reflexes, reflex spread, and ankle clonus. This pattern is likely due to lower motor neuron injury affecting the upper cervical nerve roots and plexus depressing reflexes at the biceps and brachioradialis, coupled with upper motor neuron injury to the cervico-thoracic spinal cord conferring brisk lower extremity reflexes.

Radiculopathy and plexopathy usually affect multiple nerve roots and plexus structures in the radiation field. Because they so commonly occur together, they are difficult to separate clinically. In HL survivors treated with MF radiation, radiculo-plexopathy typically, but not invariably, affects the upper cervical nerve roots (C5, C6) and upper plexus structures clinically. Weakness is most pronounced in the rhomboids, rotator cuff muscles, deltoids, and biceps. The apical location of the upper cervical nerve roots and plexus, coupled with the pyramidal shape of the thorax and protection by the clavicle of middle and lower plexus structures, may offer some explanation for this phenomenon.[30] If radiation affecting the cauda equina is given, then radiographic findings mimicking leptomeningeal tumor can sometimes be seen on gadolinium-enhanced MRI.[31]

Mononeuropathies are common in the radiation field of HL survivors. With careful evaluation, damage to several named nerves within the radiation field can be detected. Clinically, atrophy of the trapezius and sternocleidomastoid muscles suggests damage to the spinal accessory nerve. Protraction of the scapulae with weakness of the rhomboids suggests damage to the dorsal thoracic nerve. Damage to the phrenic nerve also has been described and can compound the deleterious effects of radiation to the lungs.[32]

Myopathy characterized by nemaline rods has been reported on muscle biopsy from HL survivors.[33] Myopathy is likely a major component of the atrophy and weakness observed in muscles within the radiation field, making it difficult to separate from dysfunction of other peripheral nervous system structures. Myopathic motor unit changes are often seen on needle electromyography in radiation-affected muscles.

Myelo-radiculo-plexo-neuro-myopathy in an HL survivor is not an all or none phenomenon. There is tremendous variability in how severely each segment of the peripheral neuromuscular system is affected and, thus, in the signs and symptoms with which patients present. In addition to nerves and muscles, other tissues, including ligaments, fascia, and skin, can be severely affected and contribute significantly to functional impairment.

Perhaps the most typical neuromuscular signs and symptoms seen in HL survivors is dropped head syndrome (DHS).[34] Weakness of neck extension is likely multifactorial from damage to the spinal cord, nerve roots, plexus, local nerves, and muscles. DHS is usually associated with cervical and thoracic pain. This syndrome often develops insidiously but can be precipitous in the setting of illness, injury, or other triggers. In mild cases, the patient complains of neck weakness that generally begins later in the day or with activities that require neck extension. Pain and/or tightness are common complaints. In severe cases, patients are completely unable to elevate their head.

Shoulder dysfunction is also common in HL survivors. Muscle imbalance and postural perturbations are likely contributory. The rotator cuff musculature and posterior thoracic muscles are often more compromised than the pectoral girdle muscles (which were shielded from radiation and have a multidermatomal innervation) leading to severe protraction of the shoulders and misalignment of the rotator cuff tendons within the subacromial arch. This imbalance leads to impingement and ultimately injury of the rotator cuff with subsequent inflammation, pain, restricted range of motion, and ultimately adhesive capsulitis.

TREATMENT OF RADIATION FIBROSIS SYNDROME

The primary role of the rehabilitation physician in the care of patients with RFS is the identification, evaluation, and rehabilitation of neuromuscular, musculoskeletal, pain, and functional disorders. RFS is an immortalized process that will progress indefinitely. We currently have no technology to slow or reverse this phenomenon and, therefore, RFS signs and symptoms will progress over time. Although all treatment is supportive, we have the potential to significantly improve and maintain function and quality of life in patients with RFS.

Perhaps the most important modality used to treat RFS is physical therapy (PT). HL, HNC, and other survivors often manifest weakness, postural disturbances, and other impairments that can be greatly improved with appropriate PT interventions. Patients with DHS, for instance, usually have significant myofascial restrictions of the thorax and abdomen that can be optimized with myofascial release, joint mobilization, and other manual techniques. Neuromuscular reeducation can improve balance, coordination, kinesthetic sense, and posture. Therapeutic exercise and activities can improve strength, endurance, range of motion, and flexibility.

Pain and antispasmodic medications can often benefit patients with RFS but must be carefully chosen to not interfere with or worsen medical comorbidities, such as cardiac dysfunction. For patients with cervico-thoracic pain, nerve stabilizers, such as

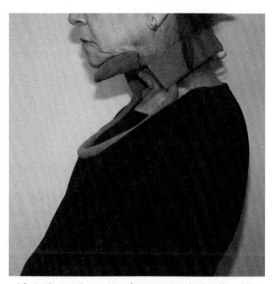

Fig. 5. HL survivor with DHS wearing a Headmaster cervical collar. (Symmetric Designs, Salt Spring Island, BC, Canada.)

pregabalin, gabapentin, duloxetine, and tricyclic antidepressants, are reasonable initial treatment options. Opioids may be required in some instances. Cervical orthotics, such as the Headmaster cervical collar (Symmetric Designs, Salt Spring Island, British Columbia, Canada), can be used to support the head, thereby decreasing fatigue, pain, and spasm (**Fig. 5**).

In addition to neuromusculoskeletal complications, cancer survivors treated with radiation are often at risk for visceral late effects. HL survivors, for instance, are at risk for secondary malignancies, cardiovascular disease, pulmonary disease, thyroid disease, infertility, premature menopause, chronic fatigue, and psychosocial issues.[35] Although these conditions are generally managed by the patient's primary care physician and/or the appropriate subspecialist, the cancer rehabilitation physician plays an important role. The physiatrist is often in a position to recognize the increased risk of visceral disorders and initiate appropriate screening. The rehabilitation physician should incorporate his or her knowledge of the patient's medical complications and treatments into the plan of care to ensure optimal efficacy and safety of given interventions. Additionally, the rehabilitation physician should coordinate care with the other clinicians involved in the patient's care.

SUMMARY

RFS is a common complication of radiation used in the treatment of cancer. Meaningful evaluation of RFS requires an understanding of how a given patient's RT was delivered, including total dose, dose per fraction, and the field treated. With this knowledge in hand, the clinician can accurately determine the structures involved in the radiation field and, thus, if the patient's signs and symptoms are in fact due to RT. Additionally, such knowledge can allow the clinician to predict which structures may ultimately become dysfunctional as a late effect of RT.

Although there is no cure for RF, the sequelae of RFS can often be improved with supportive care such as PT, medications, and bracing. A rehabilitation physician knowledgeable in the visceral late effects of RT can be instrumental in identifying and managing complications in coordination with the patient's medical team.

ACKNOWLEDGMENTS

Special thanks to Brett Lewis, MD, PhD, for generously providing many of the radiation oncology images presented in this article.

REFERENCES

1. Cancer facts & figures 2015. Available at: http://www.cancer.org/acs/groups/content/@editorial/documents/document/acspc-044552.pdf. Accessed December 29, 2015.
2. Hauer-Jensen M, Fink LM, Wang J. Radiation injury and the protein C pathway. Crit Care Med 2004;32:S325–30.
3. Stubblefield MD. Radiation fibrosis syndrome: neuromuscular and musculoskeletal complications in cancer survivors. PM R 2011;3:1041–54.
4. Cohen EE, LaMonte SJ, Erb NL, et al. American Cancer Society head and neck cancer survivorship care guideline. CA Cancer J Clin 2016;66(3):203–39.
5. Cross NE, Glantz MJ. Neurologic complications of radiation therapy. Neurol Clin 2003;21:249–77.
6. Aird EG. Radiotherapy today and tomorrow–an introduction to optimisation of conformal radiotherapy. Phys Med Biol 1989;34:1345–8.

7. Roopashri G, Baig M. Current advances in radiotherapy of head and neck malignancies. J Int Oral Health 2013;5:119–23.

8. Peng G, Wang T, Yang KY, et al. A prospective, randomized study comparing outcomes and toxicities of intensity-modulated radiotherapy vs. conventional two-dimensional radiotherapy for the treatment of nasopharyngeal carcinoma. Radiother Oncol 2012;104:286–93.

9. Laufer I, Rubin DG, Lis E, et al. The NOMS framework: approach to the treatment of spinal metastatic tumors. Oncologist 2013;18:744–51.

10. Delanian S, Lefaix JL, Pradat PF. Radiation-induced neuropathy in cancer survivors. Radiother Oncol 2012;105:273–82.

11. Pradat PF, Delanian S. Late radiation injury to peripheral nerves. Handbook Clin Neurol 2013;115:743–58.

12. Johansson AS, Erlanson M, Lenner P, et al. Late side-effects are common after treatment of Hodgkin's disease. Muscular atrophy following radiotherapy is a neglected risk. Lakartidningen 1998;95:44–7 [in Swedish].

13. Lalu T, Mercier B, Birouk N, et al. Pure motor neuropathy after radiation therapy: 6 cases. Rev Neurol 1998;154:40–4 [in French].

14. Lamy C, Mas JL, Varet B, et al. Postradiation lower motor neuron syndrome presenting as monomelic amyotrophy. J Neurol Neurosurg Psychiatry 1991;54:648–9.

15. van der Sluis RW, Wolfe GI, Nations SP, et al. Post-radiation lower motor neuron syndrome. J Clin Neuromuscul Dis 2000;2:10–7.

16. Ariji Y, Fuwa N, Tachibana H, et al. Denervation atrophy of the masticatory muscles in a patient with nasopharyngeal cancer: MR examinations before and after radiotherapy. Dentomaxillofac Radiol 2002;31:204–8.

17. Olsen NK, Pfeiffer P, Johannsen L, et al. Radiation-induced brachial plexopathy: neurological follow-up in 161 recurrence-free breast cancer patients. Int J Radiat Oncol Biol Phys 1993;26:43–9.

18. Wohlgemuth WA, Rottach K, Jaenke G, et al. Radiogenic amyotrophy. Cauda equina lesion as a late radiation sequela. Nervenarzt 1998;69:1061–5.

19. Anezaki T, Harada T, Kawachi I, et al. A case of post-irradiation lumbosacral radiculopathy successfully treated with corticosteroid and warfarin. Rinsho Shinkeigaku 1999;39:825–9 [in Japanese].

20. Gerard JM, Franck N, Moussa Z, et al. Acute ischemic brachial plexus neuropathy following radiation therapy. Neurology 1989;39:450–1.

21. Soto O. Radiation-induced conduction block: resolution following anticoagulant therapy. Muscle Nerve 2005;31:642–5.

22. Cowan DH. Vera Peters and the curability of Hodgkin disease. Curr Oncol 2008;15:206–10.

23. Pusey W. Cases of sarcoma and of Hodgkin's disease treated by exposures to X-rays: a preliminary report. JAMA 1902;38:166–9.

24. Peters MV. A study of survivals in Hodgkin's disease treated radiologically. Am J Roentgenol 1950;63:299–311.

25. Devita VT Jr, Serpick AA, Carbone PP. Combination chemotherapy in the treatment of advanced Hodgkin's disease. Ann Intern Med 1970;73:881–95.

26. Canellos GP, Rosenberg SA, Friedberg JW, et al. Treatment of Hodgkin lymphoma: a 50-year perspective. J Clin Oncol 2014;32:163–8.

27. Rosenberg SA, Kaplan HS. The management of stages I, II, and III Hodgkin's disease with combined radiotherapy and chemotherapy. Cancer 1975;35:55–63.

28. Koh ES, Tran TH, Heydarian M, et al. A comparison of mantle versus involved-field radiotherapy for Hodgkin's lymphoma: reduction in normal tissue dose and second cancer risk. Radiat Oncol 2007;2:13.

29. Giglio P, Gilbert MR. Neurologic complications of cancer and its treatment. Curr Oncol Rep 2010;12:50–9.

30. Jaeckle KA. Neurologic manifestations of neoplastic and radiation-induced plexopathies. Semin Neurol 2010;30:254–62.

31. Hsia AW, Katz JS, Hancock SL, et al. Post-irradiation polyradiculopathy mimics leptomeningeal tumor on MRI. Neurology 2003;60:1694–6.

32. Avila EK, Goenka A, Fontenla S. Bilateral phrenic nerve dysfunction: a late complication of mantle radiation. J Neurooncol 2010;103(2):393–5.

33. Portlock CS, Boland P, Hays AP, et al. Nemaline myopathy: a possible late complication of Hodgkin's disease therapy. Hum Pathol 2003;34:816–8.

34. Appels C, Goekoop R. Dropped-head syndrome due to high-dose irradiation. J Rheumatol 2009;36:2316.

35. Thompson CA, Mauck K, Havyer R, et al. Care of the adult Hodgkin lymphoma survivor. Am J Med 2011;124:1106–12.

Malignant Spinal Cord Compression

Adapting Conventional Rehabilitation Approaches

Lisa Marie Ruppert, MD[a,b,*]

KEYWORDS

- Malignant spinal cord compression • Neoplastic spinal cord injury • Rehabilitation

KEY POINTS

- Spinal tumors are classically grouped into 3 categories: extradural tumors, intradural extramedullary, and intradural intramedullary tumors.
- Localized spine pain is the most common symptom in patients with epidural spinal cord compression at time of diagnosis.
- Motor weakness is the second most common symptom in patients with epidural spinal cord compression at time of diagnosis.
- Management of spinal tumors varies according to the stability of the spine, neurologic status, and pain. Treatment options include surgical intervention, radiation therapy, and systemic treatments, such as chemotherapy and hormonal therapy.
- Principles of neurorehabilitation applied to patients with traumatic spinal cord injury are equally appropriate for patients with spinal tumors.

INTRODUCTION

When combined with medical, radiation, and surgical oncology care, rehabilitation can serve to relieve symptoms, improve quality of life, enhance functional independence, and prevent further complications in patients with malignant spinal cord compression.[1]

EPIDEMIOLOGY AND PATHOPHYSIOLOGY

Spinal tumors are classically grouped into 3 categories: extradural tumors, intradural extramedullary tumors, and intradural intramedullary tumors (**Box 1**).

Disclosure Statement: This author has noting to disclose.
[a] Department of Neurology, Rehabilitation Medicine Service, Memorial Sloan Kettering Cancer Center, Sillerman Center for Rehabilitation, 515 Madison Avenue, 5th Floor, New York, NY 10022, USA; [b] Division of Rehabilitation Medicine, Weill Cornell Medical College, 525 East 68th Street, New York, NY 10065, USA
* Department of Neurology, Rehabilitation Medicine Service, Memorial Sloan Kettering Cancer Center, Sillerman Center for Rehabilitation, 515 Madison Avenue, 5th Floor, New York, NY 10022.
E-mail address: rupperl1@mskcc.org

Phys Med Rehabil Clin N Am 28 (2017) 101–114
http://dx.doi.org/10.1016/j.pmr.2016.08.007
1047-9651/17/© 2016 Elsevier Inc. All rights reserved.

pmr.theclinics.com

Box 1
Tumors of the spine

Extradural spinal tumors

Primary malignant tumors
  Lymphoma
  Osteosarcoma
  Ewing sarcoma
  Chondrosarcoma
  Chordoma
  Sacrococcygeal teratoma
  Malignant fibrous histiocytoma
  Solitary plasmacytoma
  Fibrosarcoma

Primary benign tumors
  Vertebral hemangioma
  Giant cell tumor
  Osteochondroma
  Osteoid osteoma
  Osteoblastoma

Sources of epidural metastases
  Adult
    Prostate cancer
    Breast cancer
    Lung cancer
    Thyroid cancer
    Non-Hodgkin lymphoma
    Hodgkin disease
    Multiple myeloma
    Renal cell carcinoma
    Colorectal cancers
    Sarcoma
    Germ cell tumor
    Unknown primary
  Pediatrics
    Sarcoma: primarily Ewing sarcoma
    Neuroblastoma
    Germ cell tumors
    Hodgkin disease

Intradural extramedullary tumors

Primary malignant tumors
  Malignant nerve sheath tumors
  Hemangiopericytoma

Primary benign tumors
  Meningioma
  Schwannoma
  Neurofibroma
  Paraganglioma
  Ganglioneuroma

Sources of leptomeningeal disease
  Glioblastoma
  Central nervous system lymphoma
  Leukemia
  Lymphoma
  Breast cancer
  Lung cancer
  Melanoma

Intradural intramedullary tumors

Primary tumors
  Ependymoma
    Myxopapillary ependymoma, subependymoma
  Astrocytoma
  Hemangioblastoma
  Cavernous angioma
  Neurocytic tumors
  Oligodendroglioma
  Embryonal neoplasm
  Lipoma

Sources of intramedullary metastases
  Lung cancer
  Breast cancer
  Melanoma
  Lymphoma
  Renal cell carcinoma

Data from Kim DH, Chang UK, Kim SH, et al, editors. Tumors of the spine. Philadelphia: Saunders Elsevier; 2008, with permission; and Schiff D. Spinal cord compression. Neurol Clin 2003;21:67–86.

Extradural Tumors

Extradural (epidural) tumors refer to lesions outside of the dura mater, in the vertebral bodies, and neural arches. These tumors can be primary or secondary to metastatic disease and are more commonly malignant in nature.[2] Primary extradural tumors arise from osteoblasts, chondrocytes, fibroblasts, and hematopoietic cells. Most extradural metastases occur through hematogenous spread.[3] Direct extension of primary tumors may also lead to metastases in the spinal column. For example, prostate, bladder, and colorectal cancers may become locally aggressive and invade the lumbar or sacral epidural space.[4]

Primary and metastatic lesions may be osteolytic, osteoblastic, or mixed. Osteolytic lesions are more common in adults and with breast, lung, and thyroid cancers. Osteoblastic lesions typically occur with prostate and bladder cancers and carcinoid tumors. Mixed lytic/blastic lesions can be seen with lung, breast, cervical, and ovarian cancers.[2] Osteolytic lesions result in bone destruction greater than bone formation, whereas osteoblastic lesions result in bone deposition without breakdown of old bone first.[2]

Both osteolytic and osteoblastic lesions alter normal bone architecture and can result in deformity or collapse of the affected vertebral body. This deformity can lead to spinal instability by increasing strain on the support elements of the spine, including muscles, tendons, ligaments, and joint capsules.[4] It can also result in retropulsion of fractured bone fragments into the epidural space causing spinal cord compression.[5]

Extradural lesions (**Fig. 1**) may grow into the epidural space resulting in spinal cord compression. Epidural spinal cord compression (ESCC) results in mechanical injury to axons and myelin. ESCC also results in vascular compromise of the spinal arteries and epidural venous plexus, leading to spinal cord ischemia and/or infarction.

Depending on the underlying malignancy, 2% to 5% of patients will develop clinical signs and symptoms of ESCC during the course of their disease.[3] ESCC is most commonly diagnosed in thoracic lesions, though cadaveric studies have shown that the most common site of tumor burden in the spine is the lumbar region.[5]

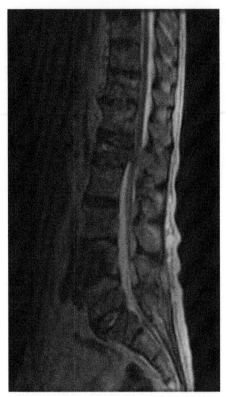

Fig. 1. Extradural tumor with epidural spinal cord compression.

Intradural Extramedullary Tumors

Primary intradural extramedullary tumors are located within the dura mater but outside of the spinal cord parenchyma. These tumors arise from peripheral nerves, nerve sheaths, and sympathetic ganglion. They are most commonly benign. Extramedullary metastases (**Fig. 2**), often referred to as leptomeningeal disease (LMD), are a relatively common complication of cancer, occurring in 3% to 8% of all patients. The most common site of involvement is the dorsal aspect of the spinal cord, particularly at the level of the cauda equina.[2]

Metastatic disease is thought to reach the leptomeninges through hematogenous spread, cerebrospinal fluid (CSF) seeding, and direct extension. CSF seeding can occur spontaneously or as a byproduct of surgical resection. Direct extension can occur along the epineurium or perineurium of spinal nerves or along veins exiting the vertebral body bone marrow.[2,6]

Similar to extradural lesions, intradural extramedullary lesions can result in spinal cord compression and vascular compromise. Vascular compromise in this setting can result not only in ischemia but also in spinal subarachnoid hemorrhage. The risk of hemorrhage is greatest in patients receiving anticoagulation therapy.[2]

Intradural Intramedullary Tumors

Primary intradural intramedullary tumors are located within the spinal cord parenchyma (**Fig. 3**) and arise from glial cells, neuronal cells, and other connective tissue

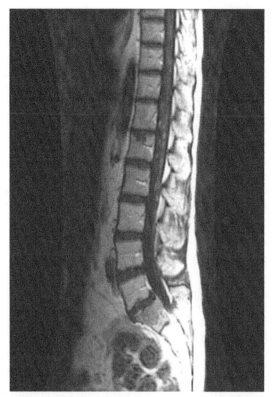

Fig. 2. Intradural-extramedullary lesion.

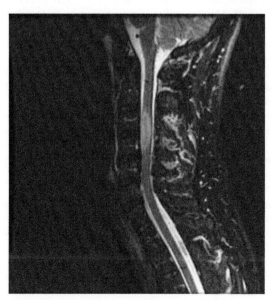

Fig. 3. Intradural-intramedullary tumor.

cells. These tumors account for 4% to 5% of all primary central nervous system tumors and are mostly benign.[2,5] Intramedullary tumors are classified as low, intermediate, or high grade based on cytology. They can be found in any region of the spinal cord, although cervical and cervicothoracic segments are slightly more favored.[2]

Intramedullary spinal cord metastases (ISCMs) are diagnosed in less than 1% of patients with cancer.[3] Metastatic lesions reach the intramedullary space either by hematogenous spread or via direct extension along leptomeninges and nerve roots or through the Virchow-Robin spaces.[3]

ISCMs usually occur in the setting of extensive metastatic disease and are rarely the first manifestation of systemic malignancy.[3] Metastatic lesions can be seen throughout the spinal cord usually as a solitary lesion. The cervical spinal cord, a vascular-rich area, is the most common site of involvement.[2]

It is generally thought that intramedullary lesions cause neurologic injury through direct compression of the surrounding spinal cord and vascular compromise.[2]

CLINICAL MANIFESTATIONS
Extradural Tumors

Pain is the most common initial symptom in patients with ESCC (89%–90%) and may precede the development of other neurologic symptoms by weeks to months. Three classically defined types of pain in the setting of extradural involvement are local, mechanical, and radicular pain. An individual with epidural involvement may be affected by one or more of these pain types.[4]

Localized pain is thought to be the result of periosteal stretching and inflammation caused by tumor growth. It is characterized as a deep gnawing or aching pain. It is often nocturnal and improves with activity and antiinflammatory medications.[4]

Mechanical pain varies with position or activity, indicates impending or established spinal instability, and characteristically occurs with transitional movements or axial loading of the spine. This pain may also be elicited by lying prone or supine, particularly in the thoracic spine. Unlike localized pain, mechanical pain is often refractory to antiinflammatory agents. Mechanical pain responds well to stabilization of the spine with bracing or surgical fixation.[3,4]

Radicular pain occurs in the setting of nerve root compression and is often described as sharp, shooting, or stabbing in nature. In the thoracic region, radicular pain is typically bilateral and described as a tight band around the chest or abdomen. In the cervical and lumbar regions, it is usually unilateral, radiating to the upper or lower extremity, respectively.[3,4]

Motor weakness results from dysfunction of pathways that include the anterior horn cells and mediate movement.[7] It is the second most common symptom of ESCC and is present in 35% to 85% of patients with metastases at the time of presentation. This weakness may be upper motor neuron, lower motor neuron, or a combination of both depending on the area of the cord involved.[4]

Sensory impairments are usually present at the time of diagnosis (60%) in individuals with ESCC but are rarely the initial symptom. The pattern of impairment depends on the spinal pathway involved. Involvement of the lateral spinothalamic tract reduces pain and temperature perception on the contralateral side of the body, one or 2 dermatomes below the level of the lesion, but rarely causes paresthesias. Bilateral lesions may effect erection, ejaculation, and orgasm.[7]

Dorsal column involvement results in loss of proprioception, vibration and touch from the ipsilateral body and information about visceral distension, and may result in paresthesias. Individuals may experience limb or gait ataxia as the result of their proprioceptive loss. Lhermitte phenomenon, an electric shock sensation that extends into the back and sometimes the limbs with changes in head or neck position, is frequently noted with dorsal column involvement in cervical and upper thoracic lesions.[3,7]

Autonomic symptoms include bowel, bladder and sexual dysfunction, loss of sweating below the lesion and orthostatic hypotension. They are unusual as an initial symptom, but are often present at the time of diagnosis. Autonomic symptoms usually correlate with the degree of motor involvement.[3,4]

Gait and truncal ataxia mimicking cerebellar involvement can be seen. This ataxia likely results from compression of the spinocerebellar tracts and can be differentiated from cerebellar lesions by the absence of dysarthria and nystagmus.[3]

Unusual signs of ESCC include the eruption of herpetic zoster at the level of cord compression, Horner syndrome with C7 to T1 involvement and neuropathic facial pain with high cervical ESCC involving the descending fibers of the trigeminal-thalamic tract.[3]

Intradural Extramedullary Tumors

Primary extradural tumors and LMD present in a similar fashion to ESCC but with a higher incidence of neurologic impairments. Approximately 70% to 90% of individuals will have pain as an initial symptom. This pain may be axial and/or radicular and worsened by recumbency. More than 60% of individuals undergoing surgical resection for LMD have some degree of weakness. Motor deficits may manifest in the absence of pain.[2]

Almost all patients will have some degree of sensory involvement. Bowel, bladder, and sexual dysfunction have been noted in 30% to 80% of individuals with LMD, usually as an early finding. LMD may present with radiculopathy, neuropathy, or in a Brown-Séquard, conus medullaris, or cauda equina pattern.[7]

Intramedullary Tumors

Intramedullary tumors may present with clinical manifestations surprisingly similar to epidural tumors. Pain, the most common initial symptom (30%–85%), may be described as radicular, posterior midline, dull, aching, and/or as paravertebral tightness and stiffness.[2]

Neurologic deficits are common and usually involve cord segments below the level of the tumor. Overall, more than 92% of patients have some degree of motor deficit on examination. Sensory deficits are seen in 62% to 87% and bowel and/or bladder dysfunction in about 70% of patients.[2]

The constellation of motor and sensory findings indicating Brown-Séquard syndrome is seen in 6% to 22% of patients. About 4% will have evidence of a Horner syndrome. Other patterns that can be seen in individuals with intramedullary tumors include central cord syndrome, conus medullaris syndrome, and cauda equina syndrome.[2,7]

Spinal Instability

Spinal instability is defined as a loss of spinal integrity as a result of a neoplastic process that is associated with movement related pain, symptomatic and progressive deformity, and/or neurologic compromise under a normal physiologic load. Factors considered when evaluating the structural stability of the spinal column include location of the lesion (Table 1), spinal alignment of the involved segment, extent of vertebral body involvement, involvement of posterior elements, bone lesion quality, overall bone mineral density, presence of multilevel contiguous and noncontiguous lesions,

Table 1			
Regions of the spine			
Region	**Segments**	**Articulations**	**Risk for Instability**
Junctional spine	Occiput–C2 C7–T2 T11–L1 L5–S1		Highest risk for instability, subject to translational forces and unique blood supply characteristics
Mobile spine	C3–C6 L2–L4		High risk for instability
Semirigid spine	T3–T10	Articulation with rib cage	Ribs provide biomechanical protection against instability
Rigid spine	S2–S5	Articulation with pelvis	Pelvis provides biomechanical protection against instability

From Fisher CG, DiPaola CP, Ryken TC, et al. A novel classification system for spinal instability in neoplastic disease: an evidence-based approach and expert consensus from the Spine Oncology Study Group. Spine 2010;35(22):E1221–9; with permission.

previous surgical intervention, cancer treatments such as radiation therapy and hormonal manipulation, degenerative changes, and presence of mechanical pain.[8]

Various scoring scales are available to assess spinal stability; the Spine Instability Neoplastic Score (SINS) is the most commonly used (**Table 2**).[9]

DIAGNOSIS

Patients with suspected spine or spinal column involvement require a thorough diagnostic workup, including a history and physical examination. History taking should include inquiries about smoking history, environmental or occupational exposures to carcinogens, travel history, recent screening examinations, and familial cancers.[4]

Physical examination should include an assessment of strength, sensation, reflexes, and sphincter function. The International Standards for Neurological Classification of Spinal Cord Injury can be used as a guide for completing this examination but not to determine prognosis.[9]

Imaging

MRI is considered the gold standard for assessing spinal involvement. MRI's resolution allows for accurate anatomic assessment of the soft tissue structures in the spine, including the intervertebral discs, spinal cord, spinal nerve roots, meninges, spinal musculature, and ligaments. Plain films are a useful screening test to identify lytic or sclerotic lesions, pathologic fractures, spinal deformities, and large masses. Computerized tomography (CT) scans provide highly detailed imaging of the osseous anatomy of the spine and degree of tumor involvement. The addition of myelography allows for assessment of spaces occupied by neural elements and identification of compressed structures. It addition to CT of the spine, patients with suspected metastatic disease should have imaging of the chest, abdomen, and pelvis to establish the extent of disease or identify the primary tumor.[4]

Serologies and Other Tests

Blood cell counts, chemistries, and cancer-specific laboratory testing, such as prostate specific antigen, breast cancer genes 1 and 2, carcinoembryonic antigen, and serum and urine protein electrophoresis, should be examined based on clinical

Table 2
Elements of the Spine Instability Neoplastic Score criteria

Element of SINS	Score
Location	
Junctional spine (occiput–C2, C7–T2, T11–L1, L5–S1)	3
Mobile spine (C3–C6, L2–L4)	2
Semirigid spine (T3–T10)	1
Rigid spine (S2–S5)	0
Pain relief with recumbency and/or pain with movement/loading of the spine	
Yes	3
No (occasional pain but not mechanical)	1
Pain-free lesion	0
Bone lesion	
Lytic	2
Mixed (lytic/blastic)	1
Blastic	0
Radiographic spinal alignment	
Subluxation/translation present	4
De novo deformity (kyphosis/scoliosis)	2
Normal alignment	0
Vertebral body collapse	
>50% collapse	3
<50% collapse	2
No collapse with >50% vertebral body involved	1
None of the above	0
Posterolateral involvement of the spinal elements (facet, pedicle, or costovertebral joint fracture or replacement with tumor)	
Bilateral	3
Unilateral	1
None of the above	0

SINS Score	
Score	
0–6	Stable spine
7–12	"Indeterminate" (possible impending) instability
13–18	Instability

The SINS score is generated by tallying each score from the 6 individual elements.
SINS scores from 7–18 warrant surgical consultation.
From Fisher CG, DiPaola CP, Ryken TC, et al. A novel classification system for spinal instability in neoplastic disease: an evidence-based approach and expert consensus from the Spine Oncology Study Group. Spine 2010;35(22):E1228; with permission.

suspicions.[4] Biopsy of an epidural lesion should be considered in patients without a prior history of cancer, unknown primary, or history of only limited stage or cured malignancy. Lumbar puncture for CSF analysis can be performed on completion of neuraxial imaging in patients with intradural involvement.[3]

ONCOLOGIC MANAGEMENT

Management of spinal tumors varies according to tumor type, treatment history, spinal stability, neurologic status, and pain intensity. Treatment options include surgical intervention, radiation therapy, chemotherapy, and hormonal manipulation.[5] Indications for surgical intervention include paraplegia lasting more than 12 to 24 hours in patients with prior radiation to the spine, spinal instability, and boney compression of the spinal cord. The primary goals for surgical management are to preserve neurologic function, reduce pain, and ensure mechanical stability.[5,10]

Surgical intervention has risks. Potential complications include instrument failure, respiratory complications, deep venous thrombosis, CSF leak, wound infection and/or dehiscence, and worsening of neurologic symptoms from vasogenic edema.[5]

Radiation therapy plays an important role in pain relief, prevention of pathologic fractures, and stabilization of neurologic function. Radiosensitive tumors include myeloma, lymphoma, and solid tumors, such as prostate and breast. Relatively radio-resistant tumors include sarcoma and renal cell carcinoma.[11]

Unfortunately radiation may also cause adverse effects, including gastrointestinal toxicity, mucositis, bone marrow suppression, and radiation-induced myelopathy. Radiation myelopathies, although uncommon, can be seen with radiation treatment of primary spine/spinal cord tumors, prophylactic radiation to prevent metastases, and when the spinal cord is included in radiation such as with colorectal cancers.[3,11]

Radiation myelopathies are generally divided into 4 subtypes, which include acute complete paraplegia/tetraplegia, lower motor neuron disease, acute transient radiation myelopathy, and chronic progressive radiation myelopathy. Acute complete radiation myelopathy is rare and presumed to be related to radiation-induced vascular damage resulting in spinal cord infarction. Lower motor neuron disease is extremely rare and presumed to result from anterior horn cell damage.[3,12]

Acute transient radiation myelopathy (ATRM) is the most common form. ATRM typically occurs 1 to 29 months after completion of radiation therapy and is hypothesized to result from demyelination of the dorsal columns. ATRM is generally associated with cervical spine irradiation but can occasionally be seen in other cord segments. Clinical manifestations include the Lhermitte sign without neurologic changes on examination. Treatment is reassurance as symptoms resolve over weeks to months.[3,12]

Chronic progressive radiation myelopathy (CPRM) occurs 9 to 15 months after radiation therapy. It is the most feared form and has been reported in 1% to 5% of patients who survive 1 year after treatment. CPRM is classically characterized by a latent period during which patients are asymptomatic. Clinical onset is usually painless and insidious. Manifestations include ascending weakness, diminished sensation, and clumsiness. A Brown-Séquard pattern of deficits has also been described. Literature suggests a steady progression of neurologic deficits over the course of weeks to months.[3,10,12]

The Pallis criteria for the diagnosis of CPRM states that the spinal cord must have been included in radiation therapy; the main neurologic deficit must be within the segment of the cord exposed to radiation; and that metastases or other primary cord lesions must be ruled out.[12]

There is no effective treatment. Corticosteroids are often tried with varying results. Anticoagulation and hyperbaric oxygen have occasionally been noted to improve or stabilize symptoms. Bevacizumab has shown benefit anecdotally.[3]

Chemotherapy is considered in the setting of highly chemosensitive tumors, such as lymphomas, neuroblastomas, and germ cell tumors. It can be used as an adjuvant therapy for metastatic disease from breast and prostate cancers and melanoma. Spinal metastases in the setting of breast and prostate cancer are also often sensitive to hormonal manipulation. However, for most patients, chemotherapy plays a limited role largely because of the slow and unpredictable response of the tumor and the urgent need to decompress the spinal cord.[5,11]

Chemotherapy-induced myelopathy is an exceedingly rare complication most associated with chemotherapeutic agents administered directly into the CSF. The exact pathogenesis is unknown; but ascending paresthesias, weakness, and sphincter dysfunction have been reported. The Lhermitte phenomenon has been noted after intravenous administration of and reflects injury to the dorsal root ganglion. This symptom is usually transient, although patients may be left with sensory ataxia after multiple cycles. There is no definitive treatment.[3]

Corticosteroids remain part of the initial treatment of spinal tumors. They reduce tumor and spinal cord vasogenic edema resulting in improvement or at least stabilization of neurologic deficits while definitive treatment is initiated. Corticosteroids also provide analgesia for pain and have direct cytotoxic effects on lymphoma and melanoma.[3]

Significant variability exists with regard to initial dose and tapering schedule. Noted side effects from steroids include hyperglycemia, increased risk of infection, gastrointestinal irritation, mood disturbances, fluid retention, impaired wound healing, and steroid myopathy.[3,5]

Bisphosphonates, which inhibit osteoclast activity and suppress bone reabsorption associated with spinal metastases, have been proven effective in reducing the risk of pathologic fractures, relieving pain, and reducing malignancy-associated hypercalcemia in metastatic breast cancer, multiple myeloma, and other cancers that produce osteolytic metastases.[11]

REHABILITATION

Benefits of rehabilitation in traumatic spinal cord injury are well established. Studies in neoplastic spinal cord injuries have shown similarly positive results and indicate a complementary role to oncologic management for this patient population.[1]

The demographic profiles (**Table 3**), mechanism of injury, and medical comorbidities of neoplastic spinal cord injuries may differ from traumatic injuries; but similar principles of neurorehabilitation can be applied. These principles aim to relieve symptoms, prevent further complications, enhance functional independence, and improve quality of life.[1]

Symptomatic Treatments

Pain is reported to be one of the most common symptoms. Determining the cause of pain is pivotal to management. Several options are available for treatment, including

Table 3
Traumatic versus neoplastic spinal cord injury: patient demographics

	Traumatic SCI	Neoplastic SCI
Sex	M > F	M = F
Age (y)	16–30	50–70
Neurologic level of injury	Tetraplegia = paraplegia	Paraplegia > tetraplegia
Severity	Complete = incomplete	Incomplete > complete

Abbreviations: F, female; M, male; SCI, spinal cord injury.
Adapted from McKinley WO, Huang ME, Brunsvold KT. Neoplastic versus traumatic spinal cord injury: an outcome comparison after inpatient rehabilitation. Arch Phys Med Rehabil 1999; 80(10):1253–7.

postural bracing (for nonsurgical or residual mechanical pain), medications, and modalities.[5]

Postural bracing can be achieved through custom and commercial orthotics and can accommodate all regions of the spine. Care should be taken when evaluating spinal alignment at involved segments with and without brace donned to ensure appropriate correction is achieved, involved segment is included within the brace, and brace is tolerated. The least restrictive brace appropriate for patients should be chosen to achieve stability while preventing further muscle weakness.

Medication management for pain may include steroids, nonsteroidal antiinflammatories, anticonvulsants, tricyclic antidepressants, and opioids.[5] Potential side effects, in the context of an individual's medical and functional status, are a key consideration for use. Physical modalities, including heat, cold, ultrasound, and electrical stimulation, may be incorporated into pain management. Caution must be used with application over areas with sensory loss. Also use caution with modalities that promote increased blood flow, as there is a potential risk of disease spread.[5]

Spasticity, Bowel/Bladder and Sexual Dysfunction

Spasticity is a common complication of upper motor neuron lesions. It may prove to be beneficial for mobility and performance of activities of daily living but may also cause pain and interfere with hygiene and function. Patients should be educated on possible benefits of spasticity and functional use of tone promoted during physical and occupational therapies. Management options for negative symptoms of spasticity include continuous passive stretching exercises, stretching splints, and oral agents, such as baclofen, tizanidine, and benzodiazepines. Intrathecal baclofen and localized treatments, such as phenol and botulinum toxin, can also be considered.

Bladder dysfunction can result in difficulty with urinary drainage and abnormalities in intravesicular pressure, increasing risk for infections, renal disease, skin breakdown, and social embarrassment. Bladder symptoms can range from frequency and urgency to complete urinary retention. A thorough neurologic examination (including sphincter function and reflexes), voiding diary, measurement of postvoid residual volumes, and urodynamic studies can be used to assess an individual's bladder pattern and aid in establishment of a bladder program.

Intermittent catheterization or indwelling catheters can be used for both upper motor neuron (detrusor overactivity with or without sphincter dyssynergia) and lower motor neuron bladder patterns (detrusor hypocontractility or a-contractility). Of note, caution must be taken in individuals with neutropenia or severe thrombocytopenia as they are at risk for infection and bleeding. Anticholinergic agents can be considered in patients with upper motor neuron patterns, whereas cholinergics and manual techniques, such as Credé and double void, can be considered in patients with lower motor neuron patterns. Depending on the severity of injury, pelvic floor physical therapy may be considered for sensory retraining, pelvic muscle/sphincter coordination, and biofeedback.

Bowel dysfunction can result in social inconvenience, embarrassment, and skin compromise. As with the bladder, a thorough neurologic assessment can help establish an individual's bowel pattern. Stool diaries, stool studies, and abdominal imaging may also be helpful. Once a pattern is established, a bowel program can be initiated to allow for control over time and place of bowel movements with desired frequency and without incontinence. Medications, such as stool softeners, oral stimulants, and contact irritants (suppositories), can be initiated for upper motor neuron (hyperreflexic) bowel patterns. Digital stimulation can also be used in place of suppository. Lower motor neuron (hyporeflexic) bowel patterns can be managed with oral bulk forming agents and manual removal of stool. Pelvic floor therapy may be considered for incomplete injuries. Caution is necessary with digital stimulation, suppository use, and manual removal in patients with neutropenia or severe thrombocytopenia.

Sexual dysfunction may be the result of the spinal cord injury, the primary cancer, attendant mood disorders, or side effects of treatment. Management should be based on the underlying cause of dysfunction. Options for sexual dysfunction related to the spinal cord injury include education, oral medications, intracavernous injection therapy, and assistive devices (vacuum device and prosthesis) pending the level of injury.[5]

Preventing Further Complications

Loss of sensation and mobility, bowel and bladder dysfunction, the catabolic state of cancer, and malnutrition can place patients at risk for skin breakdown. Pressure ulcers are preventable, and maintenance of skin integrity is vital. Education should include techniques for pressure relief, skin hygiene, and importance of nutrition.[5] Formal wound care should be initiated if breakdown occurs.

Weakness, extradural tumor involvement, hormonal manipulation, and radiation exposure place patients at risk for spinal instability even after surgical intervention. To minimize the load on the spinal column, spinal precautions should be placed on activities. These precautions may vary based on region of the spine involved but generally include no excessive flexion or extension, twisting movements, or lifting more than 10 lb. The duration of these spinal precautions depends on an individual's disease status and response to oncologic treatment. Use of bracing and physical therapy for core strengthening and postural training may also help to prevent instability.

Enhancing Functional Independence

Determination of neurologic level of injury, severity of injury, oncologic prognosis, and patient/caregiver expectations are essential to establishing realistic rehabilitation goals and determining the appropriate setting for rehabilitation efforts.

Physical and occupational therapy play a large role in these efforts. Based on neurologic and functional status, focus is placed on strengthening exercises, range of motion, sensory reintegration, transfer training, balance, wheelchair mobility, gait training, activities of daily living, and assessment for appropriate assistive devices. If indicated, upper and lower extremity bracing can be used to provide functional positioning, joint stability, compensation for weakness, and proprioceptive feedback.

During the rehabilitation course, it is important to monitor for medical comorbidities related to cancer and its treatment. These comorbidities include fatigue, cytopenias, electrolyte disturbances, vitamin deficiencies, depression, infection, and deep venous thrombosis.[5] They may require supportive care and modification of the rehabilitation care plan.

Improving Quality of Life

Studies have shown that rehabilitation efforts in individuals with malignant spinal cord compression improve function, mood, pain levels, quality of life, and survival. Incomplete injuries with the most neurologic deficits are found to benefit most.[1,5,13]

SUMMARY

As survival rates for individuals with spinal tumors improve, it becomes even more important for clinicians to be aware of the potential long-term neurologic impact of these tumors and their treatments. It is also important for clinicians to understand how to apply rehabilitation principles and practices to this patient population.

REFERENCES

1. Kirshblum S, O'Dell MW, Ho C, et al. Rehabilitation of persons with central nervous system tumors. Cancer 2001;92(4 Suppl):1029–38.
2. Kim DH, Chang UK, Kim SH, et al, editors. Tumors of the spine. Philadelphia: Saunders Elsevier; 2008.
3. Hammack JE. Spinal cord disease in patients with cancer. Continuum (Minneap Minn) 2012;18(2):312–27.
4. Sciubba DM, Gokaslan ZL. Diagnosis and management of metastatic spine disease. Surg Oncol 2006;15(3):141–51.
5. Raj VS, Lofton L. Rehabilitation and treatment of spinal cord tumors. J Spinal Cord Med 2013;36(1):4–11.
6. Clarke JL. Leptomeningeal metastasis from systemic cancer. Continuum (Minneap Minn) 2012;18(2):328–42.
7. Lin W, editor. Spinal cord medicine principles and practice. 2nd edition. New York: Demos; 2010.
8. Fisher CG, DiPaola CP, Ryken TC, et al. A novel classification system for spinal instability in neoplastic disease: an evidence-based approach and expert consensus from the Spine Oncology Study Group. Spine 2010;35(22):E1221–9.
9. Singh Chhabra H, editor. ISCoS textbook on comprehensive management of spinal cord injuries. 1st edition. New Delhi: Wolters Kluwer; 2015.
10. Schiff D. Spinal cord compression. Neurol Clin 2003;21(1):67–86, viii.
11. Sciubba DM, Petteys RJ, Dekutoski MB, et al. Diagnosis and management of metastatic spine disease. A review. J Neurosurg Spine 2010;13(1):94–108.
12. Goldwein JW. Radiation myelopathy: a review. Med Pediatr Oncol 1987;15(2):89–95.
13. Fattal C, Fabbro M, Rouays-Mabit H, et al. Metastatic paraplegia and functional outcomes: perspectives and limitations for rehabilitation care. Part 2. Arch Phys Med Rehabil 2011;92(1):134–45.

Brain Tumors and Metastases

Mary M. Vargo, MD

KEYWORDS

- Cancer rehabilitation • Brain tumor • Brain metastasis

KEY POINTS

- Brain tumors carry a high likelihood of near-term and long-term functional sequelae.
- Although primary brain malignancy comprises just 1.4% of all cancers, the incidence of brain tumor is really higher, considering that metastatic brain tumor is estimated as being at least 10 times more common than primary brain malignancy. Benign brain tumor, with incidence more than double that of malignant primary brain tumor, is also a significant group.
- Primary brain tumors occur along the full age spectrum. In fact, primary brain malignancy is the most common solid tumor in children, and data from that group inform our knowledge of long-term outcomes.
- Brain tumors encompass an extremely wide prognostic spectrum, ranging from benign brain lesions with minimal effect on life expectancy to conditions such as metastatic brain lesions and glioblastoma, which carry unfavorable prognoses.
- Many factors, such as tumor location, oncologic characteristics, and treatment effects, influence outcomes. Radiation therapy in particular has been associated with adverse long-term effects, including late (delayed onset) effects. Corticosteroid myopathy can also be a significant morbidity.

INTRODUCTION

Although malignant primary brain tumor (PBT), estimated at 24,790[1] new cases in the United States in 2016, comprises just 1.4% of all cancers, brain tumor is actually far more common when one considers benign brain tumor, with estimated incidence of more than double that, at 52,880 cases,[1] and metastatic brain tumor, which is yet more common. Estimated prevalence rate of individuals living with history of PBT is nearly 700,000.[1,2] Systematic statistical surveillance is lacking for incidence of brain metastasis, has been estimated at between 200,000 and 300,000 people per year,[2] or at least 10 times more common than primary brain malignancy, with more than

Disclosures: None.
Physical Medicine and Rehabilitation, MetroHealth Medical Center, Case Western Reserve University, 2500 MetroHealth Drive, Cleveland, OH 44109, USA
E-mail address: mvargo@metrohealth.org

Phys Med Rehabil Clin N Am 28 (2017) 115–141
http://dx.doi.org/10.1016/j.pmr.2016.08.005
1047-9651/17/© 2016 Elsevier Inc. All rights reserved.

pmr.theclinics.com

half of patients with metastatic disease presenting with multiple tumors, most commonly in the cerebrum.[3] Brain is the most common site for central nervous system (CNS) malignancy; cranial nerves, spinal cord, and cauda equina account for a collective 10% of tumors, and pituitary and pineal tumors account for 16%.[4]

PBT is seen over the entire age spectrum. Although most common in adults, with median age of 59 at diagnosis,[2] malignant brain tumor is the most common solid tumor of childhood (more than 4600 cases estimated in 2016),[2] and thus, has high representation in pediatric oncology. Seven percent of all primary CNS tumors occur in children ages 0 to 19, and another nearly 9% in young adults ages 20 to 34.[4] Brain metastasis is uncommon in children.[3]

Types of tumor vary over the age spectrum, with pilocytic astrocytomas and embryonal tumors (especially medulloblastoma) most common in childhood, pituitary tumors in late adolescence and young adulthood (ages 15–34), and meningiomas and glioblastomas through the remainder of adulthood.[4]

Prognostically, for malignant PBT, survival varies greatly, especially by type of tumor, including in some cases by their molecular markers, and also by age, with older age being less favorable. Primary malignant brain tumor of childhood averages 74% 5-year survival, but through the full age spectrum averages just 34%, and greater than age 75 averages only 6.1%.[1] Of note, malignant PBT outnumbers benign PBT in childhood (3.3:1.9, per 100,000, ages 0–19), whereas benign PBT is more common than malignant PBT in adults (17.9:8.9 per 100,000).[4] Five-year survival for benign brain tumor is 92%.[1]

Brain tumors have long been recognized as producing a high rate of disabling effects, with recognition that the creation of a "culture of hope"[5] is an important part of management. Rehabilitation needs have historically been described in upwards of 80% of individuals with CNS malignancy,[6] with multiple impairments often present.[7] Long-term effects on employment and general health have consistently been described.[8,9] Rehabilitation emphasizes individualized interdisciplinary care to address the functional impact of tumor and/or treatment-related impairments. Although the rehabilitation therapy itself is similar in approach to other neurologic disorders such as stroke or traumatic brain injury, the underlying context of the oncology-related factors must be incorporated into the clinician's perspective, so that best care and guidance can be provided. Rates of receiving rehabilitation have not been systematically studied but are generally considered to be low.[10,11]

This review follows the general outline of providing (1) a brief summary of relevant background information about brain tumors, (2) evidence for rehabilitation's significant role in the supportive care of patients with brain tumor, and related management considerations, and (3) an outline of survivorship issues. These categories should be viewed as having indistinct boundaries and rather serve as a general conceptual framework to approach patient care needs over the continuum of care.

Primary Treatment

Tumor types including incidence data, standard treatments, and prognostic information are summarized in **Table 1**. MRI with and without contrast is the diagnostic modality of choice for brain tumor.[12]

Surgery
Surgical resection is a mainstay for management of most PBT, and when feasible, for metastatic brain tumors, and has been associated with better outcomes and quality of life.[13] Guiding principles include maximal tumor removal when appropriate,

Table 1
Brain tumor types and clinical information

Tumor Type	% of PBT	Clinical and Structural Correlates	Treatment	Prognosis
Metastatic	Estimated at 10–20× incidence of all PBT; affects 8%–10% of all patients with cancer	Lung, breast, colorectal, melanoma, genitourinary 80% affect cerebral hemispheres; cerebellum 15%, brainstem 5%	Historically, WBRT; solitary brain metastasis sometimes resectable; recent trend to avoid WBRT or combine with more targeted modalities such as stereotactic radiosurgery due to acute and late effects of WBRT Chemotherapy if other modalities have failed, or for chemosensitive tumors	Life expectancy usually <6 mo but death often from other effects of the tumor Graded Prognostic Assessment categorizes patients in 4 groups with median survival ranging 2.6–11 mo Resection associated with improved survival (40 vs 15 wk) and functional outcomes (maintain independence 38 vs 8 wk)
Meningioma	36	Originate in dura	Usually surgically resectable	Usually benign, rarely anaplastic
Gliomas	27 80% of all malignant PBT	Heterogeneous molecular subtypes Headaches, focal signs, such as hemiparesis, cognitive-behavioral changes, visual field or sensory changes Fluctuating symptoms common	See below, subcategories of astrocytoma (glioblastoma, anaplastic astrocytoma, diffuse- and other low-grade astrocytoma and pilocytic astrocytoma), oligodendroglioma, ependymoma; also others (mixed glioma or oligoastrocytoma, optic glioma, gliomatosis cerebri); 75% are astrocytomas	Endothelial growth factor receptor mutations associated with poor prognosis, predispose to glioblastoma Ki-67 associated with reduced survival in anaplastic glioma p53 marker seen in up to 88% of patients with low-grade astrocytomas, unclear effect on survival

(continued on next page)

Table 1
(continued)

Tumor Type	% of PBT	Clinical and Structural Correlates	Treatment	Prognosis
Glioblastoma (grade IV)	15 55% of all gliomas and 82% of malignant gliomas	Usually cerebrum Pseudoprogression (radiographic worsening) may occur after radiation therapy May be primary or evolve secondarily from other gliomas	Surgical resection for relieving mass effect and for cytoreduction Radiation therapy TMZ Carmustine biodegradable polymers implanted into tumor bed Bevacizumab monoclonal antibody targeting angiogenesis	35% 1-y, 4.7% 5-y survival; 2-y 27% with TMZ vs 10% without Bevacizumab increases progression-free survival but not overall survival Tumors with promoter methylation of MGMT show better response to TMZ Isocitrate dehydrogenase genes 1 and 2 associated with better prognosis
Anaplastic astrocytoma (grade III)	2	Usually cerebrum Often progresses to a secondary glioblastoma	Similar to glioblastoma; surgical resection, radiation therapy; TMZ often used	Median survival 2–3 y 60% 1 y; 25.9% 5 y
Diffuse astrocytoma (grade II)	2–3	Usually cerebrum; may progress	Surgical resection; sometimes radiation therapy in adults and older children, especially if incomplete resection	72% 1 y, 47% 5 y
Pilocytic astrocytoma (grade I)	1.5	Often but not necessarily at optic pathways, thalamus, basal ganglia	Surgical resection, sometimes radiation therapy	Best when completely resectable 91% 10 y survival
Oligodendroglioma	2 6% of gliomas	Usually cerebrum Codeletion of 1p/19q chromosomes (19p to 1q translocation) associated with improved response to treatment	Surgical resection Radiation therapy Chemotherapy—procarbazine, lomustine and vincristine; TMZ under investigation	94% 1 y 79% 5 y (if anaplastic type 81%/49%)
Mixed glioma	1	Grade I or II, vary in degree astrocytoma/oligodendroglioma	Surgical resection; sometimes chemotherapy (such as TMZ), or radiation	88% 1-y, 60% 5-y survival

Tumor	Incidence	Clinical Presentation	Treatment	Prognosis
Ependymoma	2	In childhood, 90% involve brain (especially posterior fossa); in adults 60% involve spinal cord	Surgical resection, sometimes radiation or chemotherapy	82% 5-y survival. May be benign or malignant. 10%–15% may spread within CNS
Pituitary	14–15	Endocrine effects, optic pathways	Surgical resection	Usually benign, very rarely malignant
Nerve sheath tumors	8.3	Cranial nerve findings—hearing loss, vertigo, facial palsy, dysphagia, facial numbness; hydrocephalus	Monitoring vs surgical resection	Usually benign, very rarely malignant
Craniopharyngioma	0.9	Embryonic malformations of the sellar area, affect hypothalamus, pituitary (vision, hormonal; growth retardation); Obesity, cognitive deficits; hydrocephalus	Resection but can be difficult, incomplete; radiation sometimes used if incomplete resection. Shunting sometimes needed	Benign; >90% 5- and 10-y survival
Primary CNS lymphoma	2.2	Multifocal presentation common when in association with HIV	Better survival with chemotherapy, ± radiation, than resection	48% 1-y, 28% 5-y survival
Embryonal—medulloblastoma and primitive Neuroectodermal	<2; 18%–20% of childhood CNS tumors	Cognitive deficits, ataxia, facial weakness, endocrine abnormalities; Late cognitive decline may occur	Surgical resection, radiation therapy, chemotherapy	80% long-term survival in medulloblastoma, which is the most common type, and 50% in other types; Overall 82% 1 y, 61% 5 y
Leptomeningeal	5% of patients with cancer	Hematologic, lung, breast, melanoma, gastric	May include supportive care, intrathecal chemotherapy alone or ± systemic chemotherapy or radiation	Median survival 10–12 wk

Abbreviations: HIV, human immunodeficiency virus; MGMT, 06-methylguanine-DNA methyltransferase; WBRT, whole brain radiation therapy; TMZ, temozolamide.

minimization of surgical morbidity, and obtaining accurate diagnosis. When gross total resection is not feasible, other options can include stereotactic biopsy, open biopsy/debulking followed by planned observation or adjuvant therapy, and chemotherapy implants, when indicated.[12] Newer techniques such as functional imaging are increasingly incorporated to minimize morbidity.[13]

Radiation therapy

Radiation approach and dosing vary with the type of tumor. External beam radiation is most commonly used, localized to the tumor via 3-dimensional mapping. For metastatic tumor, whole brain radiation may be used. More specialized radiation therapy techniques have been developed with the goal of improved outcomes and decreased morbidity, including stereotactic radiation with gamma knife, brachytherapy (implanted radiation sources), and proton beam therapy.[13]

Radiation can have significant long-term consequences,[14] either episodic or static, and may factor highly in the differential diagnosis of a decline or lability in a patient's status. Because of correlation between radiation dose to the hippocampus and poor cognitive outcomes, hippocampal-sparing techniques are being explored in pediatric medulloblastoma.[15]

Acute radiation encephalopathy has onset days to weeks after initiation of therapy, corresponding to a time frame in which the patient may be receiving acute rehabilitation. Symptoms include headaches, lethargy, and worsening of existing focal symptoms, and respond to increase in corticosteroid dosing.[16,17]

Decline in status occurring at 1 to 6 months is known as early delayed encephalopathy, producing a somnolence syndrome, which is related to demyelination from radiation injury to oligodendrocytes, and may respond to corticosteroids.

Patients with recent radiation therapy receiving temozolomide therapy may develop a syndrome of "pseudoprogression" on imaging (with or without transient clinical worsening), in which the tumor appears larger or brighter on imaging, seen in about 25% of glioblastoma patients.[16]

Beyond 6 months to a year, late delayed encephalopathy may occur, especially after high doses exceeding 55 to 60 Gy, and typically presenting as a focal necrosis that can be life threatening.[16] Physiologically, vascular endothelial injury occurs, and damage is thought to be related to dynamic interactions between multiple cell types in the brain, including astrocytes, microglia, and neurons, with proinflammatory changes, and eventual neuronal damage related to oxidative stress.[14]

On a more chronic basis, long-term cognitive changes may be seen after radiation. Cognitive sequelae have been well described in survivors of pediatric brain tumor (see Survivorship section)[9] and have also been reported in up to 50% to 90% of adult patients with brain tumor who survive greater than 6 months after radiation.[14]

Areas of investigation into therapeutics with potential to prevent or ameliorate radiation-induced cognitive changes include anti-inflammatory agents, angiotensin-converting enzyme inhibitors, angiotensin type-1 receptor blockers, and stem cell therapies.[14] There have been reports of improvement with other agents, including pentoxyfylline, warfarin, bevacizumab, or vitamin E.[17] Symptomatically, agents such as methylphenidate, modafinil, memantine, and donepezil have been proposed.[17]

Chemotherapy

Temozolamide, the first-line agent for glioblastoma,[18] is generally well tolerated but may produce fatigue, reported to occur in more than 50% of patients, as well as constipation and headache.[19] Other protocols include combination therapy with procarbazine, lomustine and vincristine, bevacizumab (a monoclonal antibody to vascular endothelial growth factor), carmustine (bis-chloroethylnitrosourea), including implanted biodegradable polywafer form, and methotrexate (for CNS lymphoma).[13,20,21]

Novel therapies

Treatments on the horizon include NovoTTF-100A, an electrical field therapy applied via disposable transducers to the scalp, for inhibiting cell growth, and US Food and Drug Administration approved for recurrent glioblastoma. Immunotherapeutic techniques are also under investigation, including various vaccine-based approaches and oncolytic virotherapy.[13,22,23]

Corticosteroids

Corticosteroids are often needed to manage edema, especially dexamethasone, because of its relatively low mineralocorticoid (salt-retaining) activity, with starting does of 16 mg/d or more in the setting of severe symptoms, and 4 to 8 mg/d for milder symptoms.[24] Effects are typically seen within 24 to 48 hours, and taper should proceed as soon as possible, but over at least a 2-week period to avoid rebound symptoms.[24] A recent review notes that despite wide use of corticosteroids in oncology, relatively little research has been performed on optimal dosing.[25] Of note, fluorinated glucocorticoids such as dexamethasone have been implicated as more likely to cause myopathy than nonfluorinated glucocorticoids like prednisone or hydrocortisone; therefore, corticosteroids should be kept to the lowest dose that is needed and with consideration of switching from dexamethasone when feasible.[17] Symptomatic corticosteroid myopathy occurs in about 10% of patients with brain tumor receiving dexamethasone for more than 2 weeks, is most pronounced in proximal muscles of the lower limbs, and is most common in the elderly and when prolonged use of high doses is required.[26] Treatment consists of physical exercise.[27]

Supportive Care

This category contains an extremely wide range of interventions including rehabilitation interventions, management of medical complications, symptom control, psychosocial interventions (including caregiver needs), nutrition, and end-of-life comfort measures. Although thorough coverage of this topic is beyond the scope of this review, a few subtopics will be highlighted.

Acute inpatient rehabilitation

Studies of acute rehabilitation for patients with brain tumor comprise a relatively well developed area of the literature (**Table 2**) and have shown mostly consistent findings, including comparable functional improvement (usually measured by the Functional Independence Measure, or FIM)[28] and discharge to community rates as brain injury or stroke peers, with shorter or similar lengths of stay, and higher rates of discharge back to acute care.[29–41] Recently, improved functional performance was also demonstrated among a small cohort of patients with paraneoplastic cerebellar degeneration.[42] Whether the brain tumor is benign, primary malignant, or metastatic has not been demonstrated to significantly affect acute rehabilitation outcomes, and reports have been conflicting as to whether concurrent radiation therapy is favorable or detrimental to acute rehabilitation outcomes.[30,33]

Table 2
Inpatient rehabilitation outcome studies

Authors	Design	Core Results	Other Findings
Philip et al,[29] 1994	Retrospective study of 30 children ages 3–20 (mean 10) with history of PBT; follow-up data in 20 patients	Increased total WeeFIM score between rehabilitation admission and discharge ($P = .001$) and discharge to follow-up ($P = .0001$); similar pattern in subgroups of self-care, mobility, and locomotion	Significant gains in sphincter control not seen until following discharge ($P = .006$); gains in communication ($P = .01$) and social cognition ($P = .004$) became significant after discharge
O'Dell et al,[30] 1998	Retrospective, case-matched series of 40 patients with brain tumor matched with 40 TBI patients by age, gender, and admission functional status	No significant difference in FIM efficiency between TBI and BT groups (1.9 vs 1.5) or LOS (22.1 vs 17.8 d); greater total FIM increase in TBI patients (34.6 vs 25.4)	Favorable recovery patterns in meningioma, left-sided lesions, and no concurrent radiation therapy
Huang et al,[31] 1998	Retrospective case controlled comparison of 63 BT patients matched with 63 stroke patients by age, gender, and location of lesion	No difference in total FIM gains (23.6 in BT group vs 29.1 in stroke group), FIM efficiency (8.4/wk in BT group vs 7.2/wk in stroke group), or discharge to community rate (86% in BT group vs 94% for stroke group); BT with shorter LOS (25 vs 34 d, $P<.01$)	Higher admission MOB-FIM in BT group (13.6 vs 11.1, $P = .04$); lower gains in ADL-FIM score in BT group (8.3 vs 10.8, $P = .03$)
Huang et al,[32] 2001	Prospective study of 10 consecutively admitted PBT patients, reporting longitudinal data (admission, discharge, 3 mo of FIM, DRS, KPS, and FACT-BR scores, and 1-mo scores of DRS, KPS, and FACT-BR)	At 3- mo postdischarge, FIM increased 46.84 ($P<.05$), KPS 10.11 ($P<.05$), and DRS also improved significantly (F = 19.25, $P<.05$). FACT-BR improvement did not reach significance until 1 and 3 mo; 90% discharged to home; LOS = 19.4 d	The functional measures correlated with each other; QOL did not correlate significantly with functional outcomes KPS less sensitive for measuring disability than DRS or FIM
Marciniak et al,[33] 2001	Retrospective study of 132 patients, divided into 4 categories: 44 (33%) meningioma, 33 (26%) astrocytoma, 21 (16%) metastatic disease, and 33 (25%) miscellaneous PBT diagnoses	No difference in motor or cognitive FIM efficiencies by tumor type; shorter LOS in metastatic disease patients (18 d vs 21–28 d for the other categories, $P = .03$)	Better motor FIM efficiency in patients receiving radiation (1 vs 0.78, $P<.05$) Those with recurrent tumors had smaller FIM motor efficiency than those with initial presentation (0.55 vs 0.98, $P = .018$)

Study	Methods	Outcomes	Findings
Greenberg et al,[34] 2006	Retrospective comparison of patients with PBT/craniotomy due to meningioma (n = 128) or glioma (n = 40), and acute stroke (n = 1660)	Comparable functional gains per FIM points (17.9 for meningioma, 17.2 for glioma, 21.8 for stroke)	Shorter length of stay for BT patients vs stroke patients. Similar discharge to home rates, all >80%
Geler-Kulcu et al,[35] 2009	21 brain tumor (mix of benign and malignant) and 21 stroke patients, matched by side of lesion. Compared FIM, Berg Balance Score, Postural Assessment Scale for Stroke, Motor Assessment Scale	No significant difference between brain tumor and stroke patients nor brain tumor subgroups in any of the outcome measures	
Alam et al,[36] 2008	Retrospective; 188 cancer (and benign neurologic tumor) patients compared with 2801 noncancer patients; includes 72 patients with brain tumor	Patients with brain tumor more likely (25%) than brain rehabilitation controls (12%) to be transferred back to acute care (P = .004); no difference in transfer rate between benign PBT, malignant PBT, or metastatic BT; lower FIM score associated with higher risk of transfer	Infection is most common reason for transfer, compared with cardiopulmonary concerns as most common reason in controls. Only 1 of 14 patients with lung cancer (7%) with brain metastasis requires transfer
Tang et al,[37] 2008	Analysis of 63 patients with brain tumor, nearly all with malignant BT diagnoses, compared by demographic, clinical, and functional variables. GBM 18, Metastatic 25, Other 20	Estimated median survival: metastatic group, 141 d; GBM, 214 d; other, 439 d. GBM: better survival with higher FIM gain (P = .01) or low admission dexamethasone dose (P = .027); metastatic disease: better survival with higher FIM gain (P = .018), low admission dexamethasone dose (P = .012) and absence of organ metastasis (P = .003)	Metastatic disease patients had higher admit FIM score (94) vs 84 for GBM and 71 for Other patients. Metastatic disease patients had shorter LOS (P = .023) at 20 d compared with 28 d for GBM and 37 d for Other patients. No difference in discharge site

(continued on next page)

Table 2
(continued)

Authors	Design	Core Results	Other Findings
Fu et al,[38] 2010	Retrospective study of 21 high-grade and 21 low-grade astrocytoma patients, matched by tumor location, age, gender, and time period	Greater length of stay (13 vs 9 d, $P = .04$) and FIM gains (21.7 vs 13 points, $P = .02$) in the high-grade group; FIM efficiency and home discharge (90%), no difference	
Bartolo et al,[39] 2012	75 brain tumor (meningioma or glioblastoma) and 75 stroke patients, matched for age, gender, side of lesion	All outcomes (FIM, gait scores including Hauser Index, MGHFAC) improved in both groups	Meningioma patients improved more in activities of daily living ($P = .02$) and mobility ($P = .04$) than others
Roberts et al,[40] 2014	Retrospective study of newly diagnosed GBM patients, 100 who received inpatient rehabilitation (KPS 70) and 312 who did not (KPS 80); examined functional status of the rehabilitation patients and survival time of all patients	89 (93.7%) of patients improved Rehabilitation patients survived median 14.3 mo; nonrehabilitation group 17.9 mo ($P = .03$) No significant difference in survival ($P = .12$) when adjusted for age, extent of resection, and KPS	Among the rehabilitation group, age ($P = .0006$), low degree of resection ($P = .02$), and lack of Stupp regimen ($P = .05$) were associated with higher mortality
Asher et al,[41] 2014	Retrospective study of predictive factors for transfers back to acute care among 184 patients with cancer diagnoses, 90 with PBT and 110 coded as having "brain dysfunction"	17.4% transfer rate; neurosurgical complications were most common reason (31%)	Associated factors: Admission motor FIM score 35 or less (OR 4.01; $P<.001$) Presence of feeding tube or modified diet (OR 3.18; $P<.004$)

Abbreviations: BT, brain tumor; DRS, Disability Rating Scale; FACT-BR, functional assessment of cancer therapy–brain; GBM, glioblastoma multiforme; LOS, length of stay; QOL, quality of life; TBI; traumatic brain injury.

Examination of other levels of inpatient rehabilitation care, such as rehabilitation concurrent with acute oncology or neurosurgical care, or rehabilitation at a skilled nursing facility level present a relative gap in the literature. The relative lack of data for other inpatient settings is a significant concern because in order to receive acute rehabilitation, patients need to meet strict regulatory standards,[43] and some patients may be either too mildly affected or too severely affected to receive care at the acute rehabilitation setting. One study of home-based care for 121 malignant patients with brain tumor showed that function as measured by Barthel index improved in 39%, was maintained in 20%, and worsened in 44%; 72% of patients improved in at least one quality-of-life domain.[44] Studies of rehabilitation in the outpatient setting, other than cognitive rehabilitation, have been limited and are summarized in **Table 3**.[45,46]

Cognition

Cognitive function is gaining increasing attention in oncologic disease in general.[47–49] In the setting of brain neoplasm, tumor involvement itself directly affects cognition. In Brinkman's study of cognitive impairment among 224 childhood brain tumor survivors, severe cognitive impairment was seen up to 15 times more frequently than in the general population.[50] Cognitive deficits associated with brain neoplasms tend to be most pronounced in attention, memory, and executive functioning.[51]

After chemotherapy, cognitive changes may relate to effects including elevated levels of cytokines, DNA damage, neurotoxicity-related brain white matter damage, as secondary effects of fatigue or depression, and psychosomatic effects.[47] See the Radiation Therapy section for discussion of radiation effects on brain tissue, which can include both white matter and neuronal damage.

As an aside, no single brief screening tool has been recognized as effective for cancer-associated cognitive dysfunction. This concern is perhaps less pertinent to the specific clinical setting of brain tumor, where cognitive deficits may be severe, than for cancer rehabilitation in general, but is nonetheless applicable here because some patients will be high functioning and virtually all will be at risk. The Mini-Mental Status Exam (MMSE) is considered insufficiently sensitive, and full neuropsychological testing, while sometimes indicated, is too laborious for many clinical situations.[47] The Montreal Cognitive Assessment has been widely used for mild cognitive dysfunction in other clinical settings.[52] Use of computer-based cognitive screening, as sometimes used in mild brain injury[53] and dementia[54] care, has not been reported in cancer populations, including brain tumor. Function-based assessments, such as the Executive Function Performance Test[55] and Complex Task Performance Assessment,[56] hold promise. Patient-reporting tools, such as FACT-Cog or FACT-Brain,[48,57] which have a few cognitive items, may be useful from a cognitive symptom perspective. The European Organization for Research and Treatment of Cancer Quality of Life Questionnaire brain subscale, and the MD Anderson Symptom Inventory Brain Tumor Module, also are of potential utility in identifying or monitoring cognitive symptoms.[58]

Table 4 and **Table 5** describe details of studies to date on cognitive therapy[59–63] and medications[64–68] for patients with brain tumor. In general, trials of cognitive therapy have shown favorable although not always consistent results. In addition to the cognitive case series noted in the tables, there have been other case reports of effective use of cognitive strategies in this population. Based on results of 2 class II studies by Butler and colleagues,[61] Langenbahn and colleagues[51] in a recent evidence-based review have recommended cognitive rehabilitation as a practice guideline for children and adolescents treated for brain neoplasm. Virtual reality data are also emerging, with positive effects found for visual and auditory continuous concentration, short-term memory, and visual motor coordination.[63]

Table 3
Outpatient rehabilitation studies

Authors	Design	Interventions	Outcome Measures	Results
Sherer et al,[45] 1997	Retrospective case series of 13 adult PBT patients after resection, chemotherapy, and radiation therapy; assessed level of independence, vocational outcomes	Individualized outpatient speech and occupational therapy, psychology, and vocational assistance; typical quantity 5 h/d, averaging 2.6-mo duration	Independence Rating Scale, Productivity Status Rating Scale	At discharge from program: Independence improved in 6, unchanged in 6, and worse in 1 Vocational/productivity status maintained or improved in 8, unchanged in 4, and worse in 1 Treatment gains maintained at 8 mo
Khan et al,[46] 2014	Prospective trial of 106 glioma survivors, 53 in treatment group and 53 waitlist controls, allocated based on "clinical need"	Comprehensive individualized multidisciplinary rehabilitation for up to 6–8 wk, including social, psychology, occupational therapy, and physiotherapy	Outcome measure of FIM, secondary outcomes of Depression, Anxiety Distress Scale, Perceived Impact Problem Profile, and Cancer Rehabilitation Evaluation System	Treatment group with improved outcomes at 3 mo in subscales of self-care, sphincter, locomotion, mobility, and communication (all $P<.01$), and psychosocial ($P<.05$) No differences in the secondary outcome measures at 6 mo, between-group differences maintained for sphincter, communication, and cognitive subscales (all $P<.01$)

Table 4
Cognitive studies

Authors	Design	Intervention	Outcome Measures	Core Results
Locke et al,[59] 2008	19 dyads of adult patients with brain tumor and their caregivers (13 dyads completing study)	Six 50-min cognitive therapy sessions over 2 wk incorporating calendar training Six additional 50-min sessions over 2 wk for problem-solving training	Compensation Techniques Questionnaire, Post Study Feedback Questionnaire (intervention group). FACT-brain and Mayo-Portland Adaptability Inventory-4; additional measures of cognitive functioning, quality of life, caregiver burden, mood, and fatigue	Good tolerance; 88% reported using strategies including use of a calendar and specific problem-solving skills; Quality of Life Scores per Functional Assessment of Cancer Therapy-Brain did not differ between subjects and controls, nor did functional status (MPAI scores)
Gehring et al,[60] 2009	140 adult patients with low-grade and anaplastic gliomas, randomized to cognitive therapy or control group	Six weekly sessions, 2 h each, incorporating cognitive training (computer-based), and compensatory strategies	Battery of numerous neuropsychological tests and self-report questionnaires pretreatment and posttreatment and 6 mo later	Therapy group performed better on some neuropsychological measures of attention and verbal memory and reported less mental fatigue at 6 mo but not right after treatment
Butler et al,[61] 2008	108 childhood cancer survivors and 53 randomized waitlist controls, at least 1 y after treatment of CNS cancer; ages 6–17	Intervention: Cognitive therapy, up to 20 two-hour sessions	Pretesting and posttesting of academic achievement, attention, memory, learning strategies, parent/teacher attention ratings, and a self-esteem inventory	Improved academic performance in language and mathematics ($P = .003$); improved parent report of attention in daily activities ($P = .001$); improved learning strategies ($P<.001$); little effect on neurocognitive testing

(continued on next page)

Table 4
(continued)

Authors	Design	Intervention	Outcome Measures	Core Results
Zucchella et al,[62] 2013	58 adult patients with recent neurosurgery for PBT; randomization stratified by side and grade of lesion	16 one-hour cognitive therapy sessions over 4 wk, including computer exercises and metacognitive training	Neuropsychological testing within 3 d of admission to rehabilitation and at 4 wk (both groups received other usual rehabilitation)	Improvement in treatment group in all domains; compared with controls, study group performed better in some tests of attention (TMT-A), memory (RAVLT), and executive function (TMT-B)
Yang et al,[63] 2014	38 adult brain tumor (mixed benign and malignant PBT, and metastatic) patients randomized to VR training or control group	Four week VR training 30-min sessions 3 times a wk, plus computer-based cognitive therapy 30 min 5 d a wk; control group had only the computer-based cognitive training	Computerized neuropsychological tests, Korean Mini-Mental Status Examination (K-MMSE), and Korean version of the Modified Barthel Index (K-MBI)	Both groups showed improved in K-MMSE and K-MBI, in auditory continuous performance, forward digit span, forward visual span, verbal learning, and TMT-A; VR group performed better than controls in visual and auditory continuous performance tests, backward digit span, backward visual span, and TMT-A

Abbreviations: RAVLT, Rey Auditory Verbal Learning Test; TMT-A, Trail Making Test part A (attention); TMT-B, Trail Making Test part B (executive function); VR, virtual reality.

Table 5
Medication studies

Authors	Design	Intervention	Outcome Measures	Core Results
Meyers et al,[64] 1998	30 mostly adult (ages 15–70, mean 40) patients, 29 with malignant glioma	Methylphenidate, dosing levels of 10, 20, and 30 mg twice daily; patients tested at baseline and at each dosing level	Attention (digit span), HVLT, processing speed (digit symbol; TMT-A), COWA, TMT-B, motor speed and dexterity (grooved pegboard); FIM; Beck Depression Inventory; State-Trait Anxiety Inventory	Improved memory, reasoning, verbal fluency, processing speed, executive function, dexterity; lowest dosing sufficient
Thompson et al,[65] 2001	Randomized study of 32 pediatric cancer survivors, ages 6–17, 25 with history of brain tumor	Methylphenidate 0.6 mg/kg (20 mg maximum) vs placebo; testing at baseline and repeated 90 min after ingesting medication or placebo	Connors' Continuous Performance Test (CPT), California Verbal Learning Test, Visual-Auditory Learning Test	Improved sustained attention ($P = .015$) per CPT, improved overall index ($P = .008$); no difference in impulsiveness, reaction times, verbal learning, or visual auditory learning
Mulhern et al,[66] 2004 (extension of Thompson et al)	Double-blind crossover of 83 pediatric malignancy survivors—brain tumor (43) or leukemia (40), ages 6–18	Methylphenidate, in low (0.3 mg/kg, up to 20 mg/d) and moderate dosing (0.6 mg/kg, up to 40 mg/d), 3 wk each; randomized sequence of low dose, higher dose, and placebo	Weekly teacher and parent reports using the Child Behavior Checklist, and parent reports of side effects Side Effect Rating Scales	Improved parent ($P = .004$) and teacher ($P = .004$) ratings of attention; improved teacher ratings of social skills ($P = .001$), problem behaviors ($P = .045$), and academic competence ($P = .001$) No consistent advantage of low vs moderate dosing

(continued on next page)

Table 5
(continued)

Authors	Design	Intervention	Outcome Measures	Core Results
Brown et al,[67] 2013	Randomized trial of 508 adult patients with brain metastases	Memantine to 20 mg per day, vs placebo, for 24 wk, initiated within 3 d of starting whole brain radiation therapy Assessments at baseline, 8, 16, 24, and 52 wk	HVLT-R, TMT-A, (TMT-B), (COWA), and MMSE	Memantine arm with longer time to cognitive decline ($P = .01$); 8 wk ($P = .008$) and 16 wk ($P = .0041$) favorable execution function status; 24 wk favorable processing speed ($P = .0137$) and delayed recognition ($P = .0149$); trend ($P = .059$) for less decline in delayed recall
Rapp et al,[68] 2015	Randomized trial of 198 adult brain tumor survivors 6 mo after partial- or whole-brain irradiation; 66% PBT, 27% metastatic, 8% prophylactic	Donepezil (5 mg for 6 wk, 10 mg for 18 wk) vs placebo; testing at baseline, 12 and 24 wk	HVLT-R, visuomotor skills (modified Rey-Osterrieth complex figure), TMT-A, TMT-B, COWA. Digit Span Test), grooved pegboard; composite score also generated	No difference in composite scores; among subdomains, donepezil group performed better in recognition memory ($P = .027$), discrimination, ($P = .007$), both derived from HVLT-R, and motor speed and dexterity ($P = .016$); improvements greatest in setting of greater baseline cognitive deficits

Abbreviations: COWA, controlled oral word association (verbal fluency); HVLT-R, Hopkins verbal learning test-revised (verbal learning and memory); TMT-A, Trail Making Test part A (attention); TMT-B, Trail Making Test part B (executive function).

Behavioral changes have received less attention than cognitive deficits in the brain tumor literature. Simpson and colleagues,[69] investigating patient, caregiver, and clinical reports of behavioral changes in adult patients with benign or malignant PBT, using the Frontal Systems Behavioral Rating Scale, Emotional and Social Dysfunction Questionnaire, and Overt Behavior Scale, found highest reported rates of behavioral changes in individuals with seizure disorder, and lack of correlation with tumor grade, treatment modality, or depressed mood. Although "moderate agreement" was reported between patients and caregivers, caregiver reporting was generally higher (worse) and in good agreement with clinician ratings. Among patients, executive impairments were most frequently reported (51%) followed by apathy (40.5%), and anger and verbal aggression (both 27%). Among caregivers, highest reports were for apathy (59.5%), indifference (36.1%), and executive impairments (35.1%). Poggi and colleagues,[70] comparing childhood brain tumor and brain injury survivors ages 8 to 15 years, reported that in general traumatic brain injury patients were more likely to externalize problems, whereas social adjustment problems in brain tumor survivors appeared associated with internalizing problems.

Patient and caregiver psychological and supportive care needs

The supportive care needs of patients with brain tumor, especially those with high-grade malignancy, are well documented.[10,71–73] Areas that have received attention include communication and informational strategies, management of psychological stress, anxiety, and depression, caregiver needs and well-being, end-of-life supports, complementary therapies (homeopathy, vitamin or herbal supplements, meditation, and massage), sexuality, and models of care for providing a "helping system" for patients and caregivers.[71] Langbecker and Yates[10] found the highest degree of self-reported unmet supportive care needs in recently diagnosed (mean 3 months) PBT patients in the areas of physical (47.9%) and psychological (45.8%) needs, followed by health system/information needs (37.9%) and sexuality needs (34.8%).

COMMUNICATION

Communication with patients and families about brain tumor can be challenging in rehabilitation environments, because questions often arise about the tumor, including treatment and prognostic considerations, for which the primary management is typically within the domains of the neurosurgeon, medical oncologist, and/or radiation oncologist. Anecdotally, physiatrists and other rehabilitation staff may experience reluctance to discuss brain tumor treatment and prognostic issues with patients, for reasons that potentially include lack of training, lack of sufficient information about the case (ie, biopsy results not yet available, formal oncology treatment plan not yet established), concern about giving misleading information based on limited depth of medical knowledge in neuro-oncology care, and generally wishing to be circumspect within usual scope and bounds of specialty practice. In addition, the brain tumor supportive care literature shows that patients can vary in the extent of information they wish to receive,[5,74] raising further questions about how much information to convey.

Although these concerns are understandable and often appropriate, the rehabilitation setting also presents an opportunity for patients to have productive discussions with staff that are experienced in treating life-altering health issues, amid a culture of hope, support, and self-efficacy. It may be during rehabilitation that the patient becomes ready, from cognitive and/or emotional standpoints, to absorb more complex or difficult information. There are no formal guidelines on how physiatrists and other rehabilitation staff should handle communication about oncologic disease. Nonetheless, the rehabilitation physician is in a good position to use individual experience and judgment to move the patient's care and understanding forward, in therapeutic alliance with neuro-oncology staff.

Regarding patients' desire to be told information, one study found about half of the patients want all possible information, and the remainder want just "important" or "critical" information.[74] However, anxiety tends to be lower in patients who receive and understand information fully,[74] and in general, studies have shown patient dissatisfaction with communication and information provision.[71] Medical decision-making capacity must also be considered, and more systematic evaluation of cognitive status has been advocated.[71] Honesty and transparency must be balanced with compassion and maintaining a culture of hope.[5]

DEPRESSION AND ANXIETY

In the setting of malignant brain tumor, anxiety (30%–48%) and depression (5%–47%) are common and have been associated with poor quality of life.[71] Poor functional status, as measured by the Karnofsky score, has been associated with depression, and presence of preoperative depression has also been associated with decreased survival in a retrospective study of astrocytoma patients.[71,75]

Rooney and colleagues[76] note that differential diagnosis may include adjustment disorder, hypoactive delirium, cognitive impairment, and organic personality change, and that distinguishing between these entities may not be straightforward. Because the Beck Depression Inventory includes somatic items, concern has been expressed of potential to inflate depression diagnosis, with use of the Hospital Anxiety and Depression Scale proposed as being more accurate.[77] Higher rates of diagnosis are found with rating scales compared with clinical interviews.[77] Caregivers may report more depressive symptoms than patients and be more reliable in the reporting of observational behavioral symptoms.[76]

Mainio and colleagues,[75] using the Beck Depression Inventory in 77 patients with brain tumor preoperatively, found evidence of depression in 35% of patients, with associated factors of lower physical performance (Karnofsky Performance Scale [KPS] ≤ 70) and history of depression, with lower functional status continuing to be a risk factor at 3 months and 1 year.[75] Different brain tumor histologies or tumor grades have shown no consistent association with depression, nor has extent of resection, or treatment with radiation therapy or chemotherapy. Longitudinal studies suggest that patients' depression levels do change over time, but the direction of change is inconsistent.[77]

Often psychosocial interventions have been studied combined with other treatment approaches such as cognitive therapy and physical and/or relaxation exercises, limiting the ability to know which components are showing effect.[78] Improvements in depressive symptoms and quality of life have been found, but with inconsistent findings at follow-up a period of months later. Confounding factors that have been cited include disease progression, ongoing radiation therapy at time of follow-up, and access of control subjects to community supports. Kangas[78] has advocated that targeting studies toward individuals with higher distress levels may improve capacity to identify effects of treatment. Also, the psychological therapy approach traditionally emphasizes cognitive behavioral therapy, and integration of acceptance-based therapy has been proposed.

There is also a lack of data on evidence for antidepressant medication in the setting of malignant brain tumor. Bupropion and clomipramine should be avoided because of their effect of lowering the seizure threshold.[76,79] On the other hand, preclinical data exist showing that some antidepressant medications, especially serotonin reuptake inhibitors and tricyclic antidepressants, induce glioma cell death by apoptosis in cell cultures, resulting in a possible chemotherapeutic effect and survival advantage. Limited data in humans to date have given conflicting results.[76] Adequate psychosocial support as well as pharmacotherapy should be provided in appropriate patients.[26]

STRESS MANAGEMENT

Although better defined models are needed to assist patients and caregivers in dealing with stress, effectiveness of specialist nurse support has been reported.[71–73] Need for more team-based care, and better availability of psychologists or counselors, and of community supports, has been advocated.[71] Monthly telephone follow-up visits in lieu of face-to-face appointments have also been well received by patients.[80]

Organizations available to patients with brain tumor and their families include the International Brain Tumor Alliance (theibta.org), which is a global network for patient with brain tumor organizations, the National Brain Tumor Foundation (http://www.braintumor.org), the American Brain Tumor Association (http://www.abta.org), and the Children's Brain Tumor Foundation (http://www.cbtf.org).

Seizure Prophylaxis

Routine seizure prophylaxis is not recommended, although antiepileptic agents should be given when seizure has occurred, per American Association of Neurology guidelines,[81] due to multiple studies finding lack of benefit, including a recent randomized trial of perioperative anticonvulsant prophylaxis in patients undergoing brain tumor resection.[82] Enzyme-inducing medications (carbamazepine, phenytoin, phenobarbital) should be avoided due to potential for interaction with chemotherapy agents.[12,24] Phenytoin has also be associated, rarely, with risk of erythema multiforme (Steven-Johnson syndrome) in patients receiving intracranial radiation therapy.[24] Levetiracetam and other agents (topiramate, lamotrigine, valproic acid, lacosamide) are most widely used.[12]

Fatigue and Sleep

An estimated 40% to 70% of patients with brain tumor have fatigue throughout the illness trajectory, and greater than 80% of patients experience fatigue during radiation therapy, becoming worse with cumulative treatment and often persisting after radiation. Other contributing causes include underlying metabolic problems, deconditioning, depression and anxiety, or medication effects.[83] Inflammatory pathways may be involved with fatigue and sleep disturbance (See Lynn H. Gerber's article, "Cancer Related Fatigue: Persistent, Pervasive and Problematic," in this issue). In the case of brain radiation specifically, neuroinflammation has been proposed as the mechanism. Also, melatonin production can be affected, resulting in dysregulation of the "metabolic clock."[83] Management of fatigue and sleep has received limited study in brain tumor specifically, such that management is derived from other settings, such as the broader group of cancer or brain injury patients. In general, management involves evaluation for metabolic and psychiatric causes, addressing pain, adjusting medications, establishing appropriate sleep hygiene, adequate nutrition, incorporating energy conservation techniques and physical exercise, and psychosocial interventions, including cognitive-behavioral therapy for sleep.[83] From a medication standpoint, there are limited data supporting methylphenidate and modafinil for fatigue, and data for sleep medications are lacking in the brain tumor population.[83]

Headaches

Headaches have been reported in 50% to 75% of patients with brain tumor and are thought to be due to local traction on pain-sensitive structures such as arteries, veins, venous sinuses, cranial nerves, and portions of the dura.[84] Headaches might be suspected as due to brain tumor when presenting in individuals over the age of 50, with recent onset over days or months, change in headache pattern, awakening patient from sleep even when mild, exhibiting increasing intensity or frequency, consistently localized to one side, with focal symptoms, cognitive or behavioral changes, nausea and vomiting, and sometimes papilledema.[12] Emergent attention including head computed tomography is recommended for sudden severe headache, significant neurologic deterioration, status epilepticus, or repeated seizures.[12]

From a symptom-control standpoint, the main unique concern is assurance that the brain lesion has been optimally addressed. Especially in the settings of metastatic disease or radiation encephalopathy, corticosteroids may be needed. Analgesics will be needed after craniotomy, although there may be a period of time in which nonsteroidal anti-inflammatory medications are not recommended.[85] Otherwise, management is fairly empiric and can be approached in a way similar to posttraumatic headaches, matching medication to symptom pattern (ie, muscle tension, migraine, neuritic), other elements of the patient's condition (such as sleep disturbance, nausea, fatigue, and cognitive, mood or behavioral status), and frequency and timing considerations.[86,87]

Anticoagulation

Risk factors for thromboembolic disease include malignancy, immobility, as well as effects of some therapeutic agents, particularly bevacizumab.[12] Patients should be treated prophylactically during hospitalization.[12] Brain tumor does not preclude anticoagulation.[88] Inferior vena cava filters are associated with high complication rates and lack of survival advantage.[88] In the setting of recent surgery or bleeding,[88] low-molecular-weight heparin is the treatment of choice.[12] Based on PRODIGE trial findings, prophylactic anticoagulation is not routinely recommended for glioma patients in the ambulatory setting.[89]

Survivorship

For the brain tumor population, much knowledge of long-term sequelae comes from the Childhood Cancer Survivor Study database.[9] This database has provided a relatively rich picture of the long-term issues in brain tumor survivors; however, it is not entirely clear to what extent this information can be extrapolated to individuals with adult onset brain tumor, which, as already reviewed, tends to exhibit different characteristics. In addition, except perhaps for cognition, there has been little research into how to ameliorate these long-term challenges.

Cognitive outcomes Among adult survivors of childhood brain tumor, those having received targeted radiation are less likely to exhibit severe cognitive deficits than those that underwent more widespread (craniospinal) radiation.[50] History of seizures and hydrocephalus have also been found to be risk factors for adverse cognitive outcomes, including lower educational attainment, unemployment, and nonindependent living. Even those childhood brain tumor survivors with no history of cranial radiation exhibit increased frequency of memory deficits and of impaired cognitive flexibility compared with population norms. Although organization problems and emotional dysregulation are less common than other issues, they are more commonly seen in association with high-radiation therapy doses.[9]

Psychological outcomes Psychological data are more limited than cognitive; however, childhood survivor data indicate higher levels of psychological distress in brain tumor survivors, including depression and somatization, and lower expectations of future life satisfaction, than comparison groups.[90]

Vocational outcomes Adults survivors of brain and other CNS malignancies are less likely to be working than other cancer survivor groups (odds ratio [OR] 2.2), per analysis of 1433 cancer survivors 1 to 5 years after diagnosis.[8] When used, survivors of childhood brain tumor are less likely to be working in professional occupations than other cancer survivors.[91] Exposure of the temporal or frontal lobe to 50 Gy or more has been independently and statistically significantly associated with higher risk of unemployment (relative risk [RR] = 1.7) compared with siblings.[9] Besides history of radiation therapy, other risk factors for unemployment among childhood brain tumor survivors include younger age at diagnosis, female gender, lower intelligence quotient, motor impairment, and epilepsy.[92]

However, many brain tumor survivors are working, even those with less favorable disease. In one study, two-thirds of working-age glioma patients judged to be experiencing "time of everyday life" (vs "time of disease," in which life continuity was lost) were able to resume work at least on a part-time basis.[93] Factors associated with work limitations included depressive symptoms, fatigue, cognitive limitations, sleep changes, and a negative problem-solving orientation, issues which can be potentially addressed.[94]

Community integration Brinkman and colleagues[50] found brain tumor survivors tend to underreport deficits, compared with extent of cognitive deficits seen on formal testing. It is unclear whether such a response pattern relates to lack of insight into deficits, or to adaptation, such that "survivors may learn to compensate for their deficits or to avoid situations that require specific skills, thereby reducing the potential impact on daily activities." In the same study, only 27% of childhood brain tumor survivors that had received craniospinal radiation therapy were living independently, compared with 52% of those not treated with radiation.[50] One study examining life satisfaction in young adult survivors of childhood CNS tumors found that community integration, measured by the Community Integration Questionnaire, was an even stronger predictor of life satisfaction than employment.[95] This data suggest that a productive avenue for better quality of life lies not just in improving deficits but in optimizing community resources and the environment of daily living.

Physical performance and fitness A review by Ness and colleagues[96] of long-term physical performance among the Childhood Cancer Survivors Study cohort data described that childhood brain cancer survivors reported significant physical performance limitations, with OR of 4.1, compared with those who had leukemia (exceeded only by bone cancer survivors at OR 6.4). Brain tumor survivors have exhibited the highest prevalence of physical performance limitations (36.9%), followed by bone tumor survivors (26.6%).

Relatively little research has been conducted into the long-term fitness and exercise behaviors of brain tumor survivors specifically. However, numerous studies examining cancer survivors in general have indicated beneficial health outcomes,[97–99] as has research in individuals with brain disorders ranging from concussion to dementia.[100–102] Given this convergence of data from 2 relevant larger populations, brain tumor survivors may be in a particularly strong position for physical fitness to make a difference for them. Long-term survivors of childhood brain tumor have been found to be at risk for obesity, especially in the setting of younger age at diagnosis, radiation dosimetry to the hypothalamus, any endocrinopathy, extent of surgery, and highest risk with craniopharyngioma diagnosis.[103] Reduced cardiopulmonary fitness has been reported in survivors of childhood posterior fossa tumors.[104]

Ruden and colleagues[105] found exercise behaviors to be an independent predictor of survival in recurrent gliomas. Jones and colleagues[106] surveyed adult patients with brain tumor, consisting predominantly of anaplastic glioma or glioblastoma patients, finding that they were most open to exercise after completion of treatment (84% vs 47%), and that walking was the preferred form of exercise both during and after treatment. Recently, decreased risk of brain tumor mortality has been reported in association with increased energy expenditure in running and walking, as found in data from the National Runners' and Walkers' Health Studies.[107]

Because many patients with brain malignancy have received treatment with corticosteroids, physical activity is particularly important. As noted previously, exercise is the main therapy for corticosteroid myopathy.[26]

SUMMARY

The supportive care needs of patients with brain tumor, and long-term disabling effects, are high. Patients with brain tumor exhibit wide-ranging prognoses and functional implications of their disease and treatments, which must be incorporated into the rehabilitation approach. Regarding models of care, favorable data exist for acute inpatient rehabilitation and for outpatient cognitive rehabilitation (although challenges remain), both often conducted within conventional brain rehabilitation settings. Home-based rehabilitation has received limited attention, and skilled nursing facility–based care has received virtually no attention. Specialist nurses have been reported to play an important role in neuro-oncology settings, providing education as needs arise, and facilitating communication between patient or caregiver, and health care providers. Additional data are needed particularly with regard to optimizing physical activity, overall functional performance, symptom control, community integration, and employment status for those with long-term disability. Childhood-onset cancers and glioblastoma are relatively better studied than other tumor types, including metastatic brain disease.

REFERENCES

1. CBTRUS-2015 CBTRUS fact sheet. Available at: http://www.cbtrus.org/factsheet/factsheet.html. Accessed May 2, 2016.
2. American Brain Tumor Association. Brain tumor statistics. Available at: http://www.abta.org/about-us/news/brain-tumor-statistics. Accessed May 2, 2016.
3. Metastatic Brain Tumors-American Brain Tumor Association. Available at: http://www.abta.org/secure/metastatic-brain-tumor.pdf. Accessed May 2, 2016.
4. Dolecek TA, Propp JM, Stroup NE, et al. CBTRUS statistical report: primary brain and central nervous system tumors diagnosed in the United States 2005-2009. Neuro Oncol 2012;14:v1–49.
5. Salander P, Bergenheim T, Henriksson R. The creation of protection and hope in patients with malignant brain tumours. Soc Sci Med 1996;42(7):985–96.
6. Lehmann J, DeLisa JA, Warren CG, et al. Cancer rehabilitation: assessment of need, development, and education of a model of care. Arch Phys Med Rehabil 1978;59:410–9.
7. Mukand JA, Blackinton DD, Crincolli MG, et al. Incidence of neurologic deficits and rehabilitation of patients with brain tumors. Am J Phys Med Rehabil 2001; 80:346–50.

8. Short PF, Vasey JJ, Tunceli K. Employment pathways in a large cohort of adult cancer survivors. Cancer 2005;103:1292–301.

9. Armstrong GT, Liu Qi, Yasui Y, et al. Long-term outcomes among adult survivors of childhood central nervous system malignancies in the childhood cancer survivor study. J Natl Cancer Inst 2009;101(13):946–58.

10. Langbecker D, Yates P. Primary brain tumor patients' supportive care needs and multidisciplinary rehabilitation, community and psychosocial support services: awareness, referral and utilization. J Neurooncol 2016;127:91–102.

11. McCartney A, Butler C, Acreman S. Exploring access to rehabilitation services from allied health professionals for patients with primary high-grade brain tumours. Palliat Med 2011;25(8):788–96.

12. Omuro A, DeAngelis LM. Glioblastoma and other malignant gliomas: a clinical review. JAMA 2013;310(17):1842–50.

13. Sharpar S, Mhatre PV, Huang ME. Update on brain tumors: new developments in neuro-oncologic diagnosis and treatment, and impact on rehabilitation strategies. PM R 2016;8:678–89.

14. Greene-Schloesser D, Robbins ME, Peiffer AM, et al. Radiation-induced brain injury: a review. Front Oncol 2012;2:1–18.

15. Brodin NP, Rosenschöld PM, Blomstrand M, et al. Hippocampal sparing radiotherapy for pediatric medulloblastoma: impact of treatment margins and treatment technique. Neuro Oncol 2014;16(4):594–602.

16. Dropcho EJ. Neurotoxicity of radiation therapy. Neurol Clin 2010;28:217–34.

17. Lu Lee EL, Westcarth L. Neurotoxicity associated with cancer therapy. J Adv Pract Oncol 2012;3:11–21.

18. Stupp R, Mason WP, van den Bent MJ, et al, European Organisation For Research And Treatment Of Cancer Brain Tumor And Radiotherapy Groups, National Cancer Institute of Canada Clinical Trials Group. Radiotherapy plus concomitant and adjuvant temozolomide for glioblastoma. N Engl J Med 2005;352(10):987–96.

19. Thomas RP, Recht L, Nagpal S. Advances in the management of glioblastoma: the role of temozolomide and MGMT testing. Clin Pharmacol 2013;5:1–9.

20. Chinot OL, Wick W, Mason W, et al. Bevacizumab plus radiotherapy—temozolomide for newly diagnosed glioblastoma. N Engl J Med 2014;370:709–22.

21. Gilbert MR, Dignam JJ, Armstrong TS, et al. A randomized trial of bevacizumab for newly diagnosed glioblastoma. N Engl J Med 2014;370:699–708.

22. Xu L, Chow KH, Lim M, et al. Current vaccine trials in glioblastoma: a review. J Immunol Res 2014;2014:796856. Available at: http://www.hindawi.com/journals/jir/2014/796856/.

23. Wollmann G, Ozduman K, van den Pol A. Oncolytic virus therapy for glioblastoma multiforme: concepts and candidates. Cancer J 2012;18:69–81.

24. Brastianos PK, Curry WT, Oh KS. Clinical discussion and review of the management of brain metastases. J Natl Compr Canc Netw 2013;11(9):1153–64.

25. Dietrich J, Rao K, Pastorino S, et al. Corticosteroids in brain cancer patients: benefits and pitfalls. Expert Rev Clin Pharmacol 2011;4(2):233–42.

26. Wen P, Schiff D, Kesari S, et al. Medical management of patients with brain tumors. J Neurooncol 2006;80:313–32.

27. Czerwinski SM, Kurowski TG, O'Neill TM, et al. Initiating regular exercise protects against muscle atrophy from glucocorticoids. J Appl Physiol (1985) 1987;63:1504–10.

28. Kidd D, Stewart G, Baldry J, et al. The functional independence measure: a comparative validity and reliability study. Disabil Rehabil 1995;17:10–4.

29. Philip PA, Ayyangar R, Vanderbilt J, et al. Rehabilitation outcome in children after treatment of primary brain tumor. Arch Phys Med Rehabil 1994;75:36–9.
30. O'Dell MW, Barr K, Spanier D, et al. Functional outcome of inpatient rehabilitation in persons with brain tumors. Arch Phys Med Rehabil 1998;79:1530–4.
31. Huang ME, Cifu DX, Keyser-Marcus L. Functional outcome after brain tumor and acute stroke: a comparative analysis. Arch Phys Med Rehabil 1998;79:1386–90.
32. Huang ME, Wartella JE, Kreutzer JS. Functional outcomes and quality of life in patients with brain tumors: a preliminary report. Arch Phys Med Rehabil 2001; 82:1540–6.
33. Marciniak CM, Sliwa JA, Heinemann AW, et al. Functional outcomes of persons with brain tumors after inpatient rehabilitation. Arch Phys Med Rehabil 2001;82: 457–63.
34. Greenberg E, Treger I, Ring H. Rehabilitation outcomes in patients with brain tumors and acute stroke: comparative study of inpatient rehabilitation. Am J Phys Med Rehabil 2006;85:568–73.
35. Geler-Kulcu D, Gulsen G, Buyukbaba E, et al. Functional recovery of patients with brain tumor or acute stroke after rehabilitation: a comparative study. J Clin Neurosci 2009;16:74–8.
36. Alam E, Wilson RD, Vargo M. Inpatient cancer rehabilitation: a retrospective comparison of transfer back to acute care between patients with neoplasm and other rehabilitation patients. Arch Phys Med Rehabil 2008;89(7):1284–9.
37. Tang V, Rathbone M, Park Dorsay JP, et al. Rehabilitation in primary and metastatic brain tumours. Impact of functional outcomes on survival. J Neurol 2008; 255:820–7.
38. Fu JB, Parsons HA, Shin KY, et al. Comparison of functional outcomes in low- and high-grade astrocytoma rehabilitation inpatients. Am J Phys Med Rehabil 2010;89(3):205–12.
39. Bartolo M, Zucchella C, Pace A, et al. Early rehabilitation after surgery improves functional outcome in inpatients with brain tumours. J Neurooncol 2012;107: 537–44.
40. Roberts PS, Nuño M, Sherman D, et al. The impact of inpatient rehabilitation on function and survival of newly diagnosed patients with glioblastoma. PM R 2014; 6:514–21.
41. Asher A, Roberts P, Bresee C, et al. Transferring inpatient rehabilitation facility cancer patients back to acute care (TRIPBAC). PM R 2014;6:808–13.
42. Fu JB, Raj VS, Asher A, et al. Inpatient rehabilitation performance of patients with paraneoplastic cerebellar degeneration. Arch Phys Med Rehabil 2014;95:2496–9.
43. Inpatient rehabilitation facility prospective payment system, 2013. Available at: https://www.cms.gov/Outreach-and-Education/Medicare-Learning-Network-MLN/MLNMattersArticles/Downloads/MM6699.pdf.
44. Pace A, Parisi C, De Lelio M, et al. Home rehabilitation for brain tumor patients. J Exp Clin Cancer Res 2007;26(3):297–300.
45. Sherer M, Meyers CA, Bergloff P. Efficacy of postacute brain injury rehabilitation for patients with primary malignant brain tumors. Cancer 1997;80(2):250–7.
46. Khan F, Amatya B, Drummond K, et al. Effectiveness of integrated multidisciplinary rehabilitation in primary brain cancer survivors in an Australian community cohort: a controlled clinical trial. J Rehabil Med 2014;46:754–60.
47. Denlinger CS, Ligibel JA, Are M, et al. Survivorship: cognitive function, version 1.2014. J Natl Compr Canc Netw 2014;12(7):976–86.
48. Cherrier MM, Anderson K, David D, et al. A randomized trial of cognitive rehabilitation in cancer survivors. Life Sci 2013;93(17):617–22.

49. Asher A. Cognitive dysfunction among cancer survivors. Am J Phys Med Rehabil 2011;90(5 Suppl):S16–26.
50. Brinkman TM, Krasin MJ, Liu W, et al. Long-term neurocognitive functioning and social attainment in adult survivors of pediatric CNS tumors: results from the ST Jude Lifetime Cohort Study. J Clin Oncol 2016;34:1358–67.
51. Langenbahn DM, Ashman T, Cantor J, et al. An evidence-based review of cognitive rehabilitation in medical conditions affecting cognitive function. Arch Phys Med Rehabil 2013;94:271–86.
52. Nasreddine ZS, Phillips NA, Bedirian V, et al. The Montreal Cognitive Assessment, MoCA: a brief screening tool for mild cognitive impairment. J Am Geriatr Soc 2005;53(4):695–9.
53. Meehan WP, d'Hemecourt P, Collins CL, et al. Computerized neurocognitive testing for the management of sport-related concussions. Pediatrics 2012;129:38–44.
54. Saxton J, Morrow L, Eschman A, et al. Computer assessment of mild cognitive impairment. Postgrad Med 2009;121(2):177–85.
55. Baum CM, Connor LT, Morrison T, et al. Reliability, validity, and clinical utility of the executive function performance test: a measure of executive function in a sample of people with stroke. Am J Occup Ther 2008;62(4):446–55.
56. Wolf T, Morrison T, Matheson L. Initial development of a work-related assessment of dysexecutive syndrome: the Complex Task Performance Assessment. Work 2008;31(2):221–8.
57. Weitzner MA, Meyers CA, Gelke CK, et al. The Functional Assessment of Cancer Therapy (FACT) scale: development of a brain subscale and revalidation of the general version (FACT-G) in patients with primary brain tumors. Cancer 1995; 75(5):1151–61.
58. Taphoorn MJ, Sizoo EM, Bottomley A. Review on quality of life issues in patients with primary brain tumors. Oncologist 2010;15:618–26.
59. Locke DE, Cerhan JH, Wenting W, et al. Cognitive rehabilitation and problem-solving to improve quality of life of patients with primary brain tumors: a pilot study. J Support Oncol 2008;6(8):383–91.
60. Gehring K, Sitskoorn MM, Gundy CM. Cognitive rehabilitation in patients with gliomas: a randomized, controlled trial. J Clin Oncol 2009;27:3712–22.
61. Butler RW, Sahler OJ, Askins MA, et al. Interventions to improve neuropsychological functioning in childhood cancer survivors. Dev Disabil Res Rev 2008;14:251–8.
62. Zucchella C, Capone A, Codella V, et al. Cognitive rehabilitation for early post-surgery inpatients affected by primary brain tumor: a randomized, controlled trial. J Neurooncol 2013;114(1):93–100.
63. Yang S, Chun MH, Son YR. Effect of virtual reality on cognitive dysfunction in patients with brain tumor. Ann Rehabil Med 2014;38(6):726–33.
64. Meyers CA, Weitzner MA, Valentine AD, et al. Methylphenidate therapy improves cognition, mood, and function of brain tumor patients. J Clin Oncol 1998;16:2522–7.
65. Thompson SJ, Leigh L, Christensen R, et al. Immediate neurocognitive effects of methylphenidate on learning impaired survivors of childhood cancer. J Clin Oncol 2001;19:1802–8.
66. Mulhern RK, Khan RB, Kaplan S, et al. Short term efficacy of methylphenidate: a randomized, double-blind, placebo controlled trial among survivors of childhood cancer. J Clin Oncol 2004;22:4795–803.
67. Brown PD, Pugh S, Laack NN, et al. Memantine for the prevention of cognitive dysfunction in patients receiving whole-brain radiotherapy: a randomized, double-blind, placebo-controlled trial. Neuro Oncol 2013;15(10):1429–37.

68. Rapp SR, Case LD, Peiffer A, et al. Donepezil for irradiated brain tumor survivors: a phase III randomized placebo-controlled clinical trial. J Clin Oncol 2015;33(15):1653–9.
69. Simpson GK, Koh E-S, Whiting D, et al. Frequency, clinical correlates and rating of behavioral changes in primary brain tumor patients: a preliminary investigation. Front Oncol 2015;5:1–9 (article 78).
70. Poggi G, Liscio M, Adduci A, et al. Psychological and adjustment problems due to acquired brain lesion in childhood: a comparison between post-traumatic patients and brain tumor survivors. Brain Inj 2005;19:777–85.
71. Ford E, Catt S, Chalmers A, et al. Systematic review of supportive care needs in patients with primary malignant brain tumors. Neuro Oncol 2012;14:392–404.
72. Piil K, Juhler M, Jakobsen J, et al. Controlled rehabilitative and supportive care intervention trials in patients with high-grade gliomas and their caregivers: a systematic review. BMJ Support Palliat Care 2016;6:27–34.
73. Vargo M, Henriksson R, Salander P. Rehabilitation of patients with glioma. Handb Clin Neurol 2016;134:287–304.
74. Diaz JL, Barreto P, Gallego JM, et al. Proper information during the surgical decision-making process lowers the anxiety of patients with high grade gliomas. Acta Neurochir (Wien) 2009;151(4):357–62.
75. Mainio A, Hakko H, Niemela A, et al. Depression and functional outcome in patients with brain tumors: a population-based 1 year follow-up study. J Neurosurg 2005;103(5):841–7.
76. Rooney AG, Brown PD, Reijneveld JC, et al. Depression in glioma: a primer for clinicians and researchers. J Neurol Neurosurg psychiatry 2014;85:230–5.
77. Rooney AG, Carson A, Grant R. Depression in cerebral glioma patients: a systematic review of observational studies. J Natl Cancer Inst 2011;103:61–76.
78. Kangas M. Psychotherapy interventions for managing anxiety and depressive symptoms in adult brain tumor patients: a scoping review. Front Oncol 2015; 5:1–9 (article 116).
79. Alper K, Schwartz KA, Kolts RL, et al. Seizure incidence in psychopharmacological clinical trials: an analysis of Food and Drug Administration (FDA). Summary basis of approved reports. Biol Psychiatry 2007;62:345–54.
80. Sardell S, Sharpe G, Ashley S, et al. Evaluation of a nurse-led telephone clinic in the follow-up of patients with malignant glioma. Clin Oncol (R Coll Radiol) 2000; 12:36–41.
81. Sirven JI, Wingerchuk DM, Drazkowski JF, et al. Seizure prophylaxis in patients with brain tumors; a meta-analysis. Mayo Clin Proc 2004;79:1489–94.
82. Wu AS, Trinh VT, Suki D, et al. A prospective randomized trial of peri-operative seizure prophylaxis in patients with intraparenchymal brain tumors. J Neurosurg 2013;118(4):873–83.
83. Armstrong TS, Gilbert MR. Practical strategies for management of fatigue and sleep disorders in people with brain tumors. Neuro Oncol 2012;14:iv65–72.
84. Lovely MP. Symptom management of brain tumor patients. Semin Oncol Nurs 2004;20:273–83.
85. Kelly KP, Janssens MC, Ross J, et al. Controversy of non-steroidal anti-inflammatory drugs and intracranial surgery: et ne nos inducas in tentationem? Br J Anaesth 2011;107(3):302–5.
86. Lucas S. Headache management in concussion and mild traumatic brain injury. PM R 2011;3:S406–12.
87. Watanabe TK, Bell KR, Walker WC, et al. Systematic review of interventions for post-traumatic headache. PM R 2012;4:129–40.

88. Lyman GH, Khorana AA, Kuderer NM, et al. Venous thromboembolism prophylaxis and treatment in patients with cancer: American Society of Clinical Oncology Practice Guideline Update. J Clin Oncol 2013;31(17):2189–204.

89. Perry JR, Julian JA, Laperriere NJ, et al. PRODIGE: a randomized placebo-controlled trial of dalteparin low-molecular-weight heparin thromboprophylaxis in patients with newly diagnosed malignant glioma. J Thromb Haemost 2010; 8:1959–65.

90. Zeltzer LK, Recklitis C, Buchbinder D, et al. Psychological status in childhood cancer survivors: a report from the Childhood Cancer Survivor Study. J Clin Oncol 2009;27:2396–404.

91. Kirchhoff AC, Krull KR, Ness KK, et al. Occupational outcomes of adult childhood cancer survivors: a report from the Childhood Cancer Survivor Study. Cancer 2011;117:3033–44.

92. de Boer AG, Verbeek JH, vanDijk FJ. Adult survivors of childhood cancer and unemployment: a metaanalysis. Cancer 2006;107:1–11.

93. Salander P, Bergenheim T, Henriksson R. How was life after treatment of a malignant brain tumour? Soc Sci Med 2000;51(4):589–98.

94. Feuerstein M, Hansen J, Calvio L, et al. Work productivity in brain tumor survivors. J Occup Environ Med 2007;49(7):803–11.

95. Strauser DR, Wagner S, Wong AWK. Enhancing psychosocial outcomes for young adult childhood CNS cancer survivors: importance of addressing vocational identity and community integration. Int J Rehabil Res 2012;35(4):311–6.

96. Ness KK, Hudson MM, Ginsberg JP, et al. Physical performance limitations in the childhood cancer survivor study cohort. J Clin Oncol 2009;27:2382–9.

97. Ballard-Barbash R, Friedenrecih CM, Courneya K, et al. Physical activity, biomarkers and disease outcomes in cancer survivors: a systematic review. J Natl Cancer Inst 2012;104:815–40.

98. Buffart LM, Galvão DA, Brug J, et al. Evidence based physical activity guidelines for cancer survivors: current guidelines, knowledge gaps and future research directions. Cancer Treat Rev 2014;40:327–40.

99. Singh F, Newton RU, Galvão DA, et al. A systematic review of presurgical exercise intervention studies with cancer patients. Surg Oncol 2013;22:92–104.

100. Cotman CW, Berchtold NC, Christie L-A. Exercise builds brain health: key roles of growth factor cascades and inflammation. Trends Neurosci 2007;30(9):464–72.

101. Baker LD, Frank LL, Foster-Schubert K, et al. Effects of aerobic exercise on mild cognitive impairment: a controlled trial. Arch Neurol 2010;67(1):71–9.

102. Gagnon I, Galli C, Friedman D, et al. Active rehabilitation for children who are slow to recover following sport related concussion. Brain Inj 2009;23(12): 956–64.

103. Lustig RH, Post SR, Srivannaboon K, et al. Risk factors for the development of obesity in children surviving brain tumors. J Clin Endocrinol Metab 2003;88(2): 611–6.

104. Wolfe KR, Hunter GR, Madan-Swain A, et al. Cardiorespiratory fitness in survivors of pediatric posterior fossa tumor. J Pediatr Hematol Oncol 2012;34(6): e222–7.

105. Ruden E, Reardon DA, Coan AD, et al. Exercise behavior, functional capacity, and survival in adults with malignant recurrent glioma. J Clin Oncol 2011;29:2918–23.

106. Jones LW, Guill B, Keir ST. Exercise interest and preferences among patients diagnosed with primary brain cancer. Support Care Cancer 2007;15:47–55.

107. Williams PT. Reduced risk of brain cancer mortality from walking and running. Med Sci Sports Exerc 2014;46(5):927–32.

Rehabilitation in Chronic Graft-Versus-Host Disease

Sean Robinson Smith, MD[a],*, Arash Asher, MD[b]

KEYWORDS

- Chronic graft-versus-host disease • GVHD • GVHD rehabilitation
- Bone marrow transplant rehabilitation • Cancer rehabilitation

KEY POINTS

- Both the direct inflammatory effects of graft-versus-host disease (GVHD) and the treatment to suppress the disease can significantly impact function and cause pain.
- Few studies exist to guide management; the authors review the extant literature and discuss approaches that show promise based on their clinical experience.
- GVHD can affect many organ systems; this review addresses the skin/fascia and cardiac/pulmonary systems because these likely are associated with the highest degree of impairment.

INTRODUCTION

Chronic graft-versus-host disease (cGVHD) is the most common and potentially devastating complication of allogeneic (donor) hematopoietic stem cell transplantation (HSCT), often referred to as bone marrow transplantation. cGVHD occurs in 30% to 70% of patients who receive an HSCT for hematologic malignancy, and is caused by the newly donated T cells attacking highly mitotic areas of the transplant recipient's body that are considered foreign to the engrafted immune cells.[1] Most affected by cGVHD are the skin and fascia, gastrointestinal, pulmonary, hepatic, ocular, and oral mucosal organ systems. This inflammatory process can cause significant damage to the tissues affected, directly contributing to functional impairment. The treatment of cGVHD, which typically involves high-dose corticosteroids to suppress the immune system as first-line therapy, also can be destructive and necessitate rehabilitation to restore function and quality of life.[2]

Disclosure Statement: The authors have no relevant financial or commercial interests to disclose.

[a] Department of Physical Medicine & Rehabilitation, University of Michigan, 325 East Eisenhower Pkwy, Suite 100, Ann Arbor, MI 48108, USA; [b] Department of Physical Medicine & Rehabilitation, Samuel Oschin Comprehensive Cancer Institute at Cedars-Sinai Medical Center, Health Sciences, UCLA, 8700 Beverly Boulevard, AC 1109, Los Angeles, CA 90048, USA
* Corresponding author.
E-mail address: srsz@med.umich.edu

Phys Med Rehabil Clin N Am 28 (2017) 143–151
http://dx.doi.org/10.1016/j.pmr.2016.08.009
1047-9651/17/© 2016 Elsevier Inc. All rights reserved.

Although the HSCT itself requires special considerations in rehabilitation, recently transplanted patients are often pancytopenic and at increased risk for infection and bleeding events,[3] this article addresses the rehabilitation of specific impairments directly or indirectly caused by cGVHD. Furthermore, autologous HSCT, in which a person's own immune system is retransplanted into their body after myeloablation, is not discussed, as this does not cause cGVHD. Finally, acute GVHD represents a pathologically distinct process, typically occurring within the first 100 days after transplantation and affects the dermal and gastrointestinal systems, and does not impact function in the same way as cGVHD.[4] This is not directly discussed, although glucocorticoids are first-line treatment of acute GVHD, of which the side effects are addressed.

For purposes of simplicity, we have broken down this review into categories of the most physically devastating manifestations in these patients: skin/fascial and cardiopulmonary cGVHD, and the effects of steroids on muscle and bone. Manifestations of cGVHD in other organ systems, is beyond the scope of this review but a brief summary is listed in **Table 1**. For further information on the sequelae and symptomatic treatment of cGVHD beyond the measures discussed herein, the Ancillary and Supportive Care Working Group Report from the 2015 National Institutes of Health Consensus Development Project for cGVHD is recommended reading.[5]

SKIN AND FASCIAL CHRONIC GRAFT-VERSUS-HOST DISEASE

Cutaneous cGVHD is the most common manifestation of the disease, nearly 100% of people with cGVHD will develop this, and can affect one or both of the dermis and fascia.[6,7] Dermal involvement typically results in a maculopapular lichenoid rash and itself does not cause direct physical impairment; however, it is often the first sign of a cGVHD flare,[8] and may indicate that corticosteroids will soon be initiated or the dose increased.

Fascial cGVHD, on the other hand, is similar to eosinophilic fasciitis and can cause edema, fibrosis, and joint contracture.[9] Edema is often the first sign of fascial involvement, and the most common joints affected are the wrists, shoulders, and ankles, with distal joints affected first in a symmetric, bilateral fashion.[2,8] In addition to contracture, patients may develop joint destruction and skin breakdown as the upper layers of the skin become thin from the disease and corticosteroid use, and the deeper layers thicken.

When examining a patient, the progression of skin sclerosis from "moveable," that is, being able to easily compress focal areas of sclerosis, to "nonmoveable," in which

Table 1
Chronic graft-versus host disease organ involvement and common symptoms

Organ System	Symptoms
Skin (dermal)	Erythematous maculopapular rash, pain, desquamation
Skin (fascial)	Contracture, edema
Gastrointestinal	Painful cramping, watery stool
Oral	Painful lichenoid lesions, dryness, thrush, odynophagia, dysphagia
Ocular	Dryness, conjunctivitis
Vulvovaginal	Dryness, sclerosis, dyspareunia
Pulmonary	Bronchiolitis obliterans, airflow obstruction
Neurologic	Myasthenia gravis (rare), polymyositis (rare), Zoster

there is diffuse thickening that is not compressible, is a physical examination finding suggestive of chronic, difficult-to-reverse fibrosis. Sonographic measures of elasticity show promise in fibrosis assessment, although no large trials have been conducted to validate this modality.[10] Physical examination also should assess range of motion, particularly with the photographic range of motion (P-ROM) scale. This rapid, easy-to-use assessment of active range of motion at multiple joints, which can both grade the severity of involvement and monitor response to treatment, should be incorporated into the clinical assessment of all patients with fascial cGVHD[11,12] (**Fig. 1**).

Treatment for fascial cGVHD is not well understood: it is difficult to conduct large trials on such a specific manifestation of a rare disease, and most research understandably is directed at preventing and treating cGVHD, not the physical manifestations. Nevertheless, there are case series suggesting improvement in range of motion with splinting and stretching,[13,14] although it is unclear if the effects were sustained. Surgical release of contractures does not work and may make restrictions worse.[14]

In the authors' experience, interventions also must address the underlying edema and fibrosis. Occupational therapy directed at decongestive therapy, as well as compressive garments, should be a mainstay of treatment and initiated when swelling is first detected. As a corollary, it has been shown that burn patients have a lower risk of hypertrophic scarring when wearing compression garments, likely by decreasing stagnant inflammatory fluid surrounding the fascia and interstitium.[15] Modalities, such as paraffin baths[16] and phonophoresis with dexamethasone,[17] have not been studied in this population, but improve symptoms in patients with scleroderma and fasciitis, respectively, and should be considered. Iontophoresis is less likely to be

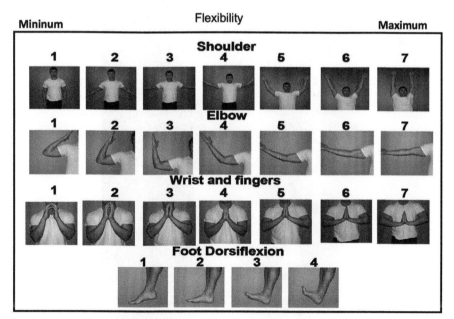

Fig. 1. The P-ROM assessment and scoring system. (*From* Carpenter PA. How I conduct a comprehensive chronic graft-versus-host disease assessment. Blood 2011;118(10):2682; with permission.)

helpful due to fibrosis impairing transit of medication, and friable skin making it difficult for the dermal patch to adhere (**Fig. 2**).

In summary, multiple approaches should be taken to restore range of motion, and early intervention is likely essential.

STEROID MYOPATHY

High-dose glucocorticoid immunosuppression puts patients at risk of developing steroid myopathy, which appears to affect at least 40% of patients who develop GVHD after HSCT, and is associated with weakness and moderate-to-severe functional impairment as measured by Functional Independence Measure (FIM) scores.[18]

The pathogenesis of steroid myopathy is complex and not fully understood. In brief, it likely involves the catabolic effects of glucocorticoids, primarily on type-2 skeletal muscle fibers, by stimulating the ubiquitin-proteasome proteolytic pathway, decreasing protein synthesis, and increasing the rate of protein metabolism.[19,20] Steroid myopathy is more frequently associated with the use of fluorinated glucocorticoid preparations, such as dexamethasone and triamcinolone than with the use of non-fluorinated preparations, such as prednisone.[21]

The risk of steroid myopathy generally increases with the dose and duration of use, with prednisone or equivalent drugs in dosages lower than 10 mg per day not typically being associated with myopathy and weakness. Instead, the use of prednisone in dosages of 40 to 60 mg per day (as often seen in treatment with cGVHD) for at least 1 month invariably results in some muscle weakness.[18,21]

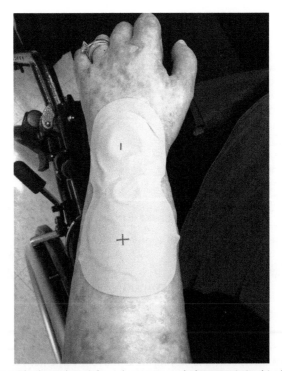

Fig. 2. A patient with dermal and fascial cGVHD and characteristic skin lesions wears an iontophoresis dermal patch.

Steroid myopathy presents as a painless proximal muscle weakness preferentially affecting the hip girdle muscles. Motor and sensory nerve conduction studies are normal, and needle electromyography is typically normal unless the myopathy is severe, when low-amplitude, short-duration motor unit action potentials can be seen in the proximal muscles.[22] Muscle enzymes (creatine phosphokinase) are normal or slightly elevated. The diagnosis is often clinical, based on the timing of the glucocorticoid exposure and the absence of other causes of myopathy, and/or by demonstrating improved strength within 3 to 4 weeks of reducing the steroid dosage.[23] Muscle biopsy may show type-II fiber atrophy.

Because reducing glucocorticoid dosing is not always an option, rehabilitation is critical, with interventions such as physical therapy, occupational therapy, and assistive devices used to help with mobility, self-care, and safety. Patients often have difficulty navigating stairs, getting up from a seated position, and have poor endurance. Limited research based on animal models suggests that resistance exercise training, when started before or during steroid administration, may attenuate subsequent muscle atrophy, with one study showing 46% less gastrocnemius atrophy.[24] These results underscore the importance of evaluating interventions like prehabilitation, which may lessen the functional decline in these patients. Exercise prescription must be individualized and tailored to each patient, given the potential comorbidities, such as contractures, neuropathy, and osteopenia.

Inpatient rehabilitation is sometimes required for patients with cGVHD and steroid myopathy who are physically incapable of being discharged home. More studies are needed regarding outcomes and optimal treatment pathways, but one preliminary study showed that patients improved significantly in motor FIM scores and most were able to discharge home in a reasonable time frame.[25]

BONE AND JOINT INVOLVEMENT

cGVHD does not directly affect bones and joints, but more than 50% of patients with cGVHD will develop low bone density, putting patients at risk for fracture, particularly when combined with sarcopenia. This is primarily due to glucocorticoid use, but patients often have other risk factors, including calcineurin inhibitor use (eg, tacrolimus), chemotherapy and radiation therapy, gonadal dysfunction, renal dysfunction, history of a hematologic malignancy for which the transplant was performed, and decreased weight-bearing activity.[26] The HSCT itself also impairs bone mineral metabolism for 6 to 12 months.[27] Bone density loss is commonly seen at the osteopenic and not osteoporotic levels, and is diagnosed with density loss at the femoral head, not the lumbar spine, as seen in postmenopausal osteopenia.[28]

Treatment is both preventive and supportive: vitamin D and calcium supplementation, and sometimes bisphosphonate therapy, is indicated.[29] Weight-bearing exercises also are essential.[30] Vertebral compression fractures must be assessed in the context of spine stability, and bracing may be required to limit flexion or extension. Oral analgesics and procedures, such as kyphoplasty, should be considered to reduce pain and improve mobility.

Avascular necrosis (AVN) is seen in 4% to 19% of HSCT survivors, with risk factors including glucocorticoid and calcineurin inhibitor use, older age, and female gender.[31,32] The most common sites of involvement are the femoral heads, humeral heads, knees, and ankles; patients frequently have more than one joint affected.[27] Advanced stages of AVN require joint replacement, but patients may not be healthy enough to undergo surgery, and rehabilitation can reduce pain and improve function in both advanced and early stages. Physical and occupational therapy, bracing, assistive mobility devices, and oral analgesics should be a mainstay of treatment. Intra-articular corticosteroid injections can reduce swelling and pain before collapse of the joint; because the condition is progressive, the benefits of pain reduction with this injection may outweigh the downside of administering more corticosteroids.

Nerve ablation for hip and knee AVN is an emerging treatment for patients who are not joint replacement candidates or who have multisite involvement. This involves diagnostic blocks and subsequent ablation to the genicular nerves (knee)[33] and branches of the obturator and femoral nerves (hip).[34,35] No studies have evaluated these in the context of patients with cGVHD/HSCT, but in the authors' experience, these procedures have been invaluable in nonoperative patients and should be considered.

CARDIOPULMONARY MANIFESTATIONS

Exercise has been studied in patients shortly after HSCT, and appears both safe and helpful even in the setting of thrombocytopenia,[36–38] but the benefits in the cGVHD population are not well known. Direct cardiac involvement of cGVHD is rare; indirect manifestations include peripheral edema in the setting of fascial or hepatic GVHD, and decreased exercise capacity due to multifactorial deconditioning. The 2-minute walk test should be a mainstay of cGVHD assessment, as recommended by the National Institutes of Health Consensus Development Project, and correlates with overall survival.[39] Exercise programs should emphasize aerobic conditioning and strengthening.

Pulmonary complications are both from direct effects of cGVHD and its treatment; the latter increases the risk of infection through immunosuppression and by steroid myopathy weakening the muscles of respiration.[40] Pulmonary cGVHD can affect up to 60% of patients, and bronchiolitis obliterans is pathognomonic. Pulmonary function tests show an obstructive process.[41] In addition to good pulmonary hygiene and patient education, pulmonary rehabilitation has been shown to provide a statistically significant benefit in patient-reported dyspnea and in 6-minute walk test distance.[42]

SUMMARY

cGVHD is an uncommon but debilitating disease, and rehabilitation professionals have a unique skillset to manage this variable and dynamic patient population. Attention must be paid to both the direct effects of the inflammatory cGVHD process, as well as the side effects of immunosuppressant medication used to treat the disease. More research is needed regarding optimal rehabilitation interventions, and physiatrists and other members of the multidisciplinary rehabilitation team should be leaders in developing supportive care models for these patients.

REFERENCES

1. Lee SJ, Flowers MED. Recognizing and managing chronic graft-versus-host disease. Hematology 2008;2008(1):134–41.
2. Smith SR, Haig AJ, Couriel DR. Musculoskeletal, neurologic, and cardiopulmonary aspects of physical rehabilitation in patients with chronic graft-versus-host disease. Biol Blood Marrow Transplant 2015;21(5):799–808.
3. Steinberg A, Asher A, Bailey C, et al. The role of physical rehabilitation in stem cell transplantation patients. Support Care Cancer 2015;23(8):2447–60.
4. Jagasia MH, Greinix HT, Arora M, et al. National Institutes of Health consensus development project on criteria for clinical trials in chronic graft-versus-host

disease: I. The 2014 diagnosis and staging working group report. Biol Blood Marrow Transplant 2015;21(3):389–401.e1.

5. Carpenter PA, Kitko CL, Elad S, et al. National Institutes of Health consensus development project on criteria for clinical trials in chronic graft-versus-host disease: V. The 2014 ancillary therapy and supportive care working group report. Biol Blood Marrow Transplant 2015;21(7):1167–87.

6. Johnson ML, Farmer ER. Graft-versus-host reactions in dermatology. J Am Acad Dermatol 1998;38(3):369–92.

7. Ballester-Sánchez R, Navarro-Mira M, Sanz-Caballer J, et al. Review of cutaneous graft-vs-host disease. Actas Dermosifiliogr 2016;107(3):183–93.

8. Filipovich AH, Weisdorf D, Pavletic S, et al. National Institutes of Health consensus development project on criteria for clinical trials in chronic graft-versus-host disease: I. Diagnosis and staging working group report. Biol Blood Marrow Transplant 2005;11(12):945–56.

9. Janin A. Fasciitis in chronic graft-versus-host disease: a clinicopathologic study of 14 cases. Ann Intern Med 1994;120(12):993.

10. Osmola-Mańkowska A, Silny W, Dańczak-Pazdrowska A, et al. Assessment of chronic sclerodermoid graft-versus-host disease patients, using 20MHz high-frequency ultrasonography and cutometer methods. Skin Res Technology 2012;19(1):e417–22.

11. Carpenter PA. How I conduct a comprehensive chronic graft-versus-host disease assessment. Blood 2011;118(10):2679–87.

12. Inamoto Y, Pidala J, Chai X, et al. Assessment of joint and fascia manifestations in chronic graft-versus-host disease. Arthritis Rheumatol 2014;66(4):1044–52.

13. Choi I-S, Jang I-S, Han J-Y, et al. Therapeutic experience on multiple contractures in sclerodermoid chronic graft versus host disease. Support Care Cancer 2009; 17(7):851–5.

14. Beredjiklian PK, Drummond DS, Dormans JP, et al. Orthopaedic manifestations of chronic graft-versus-host disease. J Pediatr Orthop 1998;18(5):572–5.

15. Sharp PA, Pan B, Yakuboff KP, et al. Development of a best evidence statement for the use of pressure therapy for management of hypertrophic scarring. J Burn Care Res 2015;37(4):255–64.

16. Sandqvist G, Åkesson A, Eklund M. Evaluation of paraffin bath treatment in patients with systemic sclerosis. Disabil Rehabil 2004;26(16):981–7.

17. Rosenbaum AJ, Dipreta JA, Misener D. Plantar heel pain. Med Clin North Am 2014;98(2):339–52.

18. Lee HJ, Oran B, Saliba RM, et al. Steroid myopathy in patients with acute graft-versus-host disease treated with high-dose steroid therapy. Bone Marrow Transplant 2006;38(4):299–303.

19. Sun L, Trausch-Azar JS, Muglia LJ, et al. Glucocorticoids differentially regulate degradation of MyoD and Id1 by N-terminal ubiquitination to promote muscle protein catabolism. Proc Natl Acad Sci U S A 2008;105(9):3339–44.

20. Schakman O, Gilson H, Thissen JP. Mechanisms of glucocorticoid-induced myopathy. J Endocrinol 2008;197(1):1–10.

21. Pereira RMR, Carvalho JFD. Glucocorticoid-induced myopathy. Joint Bone Spine 2011;78(1):41–4.

22. Paganoni S, Amato A. Electrodiagnostic evaluation of myopathies. Phys Med Rehabil Clin N Am 2013;24(1):193–207.

23. Bowyer S, Lamothe M, Hollister J. Steroid myopathy: incidence and detection in a population with asthma. J Allergy Clin Immunol 1985;76(2):234–42.

24. Lapier TK. Glucocorticoid-induced muscle atrophy. J Cardiopulm Rehabil 1997; 17(2):76–84.

25. Leung J, Smith S. Acute inpatient rehabilitation performance in chronic graft-versus-host-disease. Arch Phys Med Rehabil 2015;96(10). http://dx.doi.org/10.1016/j.apmr.2015.08.302.

26. Mcclune BL, Polgreen LE, Burmeister LA, et al. Screening, prevention and management of osteoporosis and bone loss in adult and pediatric hematopoietic cell transplant recipients. Bone Marrow Transplant 2010;46(1):1–9.

27. Mcclune B, Majhail NS, Flowers ME. Bone loss and avascular necrosis of bone after hematopoietic cell transplantation. Semin Hematol 2012;49(1):59–65.

28. Schimmer AD, Mah K, Bordeleau L, et al. Decreased bone mineral density is common after autologous blood or marrow transplantation. Bone Marrow Transplant 2001;28(4):387–91.

29. Venuturupalli SR, Sacks W. Review of new guidelines for the management of glucocorticoid induced osteoporosis. Curr Osteoporos Rep 2013;11(4):357–64.

30. Sinaki M. Exercise for patients with osteoporosis: management of vertebral compression fractures and trunk strengthening for fall prevention. PM R 2012; 4(11):882–8.

31. Mcavoy S, Baker KS, Mulrooney D, et al. Corticosteroid dose as a risk factor for avascular necrosis of the bone after hematopoietic cell transplantation. Biol Blood Marrow Transplant 2010;16(9):1231–6.

32. Enright H, Haake R, Weisdorf D. Avascular necrosis of bone: a common serious complication of allogeneic bone marrow transplantation. Am J Med 1990;89(6): 733–8.

33. Choi W-J, Hwang S-J, Song J-G, et al. Radiofrequency treatment relieves chronic knee osteoarthritis pain: a double-blind randomized controlled trial. Pain 2011; 152(3):481–7.

34. Rivera F, Mariconda C, Annaratone G. Percutaneous radiofrequency denervation in patients with contraindications for total hip arthroplasty. Orthopedics 2012; 35(3):e302–5.

35. Stone J, Matchett G. Combined ultrasound and fluoroscopic guidance for radiofrequency ablation of the obturator nerve for intractable cancer-associated hip pain. Pain Physician 2014;17(1):E83–7.

36. Rexer P, Kanphade G, Murphy S. Feasibility of an exercise program for patients with thrombocytopenia undergoing hematopoietic stem cell transplant. J Acute Care Phys Ther 2016;7(2):55–64.

37. Jarden M, Baadsgaard MT, Hovgaard DJ, et al. A randomized trial on the effect of a multimodal intervention on physical capacity, functional performance and quality of life in adult patients undergoing allogeneic SCT. Bone Marrow Transplant 2009;43(9):725–37.

38. Morris GS, Brueilly KE, Scheetz JS, et al. Adherence of stem cell transplant recipients receiving glucocorticoid therapy to an exercise-based rehabilitation program. Support Care Cancer 2011;20(10):2391–8.

39. Pidala J, Chai X, Martin P, et al. Hand grip strength and 2-minute walk test in chronic graft-versus-host disease assessment: analysis from the chronic GVHD consortium. Biol Blood Marrow Transplant 2013;19(6):967–72.

40. White AC, Terrin N, Miller KB, et al. Impaired respiratory and skeletal muscle strength in patients prior to hematopoietic stem-cell transplantation. Chest 2005;128(1):145–52.

41. Gazourian L, Rogers AJ, Ibanga R, et al. Factors associated with bronchiolitis obliterans syndrome and chronic graft-versus-host disease after allogeneic hematopoietic cell transplantation. Am J Hematol 2014;89(4):404–9.

42. Tran J, Norder EE, Diaz PT, et al. Pulmonary rehabilitation for bronchiolitis obliterans syndrome after hematopoietic stem cell transplantation. Biol Blood Marrow Transplant 2012;18(8):1250–4.

Deconstructing Postmastectomy Syndrome

Implications for Physiatric Management

Eric Wisotzky, MD[a],*, Nicole Hanrahan, MD[b],
Thomas P. Lione, DO[c], Susan Maltser, DO[d]

KEYWORDS

- Postmastectomy • Pain • Breast cancer • Cancer rehabilitation • Intercostobrachial

KEY POINTS

- Postmastectomy pain syndrome is a prevalent disorder that negatively impacts the function and quality of life of breast cancer survivors.
- The key to successful treatment of postmastectomy pain is a thorough evaluation to identify the specific anatomic structures that lead to this pain syndrome.
- After determining the anatomic cause of postmastectomy pain, there are many potential treatments, including rehabilitation, medications, injections, and other nonpharmacologic treatments.

BACKGROUND

Epidemiology of Breast Cancer

Breast cancer is the most commonly diagnosed cancer among women in the United States, irrespective of race or ethnicity, accounting for nearly 1 in 3 cancers.[1] Each year, there are more than 230,000 new cases of breast cancer in the United States and more than 40,000 deaths.[2] It is the second leading cause of cancer death among women after lung cancer and the most common cause of death from cancer among Hispanic women according to the Centers for Disease Control and Prevention. One in 8 women will develop invasive breast cancer.[3] Approximately one million new cases

The authors have no commercial or financial conflicts of interest.
[a] MedStar National Rehabilitation Network, Georgetown University School of Medicine, 102 Irving Street, Northwest, Washington, DC 20010, USA; [b] MedStar National Rehabilitation Network, 102 Irving Street, Northwest, Washington, DC 20010, USA; [c] Department of Physical Medicine and Rehabilitation, Hofstra Northwell School of Medicine, 1554 Northern Boulevard, 4th Floor, Manhasset, NY 11030, USA; [d] Cancer Rehabilitation, Department of Physical Medicine and Rehabilitation, Hofstra Northwell School of Medicine, 1554 Northern Boulevard, 4th Floor, Manhasset, NY 11030, USA
* Corresponding author.
E-mail address: eric.m.wisotzky@medstar.net

are diagnosed globally every year, and this number is expected to increase in future decades.[4] As a result, more women will likely undergo surgical procedures for the treatment of breast cancer, and the incidence of postoperative complications and pain syndromes is likely to increase.

Surgical Techniques in the Treatment of Breast Cancer

In the past several decades, the standard of care for the treatment of breast cancer involved radical mastectomy and total axillary dissection to achieve local tumor control and increase the likelihood of cure.[5] Over the years, less invasive surgical approaches have become the standard of care and include modified radical mastectomy, total (simple) mastectomy, and more recently, skin-sparing mastectomy and nipple-sparing mastectomy.[6] These less invasive surgical techniques have continued to gain favor over time. These more conservative surgical approaches have enhanced rates of local control and 5-year survival, in part due to a gradual shift from unimodal to multimodal treatment approaches.

Treatment options for patients with early stage breast cancer typically include total mastectomy or breast-conserving surgery with adjuvant radiation therapy.[7] Total mastectomy involves removal of skin, nipple, areola, breast tissue, and the fascia of the pectoralis major. Patients who have undergone total mastectomy may be candidates for immediate breast reconstruction, which is increasingly used with a skin-sparing mastectomy technique, especially for women with smaller breasts. Regardless of specific technique, all patients with invasive breast cancer should undergo sampling of axillary lymph nodes for proper staging and treatment.

Until the late 1990s, it was standard of practice for patients to undergo 2- to 3-level axillary lymph node dissection (ALND) in addition to breast-conserving treatment or mastectomy.[7] The extent of lymph node dissection can potentially be limited by the identification of the axillary sentinel lymph node(s) (SLN) using a radiolabeled isotope. Based on predictable patterns of lymphatic drainage within the breast, SLN identification limits nodal dissection and may allow for immediate completion ALND in cases with metastatic disease within the sentinel node.[7,8]

Finally, women who undergo mastectomy for the treatment or prevention of breast cancer often consider cosmetic reconstruction. Multiple surgical techniques are currently used and include single-stage reconstruction, tissue expansion followed by implant, combined autologous tissue/implant reconstruction, and autologous tissue reconstruction alone.[7] Common approaches to autologous breast reconstruction include transverse rectus abdominus muscle flap, latissimus flap, and deep inferior epigastric perforator flap. Reconstruction is deemed safe from an oncology perspective and can improve appearance, sense of femininity, and self-esteem.[7]

POSTMASTECTOMY PAIN SYNDROME
Definition

Postmastectomy pain syndrome (PMPS) refers to persistent pain following any breast surgery, not just mastectomy.[9,10] Pain has been reported following other breast procedures, including lumpectomy, breast reconstruction, augmentation, and reduction, although procedures targeting the upper outer quadrant of the breast or axilla are particularly prone to pain syndromes.[9,11,12] For a diagnosis of PMPS, pain must persist for more than 3 months postoperatively when all other causes of pain, such as infection or tumor recurrence, have been excluded[13]; however, no specific diagnostic criteria are universally accepted. Persistent pain after mastectomy was first reported during the 1970s and was characterized as a dull, burning, and/or aching sensation in the anterior chest, arm, and axilla, often worsened by movement of the shoulder.[14] There are various potential causes of PMPS, including intraoperative damage to the intercostobrachial nerve, axillary nerve, or chest wall; phantom breast pain; incisional pain; musculoskeletal pain; and pain caused by neuroma.[9,15] Although traditionally, PMPS has been defined in the literature as a neuropathic pain syndrome, the authors of this article believe this to be an inaccurate generalization. Many patients with PMPS have musculoskeletal pain syndromes with no apparent component of neuropathic pain.

Epidemiology

Reported incidence rates of PMPS have varied significantly, perhaps as a result of the absence of a formalized definition or diagnostic criteria. Most studies of chronic pain following breast surgery report an incidence ranging from 20% to 70%.[10,15,16] One study showed 44% of breast cancer survivors still with arm pain more than 4 years after breast surgery.[17] It is likely that incidence rates differ across anatomic subsets of postmastectomy pain. Therefore, more accurate and clinically relevant incidence estimates may require broad acceptance and application of subset-specific diagnoses.

An important characteristic that distinguishes PMPS subtypes and has direct import for clinical decision making is the presumed pathophysiology of the pain. Nociceptive pain occurs as a result of surgical injury and typically resolves as damaged tissue heals. Musculoskeletal pain syndromes are common nociceptive causes of PMPS, but for most, epidemiology remains uncharacterized. In contrast, neuropathic pain results from dysfunction of the nervous system and may be difficult to treat.[18] Several different types of neuropathic pain following breast surgery have been described. Phantom breast pain may occur after radical mastectomy or modified radical mastectomy and refers to the sensation of a removed breast or nipple that is painful.[17] Studies have estimated the prevalence of phantom breast pain from 13% to 44%.[17] Intercostobrachial neuralgia refers to pain related to surgical injury to the intercostobrachial nerve, which may occur following axillary dissection and is a commonly discussed cause of PMPS in the literature, although rigorous incidence estimates are lacking.[17] Neuromas are another cause of chronic pain after breast surgery and may form following injury to any nerve.[17] Neuromas can form within scars following both mastectomy and lumpectomy, although pain from neuroma may be more common following lumpectomy or in patients who have undergone concomitant ALND and radiation.[19] The prevalence of neuroma pain following breast surgery varies throughout the literature and ranges from 20% to 50%.[17] Additional causes of neuropathic pain are also possible and include damage to the intercostal, thoracodorsal, medial and lateral pectoral nerves, and long thoracic nerves.[20]

Clinical Presentation

Patients with PMPS typically present with neuropathic or musculoskeletal pain symptoms. Symptom onset may be in the immediate postoperative period, but can also occur several months after surgery and persist beyond the normal timeframe for surgical healing.[21] Pain is commonly localized to the axilla, operative site, and/or ipsilateral arm.[16,22] Patients may also experience pain in the chest wall and/or shoulder with accompanying limitations in range of motion, or decreased handgrip strength.[23]

Risk Factors

Reasons for the development of persistent pain following a mastectomy are not clearly understood and are likely multifactorial. Risk factors span clinical and demographic domains, including the severity of acute postoperative pain, adjuvant radiation,

ALND, and psychosocial factors.[10] Severe postoperative pain that becomes chronic has been studied after various surgical procedures. Persistent acute pain is thought to activate mechanisms within the central and peripheral nervous systems, leading to sensitization. This, in turn, leads to allodynia, hyperalgesia, and hyperpathia that can affect physical functioning and lead to chronic pain. In a study of 569 patients reported by Tasmuth and colleagues,[24] patients with significant postoperative pain were more likely to develop persistent ipsilateral arm pain compared with those whose pain was less severe.

Demographic risk factors
Younger age at diagnosis is associated with increased risk for PMPS.[25] Although the reason for this is poorly understood, several mechanisms have been proposed. These mechanisms include greater sensitivity to nerve damage in younger people, lower pain thresholds, and increased preoperative anxiety.[13,26] In addition, younger age may be correlated with more aggressive treatments, including a more thorough axillary dissection and adjuvant radiotherapy.[27]

Socioeconomic status has also been associated with PMPS. Patients with lower socioeconomic status, including lower annual income and educational level, are predisposed to develop higher rates of chronic pain. One explanation for this may be diagnosis at later stages of cancer, necessitating more aggressive surgical and adjuvant treatment.[28]

Treatment- and complication-related risk factors
Although it is commonly assumed that PMPS is a sequela of mastectomy, large-scale studies show no difference in PMPS rates between mastectomy and lumpectomy.[10] Rather, it is the extensiveness of ALND, damage to the intercostobrachial nerve, and adjuvant treatment that are presumed to initiate and sustain postoperative and chronic pain.[13] Tumors located in the upper outer quadrant may warrant a more extensive axillary dissection, leading to greater neuropathic pain.[29] Furthermore, the number of axillary lymph nodes dissected as well as the number and location of surgical drains may play a role.[21] Immediate reconstruction following mastectomy has not been found to effect the development of PMPS.[30]

Adjuvant radiation therapy to the axilla is another potential cause of neuropathic pain in patients with breast cancer. Pain related to radiation can occur months to years following treatment, even in those patients who undergo breast conservation surgery. Pain following radiation can present in the breast, chest wall, and ipsilateral arm.[31]

One study demonstrated that surgical complications, such as cellulitis, and the development of neuromas and seromas, do not increase the risk of developing chronic pain.

Psychosocial risk factors
In terms of psychosocial risk factors for the development of PMPS, patients with moderate postoperative pain reported significantly higher preoperative levels of depression, anxiety, sleep disturbance, and fatigue as well as lower social well-being and quality of life.[16] Almost half of all patients with cancer exhibit some elements of anxiety and depression. In one study of women with breast cancer, 50% were noted to have depression and anxiety within the first year of diagnosis.[32] In a study of 611 patients undergoing a mastectomy, preoperative catastrophizing was the only independent contributing factor to predicting clinically significant pain at 2 days after breast surgery.[29] Catastrophizing and maladaptive coping behavior may mediate postoperative pain by way of central and peripheral sensitization and impaired pain inhibition[29] (**Box 1**).

Box 1
Postmastectomy pain syndrome risk factors

- Severity of acute postmastectomy pain
- Radiation
- ALND
- Younger age
- Low socioeconomic status
- Preoperative and postoperative anxiety and depression, especially catastrophizing

CLINICAL ASSESSMENT OF POSTMASTECTOMY PAIN SYNDROME
History

Evaluation of PMPS requires a careful history and physical examination, which should focus on identifying the cause of the pain and the pain generator(s). History should include the timing of symptom onset, the type of breast surgery (mastectomy vs lumpectomy), type of reconstruction, and whether the patient had an ALND or SLN biopsy. The clinician should be aware of how many lymph nodes were removed and how many were positive for metastatic disease. In addition, the patient's tumor stage and grade should be noted. Adjuvant treatment should be included in the history, including type and duration of chemotherapy, radiation therapy, and hormonal therapy.

A careful history of the patient's pain should be taken. The distribution, duration, and quality of the pain, as well as associated symptoms such as numbness, tingling, and weakness, should be included. Phantom pain/sensations, breast pain, and/or swelling should be assessed. It is important to determine whether the patient has difficulty with shoulder motion or a history of premorbid shoulder dysfunction. Finally, the patient's psychosocial status should be evaluated, including mood, coping skills, and extent of social support. Underlying depression and anxiety should be noted and addressed. Functional history, including activities of daily living, as well as vocational and avocational activities, before and after cancer diagnosis should be assessed (**Box 2**).

Physical Examination

Physical examination includes examination of the breasts, skin, and upper extremities for any signs of cellulitis, radiation-association change, muscle atrophy, scapular

Box 2
Taking a postmastectomy pain syndrome history

- Surgical factors (timing, lumpectomy vs mastectomy, ALND vs SLN biopsy, type of reconstruction)
- Cancer pathology, stage, grade, estrogen/progesterone receptor status, metastatic disease
- Adjuvant treatments (chemotherapy, radiation, hormone therapy)
- Pain history
- Functional history
- Social status and support system
- Assess for anxiety and depression

winging, or lymphedema. The surgical incision should be evaluated for signs of wound infection, adhesions, seromas, and neuromas. The cervical and thoracic spine should be inspected for deformities and range-of-motion testing should be performed. The trapezius, serratus anterior, pectoralis muscles, rhomboids, and latissimus muscles should be palpated for potential asymmetry, trigger points, or other stigmata of myofascial dysfunction. For patients who have undergone breast reconstruction, special attention should be given to the pectoralis and lateral chest wall muscles, as well as the flap harvest sites, such as the abdomen. The axilla should be palpated for cording or masses. Shoulder girdle examination should include inspection for asymmetry, passive and active range of motion, as well as palpation and provocative testing of the rotator cuff and other musculoskeletal structures. In addition to testing strength, sensation, and deep tendon reflexes of the upper extremity myotomes and dermatomes, the neurologic examination should focus on motor testing of the muscles innervated by nerves that can be affected by surgery of the breast. These include the thoracodorsal, long thoracic, medial, and lateral pectoral nerves[7] (**Box 3**).

Diagnostic Studies

Diagnostic studies can support and supplement the history and physical examination and aid the clinician when the diagnosis is unclear. Ultrasound can be helpful in diagnosing musculoskeletal abnormality. MRI may confirm shoulder, cervical spine, or thoracic spine abnormality.[33] A chest computed tomographic scan or MRI can evaluate potential metastatic disease or brachial plexus injury. PET scanning can also be ordered if tumor recurrence or metastatic disease is suspected. Nerve conduction studies and electromyography can diagnose radiculopathy, plexopathy, mononeuropathies, polyneuropathy, or evidence of radiation fibrosis, for example, myokymia and/or myopathic motor unit action potentials.

Outcome Measures

Although standardized outcome measures in the setting of postmastectomy pain have not been clearly delineated, there are several well-established breast cancer–specific functional outcome measures. A prospective surveillance approach with functional measures for breast cancer has been proposed.[34] The authors suggested serial functional evaluations with a 6-minute walk test, chair stand, shoulder range of motion, hand grip strength, upper extremity functional index or Kwan's arm problem scale, and functional assessment of cancer therapy-breast or Breast-Q.

Box 3
Performing a postmastectomy pain syndrome physical examination

- Inspecting skin, incision, breast, cervical spine, shoulder girdle (for atrophy, asymmetry, or scapular winging)
- Palpate incision for tenderness, neuromas, and mobility
- Palpate musculature for tender/trigger points
- Palpate axilla and upper extremity for cording
- Range of motion
- Neurologic examination
- Special provocative tests depending on suspected diagnosis (eg, rotator cuff impingement signs)

POSTMASTECTOMY PAIN SYNDROME DIAGNOSTIC SUBGROUPS

The key to successful treatment of PMPS is to determine the specific pain cause or causes. The following section details pain generators that can lead to PMPS and suggested treatment approaches. Some treatments are evidence based, and some reflect anecdotal experience.

Rotator Cuff Dysfunction

Rotator cuff dysfunction, the leading cause of shoulder pain in the general population, is also a well-recognized phenomenon among breast cancer survivors. The frequency of rotator cuff–related pain among breast cancer survivors has not been rigorously estimated. Altered biomechanics have been implicated in the development of rotator cuff dysfunction, whether after mastectomy or lumpectomy. Postmastectomy scapulothoracic motion has been noted to increase disproportionately to glenohumeral motion, with subsequent rotator cuff microtrauma and tendinopathy. This is due to postoperative glenohumeral range-of-motion limitations and decreased muscle activity in the musculature affecting the scapula (serratus anterior, upper trapezius, pectoralis major, and rhomboid) ipsilateral to the carcinoma.[35] The shoulder girdle is placed in a more protracted and inferior position as a result of shortening of the pectoral muscles and associated soft tissues, thus narrowing the subacromial space available for the rotator cuff tendons.[36] Symptoms include pain, tightness, decreased function, and weakness. Kyphotic posture can also contribute to pectoralis muscle tightness, resulting in further rotator cuff impingement. It should be noted that studies have shown altered scapulothoracic motion contralateral to the cancer, explaining the occurrence of bilateral shoulder dysfunction, or even unilateral involvement of the unaffected side.

Other risk factors may contribute to rotator cuff dysfunction in patients with breast cancer. Chest wall radiation treatment contributes to muscle and soft tissue tightening; fibrosis may be a major factor in this phenomenon. Interestingly, one study demonstrated that chest wall radiation involving the pectoralis major, regardless of the presence of clinically detectable radiation fibrosis, was a significant contributor to shoulder morbidity.[37] A review of several studies involving radiotherapy demonstrated that the addition of axillary radiation places patients at increased risk for late shoulder dysfunction compared with chest wall radiation alone.[3] Lymphedema also contributes to rotator cuff tendinopathy. The incidence of shoulder pain in lymphedema patients is reported as 53% and 71% from 2 separate studies.[38,39] Increased weight of the limb and decreased joint range of motion can aggravate subacromial impingement, intrinsic tendinopathy, and/or functional overload[40] (**Fig. 1**). In addition, reports have speculated that the increased risk of cellulitis in the lymphedematous arm may decrease healing capacity of tissue and cause pathologic effects on the rotator cuff, but this has not been validated. Early management of lymphedema has been suggested given the association noted between the duration of lymphedema symptoms and, rotator cuff abnormality seen on musculoskeletal ultrasound.[37]

Anecdotally, conventional rehabilitation techniques for rotator cuff tendinopathy can be very helpful for this patient population. In addition, injection techniques including subacromial corticosteroid injection or percutaneous needle tenotomy may be considered.

Intercostobrachial Neuralgia

One of the most common causes of PMPS discussed in the literature is intercostobrachial neuralgia. The intercostobrachial nerve is a cutaneous branch of T1 and/or T2 and provides sensory innervation to the medial upper arm and lateral chest wall.

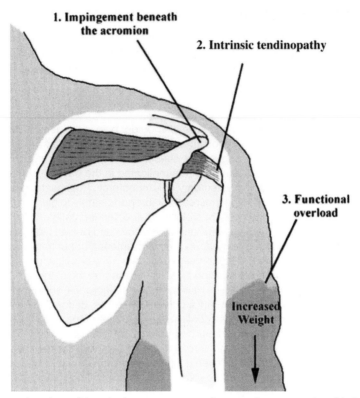

1. Impingement beneath the acromion

2. Intrinsic tendinopathy

3. Functional overload

Increased Weight

Fig. 1. Posterior view of lymphedematous arm and supraspinatus muscle with 3 possible causes of rotator cuff tendonitis. (*From* Herrera JE, Stubblefield MD. Rotator cuff tendonitis in lymphedema: a retrospective case series. Arch Phys Med Rehabil 2004;85(12):1939–42.)

This nerve is commonly sacrificed during ALND. Intercostobrachial neuralgia can be treated with nerve-stabilizing medications and desensitization techniques. Another treatment option is intercostobrachial nerve block, which has been described using ultrasound guidance.[41] The morbidity of nerve-sparing versus nerve-sacrificing surgeries is unclear. In the authors' clinical experience, intercostobrachial neuralgia is a less common cause of pain than is suggested in the literature. More often, patients report numbness in this distribution, but pain seems to be less common.

Radiation Fibrosis Syndrome

Radiation fibrosis syndrome has been defined as a myriad of musculoskeletal, neuromuscular, and other complications arising from treatment with radiation.[42] Although some degree of fibrosis is observed in most irradiated patients,[43] symptomatic radiation fibrosis is generally a late complication of radiotherapy, which can manifest months, if not years, after treatment. In general, loss of neurovascular innervation leading to atrophy is thought to be the main cause of symptoms and clinical features in irradiated patients. Virtually any type of tissue can be affected by radiation, including ligament, muscle, skin, viscera, tendon, nerve, and bone.[7] Postmastectomy patients with radiation fibrosis can experience diverse radiation-related symptoms. Sclerosis of ligaments and tendons in the radiation field may result in shortening, contracture, and loss of elasticity and subsequently decreased range of motion and loss of function.[40] Musculature of the shoulder and axilla can atrophy, leading to weakness and secondary rotator cuff dysfunction. In addition, irradiated muscles may fibrose to such an extent that a focal myopathy develops.[44] Patients with breast cancer treated with radiation also complain of muscle spasms in the chest wall, especially the pectoralis major, serratus anterior and latissimus dorsi muscles, thought to be due to ectopic activity of motor nerves. Irradiated patients may also complain of skin changes, including thickening, tightness, nipple retraction, and breast edema.[45] Radiation fibrosis syndrome is a clinical diagnosis that can be challenging to confirm exclusive of other common neuromusculoskeletal abnormalities.

Management of radiation fibrosis is geared toward functional and symptomatic treatment as well as treatment of the fibrosis. Physical and occupational therapy improve range of motion, manually release fibrotic tissue, and improve upper extremity function.

Nerve-stabilizing medications and opioids have been anecdotally reported in the literature as effective in radiation fibrosis–associated pain.[46] Botulinum toxin injection has been examined in the literature as a treatment for the muscle spasms, pain, and neuropathy associated with radiation therapy.[40] Pentoxifylline in combination with tocopherol has been validated in the treatment of radiation fibrosis. Pentoxifylline limits aberrant transforming growth factor-β activity, thereby limiting fibroblast collagen proliferation. Anti-inflammatory and immunologic effects have been posited as well. Some studies have reported effectiveness at 1200 mg/d; however, optimal treatment dose and duration continue to be researched. One study showed promising results in patients treated for up to 3 years.[41] Tocopherol in doses greater than 400 IU/d (some studies used 400 IU, some 700 IU, and some 1000 IU) has also shown promise in the treatment of radiation fibrosis, although increased all-cause mortality has also been noted with similar doses. Tocopherol is thought to scavenge radical oxygen species and decrease platelet aggregation, nitric oxide, and superoxide production in macrophages and neutrophils.[41] The combination of pentoxifylline and tocopherol has been established as safe and potentially effective in the treatment of radiation fibrosis.[41] Hyperbaric oxygen therapy has also been theorized to be effective for radiation fibrosis by stimulating angiogenesis and reducing fibroblast proliferation and tissue edema; however, small case series have reported mixed results.[41]

Chest Wall Pain

Chest wall pain in postmastectomy patients can be related to a multitude of potential causes. Pain over incision sites is a common complaint of patients with breast cancer. A study by Skov and colleagues[47] noted that 35% of women developed incisional pain after mastectomy, with 92% of these women noting that incisional pain developed within the first 3 months. This pain seems to lessen with time; in the same study, only 23% of those who had initially complained of incisional pain still had persistent discomfort, and both intensity and duration of pain had diminished as well. Pain is often due to a hypomobile incision that has adhered to the underlying chest wall. Painful scars can be treated with soft tissue mobilization and scar tissue release with a physical or occupational therapist. Silicone gel sheeting, triamcinolone cream or injection, or laser treatments may also be helpful adjuncts. If these methods are ineffective, the patient may choose to undergo elective scar resection.

Neuroma

Neuroma formation is another cause that can contribute to PMPS. It is hypothesized that this pain originates from the T4 and T5 intercostal sensory cutaneous branches that arise from the chest wall and enter the breast along with a blood vessel. These branches are often cut and cauterized during mastectomy and can cause burning, shooting pain, and point tenderness at the midaxillary line or at the inframammary fold directly inferior to the nipple.[48] Patients may benefit from nerve-stabilizing medications or desensitization techniques in physical or occupational therapy. If these methods are ineffective, perineural infiltration of these neuromas with a combination of anesthetic and corticosteroid has emerged in recent literature as a safe and potentially effective treatment. In one study, a small sample of 19 patients was treated with injections of 0.5% bupivacaine and 4 mg/mL dexamethasone at the point of maximal tenderness. All but 1 of the patients experienced relief after injection, with pain levels on the visual analogue scale decreasing from 8 to 9 to 0 to 1. Most patients required only 1 injection; however, 7 patients required 2 injections, and 1 patient required 3 injections to achieve long-term relief.[46] Ultrasound guidance can be considered for these injections to increase safety.

Postreconstruction pain syndrome

Postreconstruction pain syndrome is a term that some use (coined by Dr Michael Stubblefield) to describe a constellation of symptoms, similar to PMPS, in patients undergoing breast reconstruction, whether autologous or with implants. Pain often presents as tightness and spasm of chest wall muscles, typically the pectoralis muscles, serratus anterior, and latissimus dorsi. Studies have shown that patients with breast cancer undergoing reconstruction have pain more frequently than those without reconstruction.[49] One small case series demonstrated efficacy of botulinum toxin into the pectoralis major in patients with persistent chest wall muscular pain after breast reconstruction.[50] The authors encourage use of ultrasound guidance for these injections, especially in the setting of any underlying implant. If the implant is punctured by a needle, the results can be catastrophic and may require open surgery to replace the implant. One must also bear in mind that those undergoing 2-stage reconstruction with placement of an implant after radiation therapy develop higher rates of acute and chronic complications, including capsular contracture, as well as poorer aesthetic outcomes due to the nature of the irradiated tissue.[51]

After diagnosis via appropriate workup and imaging, several palliative treatment options have been proposed for this type of pain, including intercostal and paravertebral nerve blockade, intercostal neurolysis, serratus plane block, and thoracic nerve pulse radiofrequency ablation. For intractable cases, an intrathecal pump delivering opioid and local anesthetic may be placed in the midthoracic region after a successful screening trial has established efficacy in terms of pain relief.[52]

Axillary Web Syndrome

Axillary web syndrome, or cording, is a common phenomenon. Axillary web syndrome has been attributed to sclerosis or thrombosis of axillary lymphatics and/or veins. The syndrome can cause discomfort in the axilla and can result in decreased shoulder range of motion. The natural history is spontaneous resolution, and they may even "pop," which can be alarming to the patient, but not a cause for clinical concern. Patients should be counseled that cords may pop, so as to decrease alarm if this does occur. Resolution may be hastened by manual therapy techniques by a physical or occupational therapist.[53]

Other Musculoskeletal Pain Generators

Breast cancer survivors may experience pain from musculoskeletal structures of the neck, shoulder, chest wall, or axilla that are commonly affected irrespective of cancer treatment (**Box 4**). The causes may include cervical radiculopathy, cervical facet

---

Box 4
Postmastectomy pain syndrome diagnostic subgroups

- Rotator cuff abnormality
- Intercostobrachial neuralgia
- Chest wall pain (neuroma, postreconstruction pain, incisional pain)
- Axillary web syndrome (cording)
- Phantom breast pain
- Other musculoskeletal pain

---

arthropathy, myofascial pain syndrome, bicipital tendinopathy, shoulder osteoarthrosis, and adhesive capsulitis, among others. A recently published study demonstrated common regions for myofascial tenderness and hypersensitivity, including the upper trapezius and pectoralis major insertion.[54] A sensible rehabilitation prescription can help reduce or eliminate pain due to these anatomic structures. In addition, injections can be helpful adjuncts including trigger point injections, glenohumeral injections, bicipital tendon injections, and others, depending on the anatomic trigger of pain.

TREATMENTS FOR POSTMASTECTOMY PAIN SYNDROME
Rehabilitation

Rehabilitation protocols for patients with PMPS are highly variable. Rehabilitation prescriptions should be individualized. Four core techniques are hypothesized to be beneficial in the functional rehabilitation of PMPS: (1) restore joint mobility and prevent tendon shortening with passive mobilization techniques; (2) reduce pain with myofascial release and sustained trigger point compression; (3) address tight muscles, such as the pectoral group, with manual stretching and transverse strain; (4) strengthen shoulder girdle muscles with active and/or active-assisted mobilization.[55] A recent systematic review of these core modalities demonstrated that a multimodal approach, involving stretching and active exercises, was useful for the treatment of breast cancer pain and impaired range of motion in the upper limb. It also suggested that high-quality studies are needed to determine the effectiveness of passive mobilization, stretching, and myofascial therapy.[49] Physical and occupational therapists may benefit from attending breast cancer courses to become more comfortable with specific manual techniques.

Postmastectomy rehabilitation can usually be started in the first week after surgery, or once drains have been removed and the patient has received clearance from the surgical team. This rehabilitation includes using the affected limb to perform activities of daily living as well as gentle range-of-motion exercises. Patients can begin lifting 1- to 2-pound weights within 4 to 6 weeks postoperatively.[50] Of note, there are other evidence-based precautions during the rehabilitation of postmastectomy patients. It is important to maintain appropriate skin hygiene and avoid gross trauma to the limb and breast. Thermal therapy, laser treatment, microwave, and electrical stimulation are not recommended due to insufficient evidence supporting their use in this population.[56]

The safety of modalities among cancer populations has been controversial and requires weighing the risks and benefits in discussion with the patient's care team. A survivor's rehabilitation program should be individualized to target abnormalities noted on examination. This frequently includes scapular stabilization exercises, stretches for the chest wall muscles, and postural activities to optimize alignment.

In addition to the functional rehabilitation of the patient, a broader, multifactorial approach should be considered involving diverse health care disciplines as well as the patient and their caregivers. The authors propose that the rehabilitation team include representation from breast surgery, radiation oncology, medical oncology, physiatry, physical therapy, occupational therapy, speech and language pathology (if patient has cognitive symptoms), psychology, and social work. However, the authors recognize that these disciplines are rarely colocated outside of tertiary centers. In theory, an encompassed and collaborative approach ensures that all parties are attuned to patients' needs, allowing for the early detection and treatment of impairments.

Pharmacologic

Overall, there is a dearth of high-quality research demonstrating the efficacy of medications in the treatment of PMPS. One study noted greater relief of neuropathic PMPS with venlafaxine than placebo.[57] A retrospective review of 89 patients found improvement in neuropathic PMPS in 80% of patients on gabapentin.[58] In a small study, 8 of 15 patients treated with amitriptyline for neuropathic PMPS experienced greater than 50% pain reduction. A similarly small study of capsaicin demonstrated 5 of 13 patients experiencing greater than 50% pain relief. A randomized trial of 28 patients treated with topical lidocaine patches showed no difference between the lidocaine patch and the placebo patch.[59] Given the low-quality and limited evidence, research is needed to rigorously assess pharmacologic treatments for PMPS.

Nonpharmacologic

Transcutaneous electrical nerve stimulation (TENS) is a commonly used modality in the treatment of somatic and neuropathic pain. One study comparing TENS to a placebo treatment demonstrated no significant improvement over placebo for patients with PMPS.[60] Acupuncture has been studied in patients in the acute postoperative period after mastectomy. Patients receiving acupuncture reported reduced pain levels and improved range of motion compared with usual care during the acute postoperative period.[61]

PREVENTION OF POSTMASTECTOMY PAIN SYNDROME

Because chronic pain can develop following routine surgery, many perioperative interventions have been studied in an attempt to minimize postoperative pain and prevent the development of chronic pain.[62] Because the development of acute postoperative pain is a risk factor for chronic PMPS, perioperative pain has been targeted as a remediable contributor. Traditionally, perioperative pain management has focused on nonsteroidals, regional analgesia, and opiates, which may undertreat acute neuropathic pain.[63] Neuropathic medications that have been studied perioperatively include gabapentin, antidepressants, ketamine, N-methyl-D-aspartate (NMDA) antagonists, and local anesthetics. One Cochrane Review of the prevention of chronic pain across a spectrum of surgical procedures identified 40 randomized controlled trials (RCTs) of various perioperative pharmacologic interventions. Meta-analysis suggested a statistically significant reduction in chronic pain following treatment only with ketamine.[64] Several studies have looked at the utility of paravertebral blocks during mastectomy. Although paravertebral blocks have been established as safe and efficacious in reducing acute postoperative pain, their effect on chronic pain is unclear.[65,66] In one study, patients were treated with venlafaxine 37.5 mg/d versus gabapentin 300 mg/d versus placebo for 10 days starting the night before breast surgery. Although both medications reduced postoperative pain, only venlafaxine significantly reduced the incidence of postmastectomy pain at 6 months.[67] In another prospective study, venlafaxine 75 mg for 2 weeks beginning the evening before mastectomy with ALND was found to be effective in reducing pain in the chest wall and axilla at 6 months when compared with patients treated with placebo.[68]

Two studies evaluated gabapentin at differing doses, 1200 mg and 600 mg, perioperatively and found reduced postoperative pain and morphine requirements, although the trials did not demonstrate any long-lasting pain control.[69,70] One RCT examined the NMDA receptor antagonist amantadine in the perioperative setting. No differences were noted between the intervention and placebo group at 1, 3, and 6 months.[71]

One area of interest has been intraoperative preservation of the intercostobrachial nerve to decrease postoperative and chronic pain. Studies to date have been inconclusive. Two studies showed reduced sensory deficit but no difference in dysthesthesia, paresthesia, and shoulder pain.[72–74] For this reason, there is a lack of consensus among breast surgeons regarding the utility of intercostobrachial nerve preservation.

Psychological interventions offer techniques for coping with acute pain, and relaxation training and counseling to reduce distress. Identifying key risk factors such as catastrophizing and intervening early may prevent the development of chronic pain, although this has not been studied. Understandably, patients with breast cancer experience anxiety and depression; however, patients with higher levels of mood symptoms may be at higher risk of PMPS. For this reason, early screening followed by rapid treatment with psychological interventions, including pharmacologic agents or psychotherapy, offers the potential to improve outcomes.

SUMMARY

Postmastectomy pain is a common, debilitating complication of breast cancer treatment. Future study is warranted regarding prevention techniques, rehabilitation protocols, and pharmacologic and nonpharmacologic treatments. This review identifies specific, common anatomic generators of PMPS and guides clinicians in diagnosing the causes of pain and developing a sensible and specific treatment plan. Using this approach, clinicians will not only treat the pain but also treat its cause.[75] It is critical that patients with breast cancer undergo appropriate workup to identify remediable causes, before resigning the patient to a long-term analgesic regimen. An anatomic problem that can potentially be fixed should not be reflexively treated with chronic opioids. Patients with breast cancer deserve preservation of their function and quality of life as well as optimal cancer treatment.

REFERENCES

1. DeSantis C, Fedewa S, Sauer A, et al. Breast cancer statistics, 2015: convergence of incidence rates between black and white women. CA Cancer J Clin 2016;66:31–42.
2. Siegel R, Naishadham D, Jemal A. Cancer statistics 2013. CA Cancer J Clin 2013;63(1):11.
3. DeSantis C, Ma J, Bryan L, et al. Breast cancer statistics, 2013. CA Cancer J Clin 2014;64(1):52–62.
4. Beyaz SG, Ergönenç J, Ergönenç T, et al. Postmastectomy pain: a cross-sectional study of prevalence, pain characteristics, and effects on quality of life. Chin Med J 2016;129:66–71.
5. Mascaro A, Farina M, Gigli R, et al. Recent advances in the surgical care of breast cancer patients. World J Surg Oncol 2010;8:5.

6. Rahman GA. Breast conserving therapy: a surgical technique where little can mean more. J Surg Tech Case Rep 2011;3(1):1–4.

7. Stubblefield MD, O'Dell MW. Cancer rehabilitation, vol. 8. New York: Demos Medical Publishing; 2009. p. 105–13.

8. Cody HS, Borgen PI. State-of-the-art approaches to sentinel node biopsy for breast cancer: study design, patient selection, technique, and quality control at Memorial Sloan-Kettering Cancer Center. Surg Oncol 1999;8:85–91.

9. Macdonald L, Bruce J, Scott NW, et al. Long-term follow-up of breast cancer survivors with post-mastectomy pain syndrome. Br J Cancer 2005;92(2):225–30.

10. Gartner R, Jensen MB, Nielsen J, et al. Prevalence of and factors associated with persistent pain following breast cancer surgery. JAMA 2009;302(18):1985–92.

11. Vecht CJ, Van de Brand HJ, Wajer OJ. Post-axillary dissection pain in breast cancer due to a lesion of the intercostobrachial nerve. Pain 1989;38(2):171.

12. Wong L. Intercostal neuromas: a treatable cause of postoperative breast surgery pain. Ann Plast Surg 2001;46(5):481.

13. Meijuan Y, Zhiyou P, Yuwen T, et al. A retrospective study of postmastectomy pain syndrome: incidence, characteristics, risk factors, and influence on quality of life. ScientificWorldJournal 2013;2013:159732.

14. Wood K. Intercostobrachial nerve entrapment syndrome. South Med J 1978;71: 662–3.

15. Vilholm OJ, Cold S, Rasmussen L, et al. The postmastectomy pain syndrome: an epidemiological study on the prevalence of chronic pain after surgery for breast cancer. Br J Cancer 2008;99:604–10.

16. Belfer I, Schreiber KL, Shaffer JR, et al. Persistent postmastectomy pain in breast cancer survivors: analysis of clinical, demographic, and psychosocial factors. J Pain 2013;14(10):1185–95.

17. McCredie MRE, Dite GS, Porter L, et al. Prevalence of self-reported arm morbidity following treatment for breast cancer in the Australian Breast Cancer Family Study. Breast 2001;10(6):515–22.

18. Jung B, Ahrendt GM, Oaklander AL, et al. Neuropathic pain following breast cancer surgery: proposed classification and research update. Pain 2003;104:1–13.

19. Rosso R, Scelsi M, Carnevali L. Granular cell traumatic neuroma: a lesion occurring in mastectomy scars. Arch Pathol Lab Med 2000;124:709–11.

20. Wallace AM, Wallace MS. Postmastectomy and postthoracotomy pain. Anesth Clin North Am 1997;15:353–70.

21. Miguel R, Kuhn AM, Shons AR, et al. The effect of sentinel node selective axillary lymphadenectomy on the incidence of postmastectomy pain syndrome. Cancer Control 2001;8(5):427–30.

22. Stubblefield MD, Custodio CM. Upper-extremity pain disorders in breast cancer. Arch Phys Med Rehabil 2006;87(3 Suppl 1):S96–9.

23. Rietman JS, Dijkstra PU, Debreczeni R, et al. Impairments, disabilities and health related quality of life after treatment for breast cancer: a follow-up study 2.7 years after surgery. Disabil Rehabil 2004;26(2):78.

24. Tasmuth T, Kataja M, Blomqvist C, et al. Treatment-related factors predisposing to chronic pain in patients with breast cancer–a multivariate approach. Acta Oncol 1997;36(6):625.

25. Ip HYV, Abrishami A, Peng PWH, et al. Predictors of postoperative pain and analgesic consumption: a qualitative systematic review. Anesthesiology 2009;111(3): 657–77.

26. Fecho K, Miller NR, Merritt SA, et al. Acute and persistent postoperative pain after breast surgery. Pain Med 2009;10(4):708–15.

27. Steegers MA, Wolters B, Evers AW, et al. Effect of axillary lymph node dissection on prevalence and intensity of chronic and phantom pain after breast cancer surgery. J Pain 2008;9(9):813–22.
28. Miaskowski C, Paul SM, Cooper B, et al. Identification of patient subgroups and risk factors for persistent arm/shoulder pain following breast cancer surgery. Eur J Oncol Nurs 2014;18(3):242–53.
29. Kudel I, Edwards RR, Kozachik S, et al. Predictors and consequences of multiple persistent postmastectomy pains. J Pain Symptom Manage 2007;34(6):619–27.
30. Schreiber KL, Martel MO, Shnol H, et al. Persistent pain in postmastectomy patients: comparison of psychophysical, medical, surgical, and psychosocial characteristics between patients with and without pain. Pain 2013;154(5):660–8.
31. Tasmuth T, von Smitten K, Hietanen P, et al. Pain and other symptoms after different treatment modalities of breast cancer. Ann Oncol 1995;6(5):453.
32. Burgess C, Cornelius V, Love S, et al. Depression and anxiety in women with early breast cancer: five year observational cohort study. BMJ 2005;330(7493):702.
33. Blunt C, Schmiedel A. Some cases of severe post-mastectomy pain syndrome may be caused by an axillary haematoma. Pain 2004;108(3):294–6.
34. Campbell KL, Pusic AL, Zucker DS, et al. A prospective model of care for breast cancer rehabilitation: function. Cancer 2012;118(S8):2300–11.
35. Shamley D, Srinaganathan R, Oskrochi R, et al. Three-dimensional scapulothoracic motion following treatment for breast cancer. Breast Cancer Res Treat 2009; 118(2):315–22.
36. Stubblefield MD, Keole N. Upper body pain and functional disorders in patients with breast cancer. PM R 2014;6(2):170–83.
37. Levangie PK, Drouin J. Magnitude of late effects of breast cancer treatments on shoulder function: a systematic review. Breast Cancer Res Treat 2009;116(1): 1–15.
38. Jang D-H, Kim MW, Oh SJ, et al. The influence of arm swelling duration on shoulder pathology in breast cancer patients with lymphedema. PLoS One 2015; 10(11):e0142950.
39. Jeong HJ, Sim YJ, Hwang KH, et al. Causes of shoulder pain in women with breast cancer-related lymphedema: a pilot study. Yonsei Med J 2011;52(4): 661–7.
40. Herrera JE, Stubblefield MD. Rotator cuff tendonitis in lymphedema: a retrospective case series. Arch Phys Med Rehabil 2004;85(12):1939–42.
41. Wisotzky E, Saini V, Kao C. Ultrasound-guided intercostobrachial nerve block for intercostobrachial neuralgia in breast cancer patients: a case series. PM R 2015; 8(3):273–7.
42. Stubblefield MD, Levine A, Custodio CM, et al. The role of botulinum toxin type A in the radiation fibrosis syndrome: a preliminary report. Arch Phys Med Rehabil 2008;89(3):417–21.
43. Delanian S, Lefaix JL. Current management for late normal tissue injury: radiation-induced fibrosis and necrosis. Semin Radiat Oncol 2007;17(2):99–107.
44. Portlock CS, Boland P, Hays AP, et al. Nemaline myopathy: a possible late complication of Hodgkin's disease therapy. Hum Pathol 2003;34:816–8.
45. Yi A, Kim HH, Shin HJ, et al. Radiation-induced complications after breast cancer radiation therapy: a pictorial review of multimodality imaging findings. Korean J Radiol 2009;10(5):496–507.
46. Stubblefield MD. Radiation fibrosis syndrome: neuromuscular and musculoskeletal complications in cancer survivors. PM R 2011;3(11):1041–54.

47. Skov J, Krøner K, Krebs B, et al. Pain and dysesthesias in the mastectomy scar. Ugeskr Laeger 1990;152(42):3081–4.
48. Tang CJ, Elder SE, Lee DJ, et al. 2013 San Antonio Breast Cancer Symposium Abstract P3-10-03. Presented December 12, 2013.
49. Wallace MS, Wallace AM, Lee J, et al. Pain after breast surgery: a survey of 282 women. Pain 1996;66(2–3):195–205.
50. O'Donnell CJ. Pectoral muscle spasms after mastectomy successfully treated with botulinum toxin injections. PM R 2011;3(8):781–2.
51. Kronowitz SJ, Robb GL. Radiation therapy and breast reconstruction: a critical review of the literature. Plast Reconstr Surg 2009;124(2):395–408.
52. Gulati A, Shah R, Puttanniah V, et al. A retrospective review and treatment paradigm of interventional therapies for patients suffering from intractable thoracic chest wall pain in the oncologic population. Pain Med 2015;16(4):802–10.
53. Fourie WJ, Robb KA. Physiotherapy management of axillary web syndrome following breast cancer treatment: discussing the use of soft tissue techniques. Physiotherapy 2009;95(4):314–20.
54. Caro-Morán E, Fernández-Lao C, Díaz-Rodríguez L, et al. Pressure pain sensitivity maps of the neck-shoulder region in breast cancer survivors. Pain Med 2016 [pii: pnw064]; [Epub ahead of print].
55. De Groef A, Van Kampen M, Dieltjens E, et al. Effectiveness of postoperative physical therapy for upper-limb impairments after breast cancer treatment: a systematic review. Arch Phys Med Rehabil 2015;96(6):1140–53.
56. Harris SR, Schmitz KH, Campbell KL, et al. Clinical practice guidelines for breast cancer rehabilitation. Cancer 2012;118(S8):2312–24.
57. Tasmuth T, Härtel B, Kalso E. Venlafaxine in neuropathic pain following treatment of breast cancer. Eur J Pain 2002;6(1):17–24.
58. De Miguel-Jimeno JM, Forner-Cordero I, Zabalza-Azparren M, et al. Postmastectomy pain syndrome in our region: characteristics, treatment, and experience with gabapentin. Rev Neurol 2016;62(6):258–66 [in Spanish].
59. Cheville AL, Sloan JA, Northfelt DW, et al. Use of a lidocaine patch in the management of postsurgical neuropathic pain in patients with cancer: a phase III double-blind crossover study (N01CB). Support Care Cancer 2009;17(4):451–60.
60. Robb KA, Newham DJ, Williams J. Transcutaneous electrical nerve stimulation vs. transcutaneous spinal electroanalgesia for chronic pain associated with breast cancer treatments. J Pain Symptom Manage 2007;33(4):410–9.
61. He JP, Friedrich M, Ertan AK, et al. Pain-relief and movement improvement by acupuncture after ablation and axillary lymphadenectomy in patients with mammary cancer. Clin Exp Obstet Gynecol 1998;26(2):81–4.
62. Kehlet H, Jensen TS, Woolf CJ. Persistent postsurgical pain: risk factors and prevention. Lancet 2006;367(9522):1618–25.
63. Humble SR, Dalton AJ, Li L. A systematic review of therapeutic interventions to reduce acute and chronic post-surgical pain after amputation, thoracotomy or mastectomy. Eur J Pain 2015;19(4):451–65.
64. Chaparro LE, Smith SA, Moore RA, et al. Pharmacotherapy for the prevention of chronic pain after surgery in adults. Cochrane Database Syst Rev 2013;(7):CD008307.
65. Karmakar MK, Samy W, Li JW, et al. Thoracic paravertebral block and its effects on chronic pain and health-related quality of life after modified radical mastectomy. Reg Anesth Pain Med 2014;39(4):289–98.

66. Aufforth R, Jain J, Morreale J, et al. Paravertebral blocks in breast cancer surgery: is there a difference in postoperative pain, nausea, and vomiting? Ann Surg Oncol 2012;19(2):548–52.
67. Amr YM, Yousef AA. Evaluation of efficacy of the perioperative administration of venlafaxine or gabapentin on acute and chronic postmastectomy pain. Clin J Pain 2010;26(5):381–5.
68. Reuben SS, Makari-Judson G, Lurie SD. Evaluation of efficacy of the perioperative administration of venlafaxine XR in the prevention of postmastectomy pain syndrome. J Pain Symptom Manage 2004;27(2):133.
69. Grover VK, Mathew PJ, Yaddanapudi S, et al. A single dose of preoperative gabapentin for pain reduction and requirement of morphine after total mastectomy and axillary dissection: randomized placebo-controlled double-blind trial. J Postgrad Med 2009;55(4):257–60.
70. Fassoulaki A, Patris K, Sarantopoulos C, et al. The analgesic effect of gabapentin and mexiletine after breast surgery for cancer. Anesth Analg 2002;95(4):985–91.
71. Eisenberg E, Pud D, Koltun L, et al. Effect of early administration of the N-Methyl-D-aspartate receptor antagonist amantadine on the development of postmastectomy pain syndrome: a prospective pilot study. J Pain 2007;8(3):223–9.
72. Taira N, Shimozuma K, Ohsumi S, et al. Impact of preservation of the intercostobrachial nerve during axillary dissection on sensory change and health-related quality of life 2 years after breast cancer surgery. Breast Cancer 2014;21(2):183–90.
73. Freeman SRM, Washington SJ, Pritchard T, et al. Long term results of a randomised prospective study of preservation of the intercostobrachial nerve. Eur J Surg Oncol 2003;29(3):213–5.
74. Salmon RJ, Ansquer Y, Asselain B. Preservation versus section of intercostalbrachial nerve (IBN) in axillary dissection for breast cancer–a prospective randomized trial. Eur J Surg Oncol 1998;24(3):158–61.
75. Haig A, Grabois M. Chronic pain: cure it first, treat it second. PM R 2015;7(11):S324–5.

Rehabilitation Strategies and Outcomes of the Sarcoma Patient

Sean Robinson Smith, MD

KEYWORDS

- Sarcoma rehabilitation • Amputee rehabilitation • Cancer rehabilitation
- Desmoid rehabilitation • MPNST rehabilitation

KEY POINTS

- This familiarizes the reader with some of the sarcoma subtypes associated with loss of function, although nearly all sarcomas have deleterious potential in this regard.
- Outcomes of some of the treatment plans for lower extremity sarcoma are discussed at length; this gives an idea of the types of long-term management required, as well as what to expect from certain procedures (amputation vs limb salvage).
- Multidisciplinary approaches to rehabilitation is important, and with sarcoma it is not a "one-size-fits-all" approach due to the considerable variability in disease presentation.

INTRODUCTION

Sarcomas are tumors of mesenchymal cells that represent approximately 1% of all cancers. There are more than 70 different subtypes of this rare malignancy, each with different pathologic, molecular, and clinical features, and approximately 50% of people diagnosed with a sarcoma will die of the disease.[1] Sarcomas may arise from tissues such as bone, muscle, nerve sheaths, cartilage, or fat, making their presence potentially disruptive to the neuromusculoskeletal system and patient function. For the purposes of this article, sarcoma subtypes most likely to be associated with functional impairment are discussed, although numerous other sarcoma subtypes may have an impact on function, depending on their location, how aggressive the tumor is, and oncologic treatment rendered.

OVERVIEW

Sarcomas may manifest in different areas of the body; soft tissue sarcomas are most often located in an extremity (45%), whereas sarcomas of the bone are more likely to

Disclosure Statement: The author has no relevant financial or commercial interests to disclose. Institutional review board approval number: HUM00093618.
Department of Physical Medicine & Rehabilitation, University of Michigan, 325 East Eisenhower Parkway, Suite 100, Ann Arbor, MI 48108, USA
E-mail address: srsz@med.umich.edu

manifest in the distal femur (osteosarcoma) or the pelvis/sacrum (Ewing sarcoma).[2] The most common site of metastasis is the lung,[3] where diffuse and/or large metastatic disease may cause complications like pneumothorax or decreased volume and therefore aerobic capacity. Oncologic treatment varies depending on subtype, but typically involves a combination of surgery, chemotherapy, and radiation. Many chemotherapeutic agents used to treat sarcoma, especially bony sarcomas, are associated with increased risk of chemotherapy-induced peripheral neuropathy, such as cisplatin, which is used for osteosarcoma, and vincristine, often used for Ewing sarcoma. Doxorubicin, an anthracycline chemotherapeutic agent commonly used to treat soft tissue and bony sarcomas, does not typically cause neuropathy but is cardiotoxic and thus may have deleterious long-term effects for survivors of the disease.

Like nearly all cancers, treatment for sarcoma is determined after discussion with a multidisciplinary tumor board, in which physiatrists can play an important role. Physiatric involvement in the multidisciplinary tumor board may help with surgical decision making (amputation vs limb salvage, for example) by predicting limb and overall functional outcome with each approach. Additionally, being a part of diagnostic and treatment-planning discussions familiarizes the physiatrist with the patient; this is especially important given the considerable variation in the clinical picture of each patient with sarcoma.[4]

LOWER EXTREMITY AMPUTATION, LIMB SALVAGE, AND ROTATIONPLASTY

Sarcomas commonly affecting extremities include soft tissue sarcomas originating from skeletal muscle or fat, and bony sarcomas. Bony sarcomas are rare, but typically involve the lower extremity and include osteosarcoma and Ewing sarcoma. Chondromas require oncologic treatment similar to bony sarcomas and originate from cartilage. In the case of disease with few or no known metastases, local control with limb salvage or amputation is undertaken, each with advantages and disadvantages in terms of function and cosmesis, but with no significant differences in overall survival.[5,6] The choice of amputation versus limb salvage can be a difficult one; limb salvage is often preferred for cosmetic reasons and patients may return to independent function earlier than those undergoing amputation. Patients who opt for amputation often do so if they wish to participate in higher-impact activities including sports; patients with lower extremity limb salvage cannot participate in activities involving repetitive or heavy weightbearing or endurance exercises, such as running, whereas someone with lower extremity limb loss may be able to participate in higher-level athletic endeavors with appropriate prosthetic restoration.

Despite activity restrictions, studies have shown a benefit in function with limb salvage versus amputation. An analysis of 118 patients followed for 1 year after either lower extremity limb salvage (57%) or amputation (43%) found that patients with limb salvage had higher physical function by 1 of the 2 measurement tools used, with a more proximal amputation and presence of pain predicting lower performance. Quality of life as measured by the Short Form-36, and employment status, were equal between the groups, as was one patient-reported measure of function.[7] Another study looked at 91 adolescent and young adult patients after lower extremity sarcoma surgery, and found that patients with limb salvage again had higher Musculoskeletal Tumor Society rating scale (MSTS) scores, and that patients with rotationplasty had the overall highest function.[8] Limb salvage has also been shown to be superior to amputation specifically with regard to stair climbing.[9] Overall, limb salvage may provide a benefit in terms of everyday function, but patients who undergo amputation have similar quality of life and with prosthetic restoration have the potential to perform more physically intense activities, such as running. Given that many patients with sarcoma facing the option of limb salvage versus amputation are young and presumably in good physical shape, amputation may be preferable if a more active lifestyle is sought.

Patients undergoing limb salvage surgery may require multiple reconstructive surgeries or re-resections for local recurrence, whereas amputation is often definitive. With the advent of sophisticated external limb prostheses, patients may begin to opt for amputation more often in the future. Relative contraindications to limb salvage are tumor involvement of neurovascular structures, immature skeletal age, infection, difficulty of soft tissue reconstruction, inability to obtain sufficient tumor margins, and pathologic fracture.

Many patients requiring amputation undergo a transfemoral amputation due to disease involvement of the proximal tibia or knee joint. The residual limb may be irregular due to the tumor shape and associated bony changes, necessitating a custom rolling liner over the limb and flexible inner prosthetic liner to accommodate the shape and limb volume changes.[10] Younger patients requiring a transfemoral amputation may opt for rotationplasty, a procedure that attaches the distal lower extremity to the femur, rotates the foot, and uses the ankle to essentially replace the knee (**Fig. 1**). This provides a longer residual limb and functional joint, but is not common due to

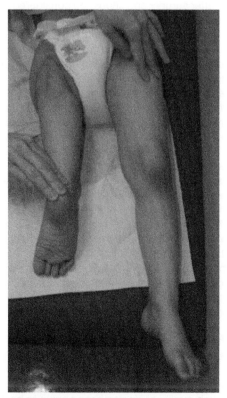

Fig. 1. A child sarcoma survivor after a rotationplasty procedure. (*From* Zachar M, Burke G, Spires MT. Prosthetic restoration and rehabilitation of the upper and lower extremity. Demos Publishing; 2013; with permission.)

complications including de-rotation, abnormal cosmesis, challenges with prosthetic fitting, and future leg length discrepancy because the growth plates may remain intact. Despite this, long-term follow-up studies have shown good outcomes in patients after rotationplasty, with leg length discrepancy and degenerative changes in the residual limb's foot contributing to lower performance.[11]

After recording a thorough history of oncologic treatment to date, clinical evaluation of the patient with sarcoma with limb salvage or patient with sarcoma treated with amputation should include an assessment for skin breakdown, signs of neuropathic or phantom limb pain (potentially worsened by chemotherapy), and musculoskeletal pain and dysfunction that may arise from limb-length disparities and altered gait mechanics. Peripheral edema and decreased reported aerobic capacity may be signs of cardiotoxicity from anthracycline administration.

In addition to a complete history and physical examination, evaluation of patients after treatment for lower extremity sarcoma should consist of one or both of the MSTS[12] and the Toronto Extremity Salvage Score (TESS)[13] questionnaires. The MSTS looks at pain, function, and emotional acceptance for both upper and lower extremity amputees. It also evaluates hand positioning, dexterity, and lifting ability specifically for upper extremity patients, and the use of supports, ability to walk, and gait quality for lower extremity patients. The TESS is a patient-reported questionnaire asking 29 (upper extremity) or 30 (lower extremity) questions regarding everyday activities. The questions are scored 1 to 5, with 5 being the maximum. Both assessment tools measure function after surgery and should be considered as outcome measures for both clinical care and research.

Rehabilitation after limb salvage should emphasize restoration of range of motion, and strengthening muscles surrounding the resected area. Patients who undergo lower extremity limb salvage procedures are typically restricted from activities such as running and jumping, but are permitted to walk, swim, and do other low-impact activities. Typically, there are no specific limitations on activity duration. Gait is invariably altered in these patients, and one analysis of 20 patients with limb salvage treated for intra-articular knee sarcomas were found to have abnormally prolonged contraction of the quadriceps and hamstring muscles 1 year postoperative, even on the unaffected limb.[14] For patients in whom bone must be resected, or who have a fracture and still undergo limb salvage, an endoprosthesis may implanted. These massive metallic prostheses, sometimes referred to as megaprostheses, may be customized to each patient and sometimes replace the entire femur (**Fig. 2**). A megaprosthesis may be able to handle loads of up to 800 lb,[15] but are at risk for structural failure[16] and still limit function, especially if the surrounding tissue was radiated and fibrosis develops. One study found that regardless of the lower extremity endoprosthesis type, patients had difficulty performing tasks requiring knee flexion and had quadriceps atrophy and restricted range of motion at the knee.[17] Outpatient rehabilitation emphasizing range of motion and strengthening, however, improves function after endoprosthethic reconstruction.[18] Despite the complex nature of the procedure, limb salvage operations were found to be overall less expensive over the long term compared with amputation.[19]

Reintegrating into the community after sarcoma surgery may be challenging,[20] but despite the differences in functional outcomes outlined previously, no long-term difference has been shown between sarcoma survivors with limb salvage, amputation, and rotationplasty with regard to quality of life, education level, marriage status, and employment,[16,21] although quality of life has been shown to be associated with functional level regardless of surgical approach.[22] For rotationplasty specifically, survivors older than 24 years had higher physical and psychosocial well-being than younger

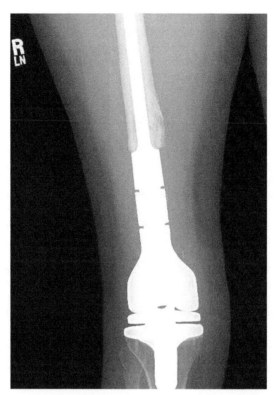

Fig. 2. Radiograph of a megaprosthesis replacing much of the right femur, knee joint, and proximal tibia.

patients, as measured by the SF-36, possibly due to having more time since the surgery to reintegrate into the community.[23]

Multidisciplinary rehabilitation can improve function in patients with sarcoma who undergo amputation.[24,25] Patients admitted for inpatient rehabilitation following sarcoma-related amputation tend to have less overall medical comorbidities than dysvascular amputees, as otherwise healthy people without medical comorbidities may develop sarcomas. Sarcoma-related amputees may tolerate prosthetic fitting much earlier due to good tissue healing, even immediately postoperative.[26]

Acute inpatient rehabilitation outcomes at the University of Michigan of 15 adults after lower extremity sarcoma–associated amputation between September 2010 and May 2014, published for the first time in this article, show that patients gained on average more than 16 Functional Independence Measure (FIM) points during their stay, at a clip of 2 points per day. Gains were primarily in motor scores, and the average length of stay was approximately 11 days. Most patients were discharged directly home, and most patients with above- or below-knee amputations were community ambulators with a prosthetic limb at 6 months postoperative. The average age of the cohort was 61, suggesting that younger patients were able to discharge home without inpatient rehabilitation. In contrast, dysvascular amputees, n = 136, admitted to the University of Michigan Acute Inpatient Rehabilitation unit during that period gained only 13 total, and 1.1 FIM points per day during an average length of stay of approximately 15 days. This suggests that patients with sarcoma may gain function more quickly than dysvascular amputees, possibly due to having fewer chronic comorbidities. Inferential statistical analysis could not be performed due to the vast difference in cohort size (15 sarcoma vs 136 dysvascular amputees). The data were for initial rehabilitation stays; patients re-admitted for various reasons were not included. See **Table 1** for full detail.

DESMOID TUMORS: SPACE-OCCUPYING BENIGN LESIONS

Desmoid tumors are sarcomas composed of spindle cells and that are rarely metastatic, but may be locally aggressive and difficult to treat. They typically appear in the abdominal wall, mesentery, or extremity and may cause focal muscle spasm, pain, and joint contracture.[27] (**Fig. 3**) Multiple, small desmoid tumors may also occur and affect different body parts, including the plantar fascia. Because of a high rate of recurrence, surgery is not typically performed unless the desmoid is near a vital structure, and oncologic treatment may consist of long-term anti-inflammatory medication, tyrosine kinase inhibitors, or aromatase inhibitors, the latter of which may cause significant pain.[28]

Given that patients have an unresectable mass that is causing pain, rehabilitation should be a standard component of patient care,[29] and must focus on maintaining or restoring function, alleviating muscle spasm, patient education to avoid injury, and addressing the psychosocial impact of the symptoms. Large rehabilitation studies

Table 1		
Outcomes of first-time acute inpatient rehabilitation for sarcoma-associated lower extremity amputation		
Variable	**Sarcoma**	**Dysvascular**
Number	15	136
Age	61.1	NR
Gender	10 m, 5 f	93 m, 43 f
LOS	10.9	15.3
Adm motor FIM	46.1	39.4
Adm cog FIM	30.6	28.5
DC motor FIM	59.2	51.1
DC cog FIM	33.8	29.8
FIM gain (total)	16.3	13.0
FIM eff	2.0	1.1
Amputation level	1 BKA 7 AKA 7 HD	NR
Discharge location	12 Home 2 SAR 1 Medical	NR
Community BKA/AKA prosthetic use		
At 3 mo	3/8	NR
At 6 mo	5/8	NR

Abbreviaitons: Adm, admission; AKA, above-knee amputation; BKA, below-knee amputation; cog, cognitive; DC, discharge; eff, efficiency; f, female; FIM, functional independence measure score; HD, hip disarticulation; m, male; Medical, acute medical service; NR, not recorded; SAR, subacute rehabilitation.

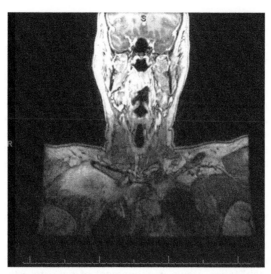

Fig. 3. Coronal MRI of a desmoid tumor in the right anterior chest wall.

have not been conducted given the rarity and variability of the disease, but case reports and small studies have shown benefit with nerve-stabilizing agents[30] and botulinum toxin injections[31] for the neuromuscular effects exerted by the desmoid via stretching surrounding tissue as it slowly grows. In this author's experience, a combination of gabapentin or pregabalin, botulinum toxin for localized pain, occasional opioids, and aggressive physical and/or occupational therapy are often required. Patients with well-controlled pain and optimal function should still be evaluated every 6 to 12 months given that the tumor will often grow over time.

MALIGNANT PERIPHERAL NERVE SHEATH TUMORS: DYNAMIC NEUROLOGIC DEFICITS

Malignant peripheral nerve sheath tumors (MPNST) are rare in the general population and more common in patients with neurofibromatosis type 1.[32] These are tumors within nerve sheaths and may cause pain, weakness, numbness, and tingling along the distribution of the nerve on which they originate. As they grow, they may compress vital structures including the spinal cord for MPNSTs that arise proximally. MPNSTs are most often found in the lower extremity, including the sciatic nerve, and are typically treated with surgical resection with or without adjuvant radiation therapy. Damage to the nerve from the tumor itself, surgery, or radiation can cause debilitating pain and weakness. In the case of radiation-induced nerve injury, symptoms may progress over time, necessitating ongoing surveillance of the patient's pain and function.

Physiatrists should play a vital role in the care of these patients, as management often requires neuropathic pain control, orthotic and assistive device prescription, and strengthening programs. Patients often have multiple MPNSTs at a time, with multiple areas of pain and weakness. The clinical picture is a dynamic one, as neurologic deficits tend to progress as the disease or damage from radiation advances. For large MPNSTs, amputation may be required.

SURVIVORSHIP CONSIDERATIONS

Much of the existing sarcoma-related survivorship research pertains to patients after lower extremity surgery and is described previously. Other important considerations include aerobic capacity and physical activity level in patients who received anthracy-cline chemotherapy, radiation fibrosis in patients treated definitively with limb salvage and radiation therapy and who may develop contractures years later, and the transi-tion of care as childhood survivors become adults. In addition to primary care pro-viders, physiatric collaboration with CardioOncology may be important.

Sarcoma survivorship clinics are becoming increasingly common and provide an opportunity for physiatric involvement.[33] Patients should be made aware of the possible late effects of the treatment they received, sometimes several years earlier, and multidisciplinary services to treat the physical, cognitive, and psychosocial defi-cits they may face should be made available. Survivorship Care Plans and clinics pro-vide an opportunity to educate patients about these long-term issues.

SUMMARY

Sarcomas are rare tumors and are typically only managed in large volumes at major academic medical centers. Nevertheless, as experts in neuromusculoskeletal anat-omy and comprehensive approaches to improving patient function, physiatrists are uniquely suited to manage the often-complex sarcoma-associated morbidity. As the field of cancer rehabilitation grows, management of patients with sarcoma should be considered an essential component of practice.

REFERENCES

1. Singer S, Tap WD, Crago AM, et al. Soft tissue sarcoma. In: DeVita V, Lawrence T, Rosenberg S, editors. Cancer: principles and practice of oncology. 10th edition. Wolters Kluwer Health; 2015. p. 1253–91. Print.
2. Wold LE, Unni KK, Sim FH, et al. Atlas oforthopedic pathology. Philadelphia: Saunders; 2008. p. 179.
3. Heare T, Hensley MA, Dell'Orfano S. Bone tumors: osteosarcoma and Ewing's sarcoma. Curr Opin Pediatr 2009;21(3):365–72.
4. Siegel G, Biermann JS, Chugh R, et al. The multidisciplinary management of bone and soft tissue sarcoma: an essential organizational framework. J Multidiscip Healthc 2015;8:109–15.
5. Rougraff BT, Simon MA, Kniesl JS, et al. Limb salvage compared with amputation for osteosarcoma of the distal end of the femur. A long-term oncological, func-tional, and quality-of-life study. J Bone Joint Surg Am 1994;76:649–56.
6. Kong C-B, Song WS, Cho WH, et al. Local recurrence has only a small effect on survival in high-risk extremity osteosarcoma. Clin Orthop Relat Res 2011;470(5): 1482–90.
7. Aksnes LH, Bauer HCF, Jebsen NL, et al. Limb-sparing surgery preserves more function than amputation: a Scandinavian sarcoma group study of 118 patients. J Bone Joint Surg Br 2008;90(6):786–94.
8. Ginsberg JP, Rai SN, Carlson CA, et al. A comparative analysis of functional out-comes in adolescents and young adults with lower-extremity bone sarcoma. Pe-diatr Blood Cancer 2006;49(7):964–9.
9. Bekkering WP, Vlieland TPV, Koopman HM, et al. Functional ability and physical activity in children and young adults after limb-salvage or ablative surgery for lower extremity bone tumors. J Surg Oncol 2011;103(3):276–82.
10. O'Donnell RJ, DuBois SG, Haas-Kogan, DA. Sarcomas of bone. In: DeVita V, Lawrence T, Rosenberg S, et al, editors. DeVita, Hellman, and Rosenberg's Can-cer principles & practice of oncology. 10th edition; 2014. p. 1292–313.

11. Benedetti MG, Okita Y, Recubini E, et al. How much clinical and functional impairment do children treated with knee rotationplasty experience in adulthood? Clin Orthop Relat Res 2016;474(4):995–1004.
12. Enneking WF, Dunham W, Gebhardt MC, et al. A system for the functional evaluation of reconstructive procedures after surgical treatment of tumors of the musculoskeletal system. Clin Orthop Relat Res 1993;(286):241–6.
13. Davis AM, Wright JG, Williams JI, et al. Development of a measure of physical function for patients with bone and soft tissue sarcoma. Qual Life Res 1996; 5(5):508–16.
14. Carty CP, Bennett MB, Dickinson IC, et al. Electromyographic assessment of gait function following limb salvage procedures for bone sarcoma. J Electromyogr Kinesiol 2010;20(3):502–7.
15. Bini SA, Johnston JO, Martin DL. Compliant prestress fixation in tumor prostheses: interface retrieval data. Orthopedics 2000;23:707–11.
16. Henderson ER, Groundland JS, Pala E, et al. Failure mode classification for tumor endoprostheses: retrospective review of five institutions and a literature review. J Bone Joint Surg Am 2011;93:418–29.
17. Carty CP, Dickinson IC, Watts MC, et al. Impairment and disability following limb salvage procedures for bone sarcoma. Knee 2009;16(5):405–8.
18. Lopresti M, Rancati J, Farina E, et al. Rehabilitation pathway after knee arthroplasty with mega prosthesis in osteosarcoma. Recenti Prog Med 2015;106(8): 385–92 [in Italian].
19. Grimer RJ, Carter SR, Pynsent PB. The cost-effectiveness of limb salvage for bone tumours. J Bone Joint Surg Br 1997;79(4):558–61.
20. Parsons JA, Eakin JM, Bell RS, et al. "So, are you back to work yet?" Reconceptualizing 'work' and 'return to work' in the context of primary bone cancer. Soc Sci Med 2008;67(11):1826–36.
21. Nagarajan R, Neglia JP, Clohisy DR, et al. Education, employment, insurance, and marital status among 694 survivors of pediatric lower extremity bone tumors: a report from the childhood cancer survivor study. Cancer 2003;97(10):2554–64.
22. Robert RS, Ottaviani G, Huh WW, et al. Psychosocial and functional outcomes in long-term survivors of osteosarcoma: a comparison of limb-salvage surgery and amputation. Pediatr Blood Cancer 2010;54:990–9.
23. Forni C, Gaudenzi N, Zoli M, et al. Living with rotationplasty: quality of life in rotationplasty patients from childhood to adulthood. J Surg Oncol 2012;105(4): 331–6.
24. Kauzlarić N, Kauzlarić K, Kolundžić R. Prosthetic rehabilitation of persons with lower limb amputations due to tumour. Eur J Cancer Care 2007;16(3):238–43.
25. Punzalan M, Hyden G. The role of physical therapy and occupational therapy in the rehabilitation of pediatric and adolescent patients with osteosarcoma. Cancer Treat Res 2009;152:367–84.
26. Folsom D, King T, Rubin JR. Lower-extremity amputation with immediate postoperative prosthetic placement. Am J Surg 1992;164(4):320–2.
27. Fong Y, Rosen PP, Brennan MF. Multifocal desmoids. Surgery 1993;114:902–6.
28. Henry NL, Giles JT, Ang D, et al. Prospective characterization of musculoskeletal symptoms in early stage breast cancer patients treated with aromatase inhibitors. Breast Cancer Res Treat 2007;111(2):365–72.
29. Ghert M, Yao X, Corbett T, et al. Treatment and follow-up strategies in desmoid tumours: a practice guideline. Curr Oncol 2014;21(4):e642–9.
30. Mathew D, Jeba J, George R, et al. Neuropathic pain due to fibromatosis: does anticancer treatment help? Indian J Palliat Care 2011;17(3):245–7.

31. Fusaro I, Orsini S, Bellenghi C, et al. Treatment of scapula dyskinesia with botulin toxin: two case reports. Musculoskelet Surg 2010;94(Suppl 1):S95–8.
32. Evans DGR. Malignant peripheral nerve sheath tumours in neurofibromatosis 1. J Med Genet 2002;39(5):311–4.
33. Smith SR, Reish AG, Andrews C. Cancer survivorship: a growing role for physiatric care. PM R 2015;7(5):527–31.

Alternative Exercise Traditions in Cancer Rehabilitation

Kathryn J. Ruddy, MD, MPH[a], Daniela L. Stan, MD[b],
Anjali Bhagra, MBBS[b], Mary Jurisson, MD[c],
Andrea L. Cheville, MD, MSCE[c],*

KEYWORDS

- Cancer • Rehabilitation • Alternative exercise traditions

KEY POINTS

- Cancer survivors are physically and mentally vulnerable because of the emotional strain caused by a cancer diagnosis and the physical and mental side effects of oncologic therapies.
- Alternative exercise traditions (AETs) offer the potential to improve diverse outcomes among cancer survivors by reducing adverse symptoms and mood disorders, and by enhancing function.
- AETs' affordability and accessibility, as well as their capacity to simultaneously span social, physical, and psycho-emotional domains may address deficits in current disease-focused care delivery models.
- Despite AETs' many benefits, clinician enthusiasm may be low due to extensive heterogeneity across and within AETs, limited individualization, and inconsistent instructor/practitioner expertise.
- Systematic reviews and meta-analyses have concluded that AETs have beneficial effects among cancer populations but consistently identify a high risk of bias in most trials.

INTRODUCTION

Alternative exercise traditions (AETs), such as Pilates, yoga, Tai Chi Chuan, Qigong, and various forms of dance, have been extensively promoted as methods of rehabilitation after cancer treatment. There are compelling reasons for this trend, as the putative and empirical benefits of these traditions are extensive. However, many remain

[a] Department of Oncology, Mayo Clinic, 200 First Street, SW, Rochester, MN 55905, USA;
[b] Department of General Internal Medicine, Mayo Clinic, 200 First Street, SW, Rochester, MN 55905, USA; [c] Department of Physical Medicine and Rehabilitation, Mayo Clinic, 200 First Street, SW, Rochester, MN 55905, USA
* Corresponding author.
E-mail address: Cheville.andrea@mayo.edu

Phys Med Rehabil Clin N Am 28 (2017) 181–192
http://dx.doi.org/10.1016/j.pmr.2016.08.002
1047-9651/17/© 2016 Elsevier Inc. All rights reserved.

underresearched, and the attributes assumed to mediate their beneficial effects inadequately specified. Clinicians face the challenge of directing motivated and inquisitive survivors in their efforts to negotiate a dynamic landscape of staggering diversity. This article outlines the needs of cancer survivors that may be addressed through AETs, the pros and cons of common AETs, the current supportive evidence, and how clinicians may help survivors to identify beneficial and safe AETs.

HOW ALTERNATIVE EXERCISE TRADITIONS CAN BENEFIT CANCER POPULATIONS

Cancer survivors are physically and mentally vulnerable because of the emotional strain caused by a cancer diagnosis and the physical and mental side effects of oncologic therapies. Arduous treatments, such as surgery, chemotherapy, and radiation, often cause a variety of symptoms that can interfere with functioning and cause distress. Strong associations have been reported between functional degradation and specific symptoms, including fatigue, sleep disturbance, hormonally induced symptoms, and mood disorders.[1,2] In fact, reports suggest that symptoms, in concert with accumulated mild impairments, are the primary drivers of cancer-associated disablement. Although some survivors recover quickly from treatment toxicities, others suffer treatment-related symptoms for years, and some never fully recover.

Physical toxicities that can be long-lasting and have substantial impact on quality of life (QOL) include (but are not limited to) (1) lymphedema, often caused by surgery and/or radiation; (2) neuropathy, caused by certain types of chemotherapy (eg, the taxanes and platinums that are used to treat many solid tumors, most medications used for multiple myeloma, and the plant alkaloids that are active against many hematologic cancers as well as solid tumors); (3) fatigue, common after nearly all types of cancer treatments; (4) hot flashes and arthralgias, which can be caused by antiestrogen therapies and by chemotherapy-related ovarian damage; and (5) biomechanical dysfunction.

Lymphedema is a chronic condition that affects more than 10% of breast cancer survivors, and also can be problematic after treatment for skin, gynecologic, urologic, colorectal, and head and neck cancers.[3] Neuropathy frequently causes longstanding numbness and tingling in survivors.[4] In one study, severe neuropathy was present in 19% of recipients of standard doses of oxaliplatin 18 months after treatment for colorectal cancer. In another study, severe neuropathy of the hands was reported by 27% of breast cancer survivors 6 to 24 months after paclitaxel-based chemotherapy, and severe neuropathy of the feet was reported by 25%.[5] Fatigue also is a major issue after cancer treatment. A study of 1294 breast, prostate, and colorectal cancer survivors found that 29% reported significant fatigue (defined as having FACT-F [Functional Assessment of Cancer Therapy: Fatigue] scores $\leq$34), and fatigue was associated with more physical symptom burden, depression, comorbidity, and disability.[6] Furthermore, hot flashes and arthralgias are both bothersome in more than a quarter of the hundreds of thousands of breast cancer survivors who are taking endocrine therapy in the United States currently.[7]

Sleep disturbances, anxiety, and depression are common in cancer survivors as well.[8] One recent study showed that 39% of breast cancer survivors and 25% of prostate cancer survivors suffered insomnia 18 months after a curative surgery.[9] In another study, 21% of adult cancer survivors were anxious and 13% were depressed 1 year after a cancer diagnosis.[10] Depression was more likely in those with insufficient physical activity, possibly reflecting bidirectional causality. In addition, depression and anxiety can both cause sleep disturbances, and many other symptoms (including pain due to local cancer therapies or chemotherapy-induced peripheral neuropathy) can contribute to both insomnia and depression.

In addition to engendering symptoms, cancer therapies also can focally disrupt the biomechanics of discrete body parts or whole segments leading to compromised strength, flexibility, and coordination.[11,12] Surgery, in addition to removing or reorganizing anatomy, may result in lasting soft tissue contractures and may blunt or distort afferent sensory information. Patients' recovery from cancer surgeries is frequently interrupted by the initiation of chemotherapy and/or radiation therapy within weeks after their operations. The sequence and timing of anticancer therapies has been dictated by their impact on progression-free and overall survival rather than their potential to disable. Radiation alone or after surgery may incite progressive fibrosis; that is, scarification of connective tissues, and may contribute to the denervation of functionally vital muscle groups.[13,14]

Unfortunately, biomechanical dysfunction, lymphedema, neuropathy, fatigue, hot flashes, insomnia, anxiety, and depression are difficult to treat, and all may substantially impair daily functioning and QOL. Better management strategies are needed for long-term physical toxicities and emotional distress in cancer survivors. Improvements in dynamic posture, isometric strengthening, flexibility, kinesthetic awareness, and balance may help improve physical and mental health in cancer survivors. These health benefits may be particularly important for those suffering QOL impairments due to long-term treatment toxicities. In addition, for certain cancers (eg, breast cancer and colorectal cancer), some data suggest that physical activity reduces risk of recurrence.[15–17]

ALTERNATIVE EXERCISE TRADITIONS MAY BE AN ACCESSIBLE MEANS OF ADDRESSING FUNCTION-DEGRADING SYMPTOMS AND IMPAIRMENTS

Current health care delivery models, with their disproportionate emphasis on disease management, either neglect function-degrading symptoms or promote referrals to multiple specialists. The former is clearly unsatisfactory, and the latter approach is costly, not patient-centric, disjointed, and often ineffective in realizing the lasting behavioral changes that are required for functional restoration and symptom control. The consequences of our current system's shortcomings are not trivial, as they contribute to the well-characterized persistence of symptoms and impairments among cancer survivors that degrade their ability to resume gainful employment and reengage in defining life roles.[18]

AETs have emerged as a potential means to address the deficits in current delivery models. These traditions have a number of characteristics that positively distinguish them from allopathic delivery mechanisms. Perhaps most notable are accessibility and affordability. Allopathic delivery has been shaped by fee-for-service reimbursement, which generally requires 1:1 visits with certified, licensed practitioners. Such visits are expensive, exceeding out-of-pocket affordability for many survivors. Both commercial and federal payers have endeavored to contain costs by capping the number of clinic visits, as is now common with physical therapy (PT). Most AETs, in contrast, are delivered via group classes or 1:1 lessons priced to attract even patients with middle to low socioeconomic status. Additionally, many health clubs, including local YMCAs and employer-sponsored work site gyms, now offer AET classes. Free-standing dance and yoga studios are common in even small to mid-sized towns.

An additional distinguishing feature of AETs is their potential to simultaneously address needs spanning multiple domains, including social, physical, and psycho-emotional. The social support and community that develops naturally in many group classes counters the feelings of isolation that are experienced by many cancer survivors.[18] The mindfulness dimension of yoga, Tai Chi, and chi gong has been shown to relieve stress, dysphoria, and anxiety in some cancer populations.[19] From a physical impairment perspective, AETs offer the salient benefits of promoting integrated whole body movement and concurrently enhancing strength, coordination, balance, posture, and flexibility. Last, many survivors grapple with the somewhat paradoxic drives to do everything possible to prevent recurrence or progression of their cancer and to concurrently demedicalize their lives. Many AETs normalize rather than pathologize the sequelae of cancer and its treatment by focusing on balance, wellness, and vitality.

From a more concrete and biomechanical viewpoint, AETs also offer unique benefits relative to conventional therapeutic exercise. The aforementioned benefit of concurrently addressing strength, coordination, posture, and flexibility that characterizes most AETs also promotes the subtler and arguably more essential attribute of kinesthetic awareness. Almost without exception, cancer survivors' bodies have been altered by treatment, generally in ways that undermine their ability to maintain adaptive biomechanics for static and dynamic body positioning. The underlying mechanisms are complex and beyond the scope of this article. In brief, afferent input to the central nervous system (CNS) may become attenuated or distorted, thereby undermining proprioception and the more rostral CNS mechanisms that maintain posture and healthy biomechanics. As a consequence, survivors may lose the ability to recognize when muscle groups fatigue, and begin to use compensatory, potentially maladaptive, motor patterns to complete an activity.

AETs often incorporate several strategies that enhance kinesthetic awareness. First, many begin with simple, supported movements that become progressively more complex. This is true of ballet, which progresses from barre to floor work, and from isolated, rudimentary to full-body, integrated movements. The progression allows practitioners to work on sustaining postural alignment before having to negotiate balance and 3-dimensional movement. Second, the mindfulness or conscious awareness of body emphasized by many AETs helps practitioners to increase their sensibility of adaptive versus aberrant body positioning. With practice, as their sensibility grows, participants consciously and, eventually, subconsciously correct themselves. Third, many AETs have developed well-delineated strategies that allow new practitioners to become sensitized to when their body is properly versus improperly aligned. Iyengar yoga is an exemplar in this regard, as it makes extensive use of "props," for example, ropes, blocks, and bolsters, to enable practitioners to experience optimal positioning even when they may lack the strength and flexibility to maintain it independently. Last, many AETs are performed with mirrors, and even videotaping, to provide visual feedback that supplements an instructor's corrections and a practitioner's inherent sense of proper body positioning. Dance studios invariably have mirrors on more than 1 full wall to promote visually guided self-correction. Once students learn what proper alignment and biomechanics look like, they can begin the process of internalizing what they feel like. The intent is that practitioners will eventually become independent of the visual "crutch" of the mirror so that they can consciously, based on sensation alone, self-correct their posture and movement pattern.

CURRENT LIMITATIONS TO THE CLINICAL INTEGRATION OF ALTERNATIVE EXERCISE TRADITIONS

Why are all cancer survivors not systematically directed to AETs? One obstacle is the extensive heterogeneity across and even within AETs. Yoga, for example, may involve the passive and supported maintenance of static reclining postures, as in restorative

Iyengar yoga, or the profoundly strenuous and dynamic movements of Ashtanga yoga. The potential benefits and harms of these 2 extremes of the yogic spectrum differ radically. The variance of other AETs may not be as marked as yoga; however, physical intensity is but one source of heterogeneity.

An additional concern is that the one-size-fits-many nature of AET classes undermines an instructor's capacity to individualize dose, type, frequency, and intensity, which are cornerstones of effective therapeutic exercise. Reports increasingly indicate that specific parameters critically determine whether and to what extent an AET will affect a particular outcome, for example, function, QOL.[20] This evidence suggest that, to reliably benefit cancer survivors, AETs may require a degree of rigor comparable to the quantification that has become standard for medically directed aerobic training. Inconsistencies that have emerged in the relative capacity of different AETs to affect different outcomes argue strongly that their nonspecific prescription in the hope of general benefit or other similarly vague goals is inappropriate. As with any other therapeutic modality, discreet therapeutic targets should be defined and administration of the appropriate AET individualized to realize these goals.

Inconsistencies in AET practitioner expertise and certification, as well as the extent of practitioner familiarity with vulnerabilities unique to cancer populations, are also problematic. Some AETs are distinguished by highly structured, incremental training programs linked to rigorous certifications; however, these tend to be the exception. Iyengar yoga is an exemplar of such an approach. Instructors pursue a systemized training pathway divided into formal levels of expertise.

EVIDENCE IN CANCER

Most of the concerns regarding the pragmatic delivery of AETs are likely remediable through relatively inexpensive training and standardization approaches. However, such remediation would not be a trivial undertaking, and the allocated resources should be commensurate with the probability that standardized, high-quality AETs will improve key outcomes among cancer survivors. At this juncture, an extensive literature of inconsistent quality that spans diverse cancer populations frustrates efforts to precisely determine the effect size of any specific AET in improving a specific outcome. Details of delivery make a difference, and too often these are limitedly described. Perhaps most frustrating is the dearth of effort to accurately and consistently distinguish how AETs systematically differ from the exercise and movement approaches that are reimbursed by payers and well integrated into allopathic care pathways (eg, PT). The paragraphs that follow briefly describe and outline the current level of evidence of common AETs.

Qigong and Tai Chi

Qigong is a term that includes "Qi" interpreted as "energy" and "gong," which implies learning with attention and acquiring skill. Qigong then implies skillful cultivation of life energy in a movement-based, embodied contemplative practice. Qigong movement exercises can be part of a general program of health enhancement, a sport or martial art, such as Tai Chi, or a traditional Chinese medical treatment. Qigong aims to align the body, breath and mind in a holistic approach to nurture health and well-being. There are many kinds of breathing in Qigong practice that include concepts of chest and abdominal breathing, "fetal breathing," patterns of inhalation and exhalation, "anus lifting" or pelvic diaphragm breathing, and breathing during vocalization. Mind exercises cultivate focus and attention, tranquility and imagery in stillness, or during specific movements.

Qigong movement exercises can be prescribed for specific symptoms or may include a traditional set of movements such as "The Eight Pieces of Brocade," tones such as the "Six Healing Sounds," or patterns of self-administered massage, breath, or thought. Medical Qigong also can involve treatments by the practitioner, such as types of "external Qigong." Qigong exercise usually involves coordination of postures, movements, breath, intention, and environmental awareness. Exercises are suitable for diverse cancer populations as they may be performed lying, sitting, or standing, and be completely still, or slowly, abruptly, or explosively moving.

Tai Chi Chuan, the most well-known of the Chinese internal martial arts, refers to the balanced emergence of extreme opposites (yin and yang) from stillness or nothingness alluded to in the Tai Chi symbol. Tai Chi is also interpreted as "supreme/extreme ultimate." "Quan," or Chuan, refers to "fist" or fighting. So Tai Chi Chuan means "supreme ultimate fist/fighting" or "Yin-yang fighting." The traditional curriculum includes 3 main elements: still and moving exercises; practice of "form," a memorized sequence of movements with self-defense applications; and application of these forms in types of sparring or practice fighting referred to as "push hands."

Both Qigong and Tai Chi Chuan offer unique potential benefits for cancer survivors. Managing existential anxiety is a challenge both to those facing potentially fatal disease and those facing a personal physical attack. The physical requirements for the economical, adaptive movements of self-defense; postural control, flexibility, coordination, agility, strength, awareness, and quick reaction time; are also necessary for everyday life, particularly when living with cancer, and its treatments and effects. Qigong and Tai Chi Chuan are generally practiced in groups that promote socialization and feelings of connection. Some Qigong and Tai Chi practices are purported to promote a shift from sympathetic to parasympathetic dominance, similar to mindfulness practices, and are therefore sometimes referred to as "moving meditation."[21]

An extensive literature has accrued estimating the effect of Qigong and Tai Chi on diverse patient reported outcomes, including fatigue, pain, sleep quality, and QOL. As with other AETs, diversity of protocol specification, or a lack of precise specification, hampers the formulation of general conclusions regarding overall effectiveness. Additionally, efforts to address barriers to participation, namely length and complexity of curricula and a dearth of trained teachers, have produced simpler curricula for specific populations, with accelerated teacher certifications. This well-intentioned process may inadvertently lead to loss of critical elements of practice and should be considered when evaluating literature on effectiveness. Systematic reviews and meta-analyses have differed in their findings, with a recent meta-analysis concluding that Tai Chi and Qigong had no effect on the QOL of breast cancer survivors, although Tai Chi did improve their vital capacity.[22] Slightly earlier systematic reviews, with more restrictive inclusion criteria, concluded that Qigong/Tai Chi had positive effects on the QOL, fatigue, immune function, and cortisol levels of cancer survivors.[22,23] All 3 reports emphasized a high risk of bias in most trials related to a lack of blinding, poor allocation concealment, and incomplete outcome data.

Yoga

Yoga is the most scientifically studied and the most popular mind-body practice, with 9.5 million people practicing yoga in the United States in 2012,[23] although only 15% use it for a health condition. It consists of a series of postures (asanas) that are combined with a deep diaphragmatic breathing (pranayama) and meditative techniques, with the purpose of creating a union between the mind and the body.

Studies of yoga in cancer survivors have preponderantly involved survivors of breast cancer. Although systematic reviews and meta-analyses concluded that there was benefit from yoga for fatigue, distress, anxiety, depression, and QOL,[24–26] the evidence is weak due to the heterogeneous nature of the yoga interventions (type and dose), as well as the methodological flaws of the studies (eg, small sample sizes or the lack of an active control group). Small effect sizes for some of the outcomes in these studies could be attributed to the inclusion of asymptomatic patients (which might dilute a potential benefit).

The more contemporary studies of yoga in cancer survivors benefit from a stronger methodology: a trial of 410 cancer survivors with insomnia randomly assigned to 4 weeks of yoga versus standard of care demonstrated a significant improvement in sleep quality and a reduction in the use of sleep medications in the yoga group.[27] Another study of yoga versus stretching versus wait-list interventions in breast cancer survivors (n = 163) undergoing radiation therapy noted a significant improvement in the cancer-related fatigue in the yoga and the stretching groups compared with the wait-list group[27]; the physical component of QOL improved significantly in the yoga group compared with the other groups, whereas the mental component of QOL and the sleep quality did not differ between groups in this study. Yoga also was shown to improve cognitive function at 3 months after completion of a 12-week yoga intervention, as compared with a wait-list group.[28]

The caregivers of patients with cancer are also affected by distress, fatigue, insomnia, and a reduced QOL,[29,30] and they might benefit from yoga interventions.[31] In one study of patients with lung cancer and their caregivers undergoing Tibetan yoga therapy as a couple, there were benefits in the patients' spiritual well-being, benefit finding, sleep, and depressive symptoms, as well as significant improvement in the caregivers' fatigue and anxiety and a trend toward improvements in sleep.[32]

Yoga might be an alternative to more strenuous physical exercise routines in cancer survivors, especially for patients experiencing side effects of treatments, given its versatility and adaptability to each person's level of activity and mobility. Patients with fatigue or discomfort can perform a gentle yoga intervention, such as restorative yoga, whereas those looking for a fitness routine can choose from a variety of more physical forms, such as Ashtanga or hatha yoga. In addition, given the potential psychological and sleep benefits, yoga might be an ideal addition to an overall wellness plan for cancer survivors.

Pilates

The Pilates method, established in the 1920s by the German body builder Joseph Pilates, combines physical exercise with mind-body techniques inspired from yoga and martial arts, as well as from Zen meditation and the Greek and Roman philosophies of achieving mental and physical perfection.[33,34] Pilates coined the term "contrology," defined as the complete coordination of the mind and the body, and adopters of the Pilates method claim that it promotes total coordination and revitalization of the mind, body, and spirit. Pilates is performed usually on a mat, but chair Pilates on a special MVe fitness chair and Reformer Pilates on a spring apparatus are also popular. Although already a popular fitness method, with 8.5 million Americans practicing Pilates,[35] scientific evidence of benefit in disease states remains limited to patients suffering from musculoskeletal diseases, such as low back pain, ankylosing spondylitis, and scoliosis. The evidence of benefit in cancer is scarce, with only 2 randomized controlled trials (RCTs), both in breast cancer survivors. The study by Eyigor and colleagues[36] in Turkey randomized 52 breast cancer survivors post-mastectomy to Mat Pilates versus a home-exercise program, comparing their walking endurance, spine flexibility, fatigue, depression, and QOL. The Pilates method was superior to the home exercise only for the walking endurance. Another RCT assessing muscular endurance in 26 breast cancer survivors compared Pilates on the MVe Fitness Chair with traditional resistance training and a control group; this study found similar improvements in the muscle endurance for the 2 active groups, whereas the control group showed no change.[37]

Smaller uncontrolled pilot studies of Pilates Mat exercises in breast cancer survivors did show significant improvements in QOL and shoulder function.[38] One of these studies noted increased volumes of the limb on the operated side after the Pilates intervention, thus raising concerns that Pilates might contribute to lymphedema.[39]

Larger, randomized controlled studies are needed, preferably in symptomatic patients, before Pilates can be considered a safe and beneficial intervention for rehabilitation in cancer survivors. Further investigation into the potential risk for lymphedema is required, and consideration should be given to using modifications for the arm exercises in cancer survivors who have had axillary node surgery or radiation.

Dance Traditions

An extensive literature ranging from opinion pieces and small studies to systematic reviews suggest that dance in its many forms may improve cancer survivors' functional, psycho-emotional and social well-being, and may even reduce primary and secondary cancer risk.[40–43] Reports additionally suggest that dance may alleviate adverse cancer-related symptoms, such as anxiety and fatigue.[44,45] A challenge to interpreting the literature is the diversity of dance traditions and the heterogeneity of their participation requirements. For example, Dance/Movement Therapy (DMT) was developed as a therapeutic modality to address psycho-emotional, developmental, and physical problems.[46] This distinguishes DMT from social and couples dance forms, including folk, contra, swing, and square dance, that developed organically and include simple movements that can be easily learned. In contrast, performance dance forms, ballet, modern dance, belly dance, and flamenco, include far more complex and demanding movements that may take years to master. A barrier to interpreting the literature is the lack of an established taxonomy that distinguishes the social, physical, and psychological attributes of these different dance forms. Their defining characteristics may critically mediate dance's beneficial effects, and research is critically needed to develop more effective and targeted interventions.

The therapeutic dance literature specific to cancer is less marked by the common shortcomings of limited detail regarding instructor type and skill, instructional emphases, and distinctions between dance traditions. Several small studies found beneficial effects with DMT across multiple domains. For example, a small pilot study (n = 35) that compared The Lebed Method of DMT to wait-list control among breast cancer survivors found significant intergroup differences favoring the intervention with respect to shoulder range of motion, body image, and overall QOL as assessed with the FACT-B.[47] A similarly small (n = 49) study of a mindfulness-based DMT program among breast cancer survivors showed improved QOL via decreased fear of recurrence and increased mindfulness.[48] An additional DMT study was positive but provided insufficient detail for meaningful interpretation.[49] Despite these positive results, a recent systematic review from the Cochrane group concluded that DMT may have a beneficial effect solely on QOL, somatization, and vigor, and that there is insufficient evidence of DMT's effect on symptoms, mood, and body image.[50] Folk dance traditions also appear to offer similar potential benefits to cancer survivors spanning multiple domains. Two nonrandomized studies, one using Greek traditional dance (n = 27)[48] and a second using belly dance (n = 114),[51] detected significant improvements in physical function and mood.

Dance as therapy is distinguished by several additional characteristics that may enhance the well-being of specific cancer survivor subgroups. First, dance appeals to children and adolescent survivors.[52] However, the Bristol Girls Dance Study that randomized adolescents to an after-school dance intervention underpinned by self-determination theory found consenting participants had disproportionately high baseline activity levels. This suggests that additional targeting may be needed to successfully engage young sedentary survivors.[53] Second, dance has the potential to be culturally relevant to many ethnic subgroups, as most have established dance traditions. A study of Native Pacific and Hawaiian islanders found Hula dancing to be an effective means of increasing recreational activity levels among sedentary women.[54] Last, dance uses the body as an expressive and aesthetic medium, and, therefore, has been highlighted as a means to enhance survivors' body image.[52,55]

THE PHYSICIAN'S ROLE IN COUNSELING, DIRECTING, AND PRESCRIBING ALTERNATIVE EXERCISE TRADITIONS

Integrative oncology is both a science and a philosophy that focuses on the complex health of patients with cancer and proposes an array of approaches to accompany the conventional therapies to facilitate health and promote overall wellness in patients with cancer.[56] Many patients with cancer ask their oncology providers about complementary therapies that may improve their cancer-related prognoses or health-related QOL. Most oncologists feel comfortable recommending exercise, but the focus of this recommendation is often traditional exercise, such as walking or weight lifting. As data accumulate with regard to the mental and physical benefits of integrated or alternative exercise and dance traditions, it will be important to educate health care providers about what these entail and how to talk to patients about incorporating these practices into their comprehensive survivorship plans. Previous studies have shown that clinician counseling regarding smoking cessation and traditional exercise programs can have a positive impact on patient behavior,[16,57] so clinicians who inform patients about nontraditional ways to be active also may increase the likelihood that survivors will initiate and continue with these exercises.

Health care providers vary greatly in their receptivity to integrative therapies, likely related to their personal and professional experience with these practices. An evaluation of referral practices within an integrated practice network including medical doctors, chiropractors, and Complementary and Alternative Medicine (CAM) providers revealed that only 20% of the medical doctors were responsible for most of the referrals to integrative therapies, that there was a preference toward certain CAM providers (3 of them received almost half of the referrals) and that the most common CAM referrals were to acupuncture (>1000 visits), whereas homeopathy, osteopathy, massage therapy, and therapeutic yoga each had fewer than 100 visits.[58] These referral patterns were mostly driven by the patients (75%) rather than providers.

Additional research on the risks and benefits, optimal frequencies, and disease-related impacts will help inform these conversations.

REFERENCES

1. Cheville AL, Yost KJ, Larson DR, et al. Performance of an item response theory-based computer adaptive test in identifying functional decline. Arch Phys Med Rehabil 2012;93:1153–60.
2. Cheville AL, Dose AM, Basford JR, et al. Insights into the reluctance of patients with late-stage cancer to adopt exercise as a means to reduce their symptoms and improve their function. J Pain Symptom Manag 2012;44:84–94.

3. Paskett ED, Dean JA, Oliveri JM, et al. Cancer-related lymphedema risk factors, diagnosis, treatment, and impact: a review. J Clin Oncol 2012;30:3726–33.

4. Hershman DL, Lacchetti C, Dworkin RH, et al. Prevention and management of chemotherapy-induced peripheral neuropathy in survivors of adult cancers: American Society of Clinical Oncology clinical practice guideline. J Clin Oncol 2014;32:1941–67.

5. Hershman DL, Weimer LH, Wang A, et al. Association between patient reported outcomes and quantitative sensory tests for measuring long-term neurotoxicity in breast cancer survivors treated with adjuvant paclitaxel chemotherapy. Breast Cancer Res Treat 2011;125:767–74.

6. Jones JM, Olson K, Catton P, et al. Cancer-related fatigue and associated disability in post-treatment cancer survivors. J Cancer Surviv 2016;10:51–61.

7. Cella D, Fallowfield L, Barker P, et al. Quality of life of postmenopausal women in the ATAC ("Arimidex", tamoxifen, alone or in combination) trial after completion of 5 years' adjuvant treatment for early breast cancer. Breast Cancer Res Treat 2006;100:273–84.

8. Pachman DR, Barton DL, Swetz KM, et al. Troublesome symptoms in cancer survivors: fatigue, insomnia, neuropathy, and pain. J Clin Oncol 2012;30:3687–96.

9. Savard J, Ivers H, Savard MH, et al. Cancer treatments and their side effects are associated with aggravation of insomnia: results of a longitudinal study. Cancer 2015;121:1703–11.

10. Boyes AW, Girgis A, D'Este CA, et al. Prevalence and predictors of the short-term trajectory of anxiety and depression in the first year after a cancer diagnosis: a population-based longitudinal study. J Clin Oncol 2013;31:2724–9.

11. Shamley D, Lascurain-Aguirrebena I, Oskrochi R. Clinical anatomy of the shoulder after treatment for breast cancer. Clin Anat 2014;27:467–77.

12. Stubblefield MD, Keole N. Upper body pain and functional disorders in patients with breast cancer. PM R 2014;6:170–83.

13. Stubblefield MD. Radiation fibrosis syndrome: neuromuscular and musculoskeletal complications in cancer survivors. PM R 2011;3:1041–54.

14. Delanian S, Lefaix JL, Pradat PF. Radiation-induced neuropathy in cancer survivors. Radiother Oncol 2012;105:273–82.

15. Holmes MD, Chen WY, Feskanich D, et al. Physical activity and survival after breast cancer diagnosis. JAMA 2005;293:2479–86.

16. Pinto BM, Frierson GM, Rabin C, et al. Home-based physical activity intervention for breast cancer patients. J Clin Oncol 2005;23:3577–87.

17. Meyerhardt JA, Giovannucci EL, Holmes MD, et al. Physical activity and survival after colorectal cancer diagnosis. J Clin Oncol 2006;24:3527–34.

18. Bennion AE, Molassiotis A. Qualitative research into the symptom experiences of adult cancer patients after treatments: a systematic review and meta-synthesis. Support Care Cancer 2013;21:9–25.

19. Mackenzie MJ, Carlson LE, Ekkekakis P, et al. Affect and mindfulness as predictors of change in mood disturbance, stress symptoms, and quality of life in a community-based yoga program for cancer survivors. Evid Based Complement Alternat Med 2013;2013:419496.

20. Carayol M, Bernard P, Boiche J, et al. Psychological effect of exercise in women with breast cancer receiving adjuvant therapy: what is the optimal dose needed? Ann Oncol 2013;24:291–300.

21. Sun FL, Yan YA. Effects of various qigong breathing pattern on variability of heart rate. Zhongguo Zhong Xi Yi Jie He Za Zhi 1992;12:527–30, 516. [in Chinese].

22. Tao WW, Jiang H, Tao XM, et al. Effects of acupuncture, tuina, tai chi, qigong, and traditional Chinese medicine five-element music therapy on symptom management and quality of life for cancer patients: a meta-analysis. J pain symptom Manag 2016;51:728–47.

23. Use of complementary health approaches in the United States. Available at: https://nccih.nih.gov/research/statistics/NHIS/2012/mind-body. Accessed August 11, 2016.

24. Sadja J, Mills PJ. Effects of yoga interventions on fatigue in cancer patients and survivors: a systematic review of randomized controlled trials. Explore (NY) 2013; 9:232–43.

25. Buffart LM, van Uffelen JG, Riphagen II, et al. Physical and psychosocial benefits of yoga in cancer patients and survivors, a systematic review and meta-analysis of randomized controlled trials. BMC Cancer 2012;12:559.

26. Sharma M, Haider T, Knowlden AP. Yoga as an alternative and complementary treatment for cancer: a systematic review. J Altern Complement Med 2013;19: 870–5.

27. Mustian KM, Janelsins M, Peppone LJ, et al. Yoga for the treatment of insomnia among cancer patients: evidence, mechanisms of action, and clinical recommendations. Oncol Hematol Rev 2014;10:164–8.

28. Derry HM, Jaremka LM, Bennett JM, et al. Yoga and self-reported cognitive problems in breast cancer survivors: a randomized controlled trial. Psychooncology 2015;24:958–66.

29. Braun M, Mikulincer M, Rydall A, et al. Hidden morbidity in cancer: spouse caregivers. J Clin Oncol 2007;25:4829–34.

30. Swore Fletcher BA, Dodd MJ, Schumacher KL, et al. Symptom experience of family caregivers of patients with cancer. Oncol Nurs Forum 2008;35:E23–44.

31. Martin AC, Keats MR. The impact of yoga on quality of life and psychological distress in caregivers for patients with cancer. Oncol Nurs Forum 2014;41: 257–64.

32. Milbury K, Chaoul A, Engle R, et al. Couple-based Tibetan yoga program for lung cancer patients and their caregivers. Psychooncology 2015;24:117–20.

33. Levine B, Kaplanek B, Scafura D, et al. Rehabilitation after total hip and knee arthroplasty: a new regimen using Pilates training. Bull NYU Hosp Jt Dis 2007;65: 120–5.

34. Shand D. Pilates to pit. Lancet 2004;363:1340.

35. Available at: http://www.statista.com/statistics/191616/participants-in-pilates-training-in-the-us-since-2006/. Accessed August 11, 2016.

36. Eyigor S, Karapolat H, Yesil H, et al. Effects of Pilates exercises on functional capacity, flexibility, fatigue, depression and quality of life in female breast cancer patients: a randomized controlled study. Eur J Phys Rehabil Med 2010;46:481–7.

37. Martin E, Battaglini C, Groff D, et al. Improving muscular endurance with the MVe Fitness Chair in breast cancer survivors: a feasibility and efficacy study. J Sci Med Sport 2013;16:372–6.

38. Keays KS, Harris SR, Lucyshyn JM, et al. Effects of Pilates exercises on shoulder range of motion, pain, mood, and upper-extremity function in women living with breast cancer: a pilot study. Phys Ther 2008;88:494–510.

39. Stan DL, Rausch SM, Sundt K, et al. Pilates for breast cancer survivors. Clin J Oncol Nurs 2012;16:131–41.

40. Aktas G, Ogce F. Dance as a therapy for cancer prevention. Asian Pac J Cancer Prev 2005;6:408–11.

41. Whiteker JS. Flash mob dance: empowering survivors. Clin J Oncol Nurs 2010; 14:679–80.

42. Archer S, Buxton S, Sheffield D. The effect of creative psychological interventions on psychological outcomes for adult cancer patients: a systematic review of randomised controlled trials. Psychooncology 2015;24:1–10.

43. Butler M, Snook B, Buck R. The transformative potential of community dance for people with cancer. Qual Health Res 2015. [Epub ahead of print].

44. Sturm I, Baak J, Storek B, et al. Effect of dance on cancer-related fatigue and quality of life. Support Care Cancer 2014;22:2241–9.

45. Boehm K, Cramer H, Staroszynski T, et al. Arts therapies for anxiety, depression, and quality of life in breast cancer patients: a systematic review and meta-analysis. Evid Based Complement Alternat Med 2014;2014:103297.

46. Payne H. Introduction. In: Payne H, editor. Dance movement therapy; theory and practice. New York: Routledge; 1992. p. 1–17.

47. Sandel SL, Judge JO, Landry N, et al. Dance and movement program improves quality-of-life measures in breast cancer survivors. Cancer Nurs 2005;28:301–9.

48. Crane-Okada R, Kiger H, Sugerman F, et al. Mindful movement program for older breast cancer survivors: a pilot study. Cancer Nurs 2012;35:E1–13.

49. Mannheim EG, Helmes A, Weis J. Dance/movement therapy in oncological rehabilitation. Forsch Komplementarmed 2013;20:33–41 [in German].

50. Bradt J, Shim M, Goodill SW. Dance/movement therapy for improving psychological and physical outcomes in cancer patients. Cochrane Database Syst Rev 2015;(1):CD007103.

51. Szalai M, Levay B, Szirmai A, et al. A clinical study to assess the efficacy of belly dancing as a tool for rehabilitation in female patients with malignancies. Eur J Oncol Nurs 2015;19:60–5.

52. Cohen SO, Walco GA. Dance/movement therapy for children and adolescents with cancer. Cancer Pract 1999;7:34–42.

53. Jago R, Edwards MJ, Sebire SJ, et al. Bristol girls dance project: a cluster randomised controlled trial of an after-school dance programme to increase physical activity among 11- to 12-year-old girls. Public Health Res 2016;4(6).

54. Kaholokula JK, Look M, Mabellos T, et al. Cultural dance program improves hypertension management for native Hawaiians and Pacific islanders: a pilot randomized trial. J Racial Ethn Health Disparities 2015. [Epub ahead of print].

55. Ho RT, Lo PH, Luk MY. A good time to dance? A mixed-methods approach of the effects of dance movement therapy for breast cancer patients during and after radiotherapy. Cancer Nurs 2016;39:32–41.

56. Deng GE, Frenkel M, Cohen L, et al. Evidence-based clinical practice guidelines for integrative oncology: complementary therapies and botanicals. J Soc Integr Oncol 2009;7:85–120.

57. Schauer GL, Wheaton AG, Malarcher AM, et al. Health care provider screening and advice for smoking cessation among smokers with and without COPD: 2009-2010 National Adult Tobacco Survey. Chest 2016;149(3):676–84.

58. Coulter ID, Singh BB, Riley D, et al. Interprofessional referral patterns in an integrated medical system. J Manipulative Physiol Ther 2005;28:170–4.

Electrodiagnosis in Cancer Rehabilitation

Christian M. Custodio, MD[a,b,]*

KEYWORDS

- Electrodiagnosis • Radiculopathy • Plexopathy • Neuropathy
- Paraneoplastic syndrome • Cancer rehabiliation

KEY POINTS

- The patient with cancer is prone to peripheral nervous system injury at multiple anatomic levels.
- A wide variety of nerve injuries can be caused by cancer and its treatments, either by direct effects from tumors, cancer treatment effects, paraneoplastic effects, or indirect effects associated with cancer symptoms.
- Electrodiagnostic studies are an invaluable tool in the evaluation of neuromuscular disorders in the cancer patient population.

INTRODUCTION

Neuromuscular complications related to cancer are common. Cancer can directly affect the peripheral nervous system at any level via numerous mechanisms, including direct nerve compression or infiltration, hematogenous or lymphatic spread, meningeal dissemination, or perineural spread. Paraneoplastic syndromes often manifest with neuromuscular dysfunction, as can cancer-associated medical complications, such as infections, weight loss, or malnutrition. Acquired neuropathies can result from effects of cancer treatment itself, be it surgery, chemotherapy, radiation therapy, hematopoietic stem cell transplantation, or immunologic therapy. Patients may also have pre-existing neurologic conditions, such as diabetic or hereditary neuropathies, that can be exacerbated by cancer or its related treatments. Often, a combination of processes can be present.

Electrodiagnostic studies, including nerve conduction studies (NCS) and needle electromyography (EMG), are invaluable tools for assessing neuromuscular function

[a] Rehabilitation Medicine Service, Department of Neurology, Memorial Sloan Kettering Cancer Center, 1275 York Avenue, New York, NY 10065, USA; [b] Division of Rehabilitation Medicine, Weill Cornell Medicine, 525 East 68th Street, New York, NY 10065, USA
* Rehabilitation Medicine Service, Department of Neurology, Sillerman Center for Rehabilitation, Memorial Sloan Kettering Cancer Center, 515 Madison Avenue, 5th Floor, New York, NY 10022.
E-mail address: custodc1@mskcc.org

Phys Med Rehabil Clin N Am 28 (2017) 193–203
http://dx.doi.org/10.1016/j.pmr.2016.08.010
1047-9651/17/© 2016 Elsevier Inc. All rights reserved.

in patients with cancer. Electrodiagnosis can confirm a suspected neuropathic or myopathic process as well as rule out other possibilities. It can detect subclinical neuropathies, which can inform clinical decision making regarding use of neurotoxic chemotherapeutic agents. They can help with localizing lesions and determining pathophysiology, chronicity, and severity, which in turn can aid the cancer physiatrist in determining prognosis for recovery and the utility of future rehabilitation interventions. Finally, the information obtained with electrodiagnostic testing can help guide the oncology team with regards to surgery, chemotherapy, or radiation therapy planning.

Electrodiagnosis should be thought of as an extension of the history and physical examination, with the expected clinical and NCS/EMG findings dependent on the location, distribution, and pathophysiology of the neurologic lesion. Any and all levels of the peripheral nervous system can be affected by cancer and its treatments, including spinal roots, brachial or lumbosacral plexus, peripheral axons and/or myelin sheaths, the neuromuscular junction, and muscle fibers. Because of the variety of mechanisms of injury and wide scope of clinical presentation, the true incidence and prevalence of neuromuscular disorders in patients with cancer are unknown. However, it is estimated that approximately one-third of adult patients with chronic cancer pain, across all tumor types and stages, are thought to have cancer-related neuropathic pain.[1]

RADICULOPATHY

After disc disease and spinal stenosis, tumors involving the spine and spinal cord are the most common causes of radiculopathy.[2] All tumor types can metastasize to the spine, although the most common primary malignancies that do so include breast, lung, prostate, colon, thyroid, and kidney. Common primary malignant spinal tumors include multiple myeloma, plasmacytoma, and Ewing and osteogenic sarcoma. Single- or multilevel radiculopathies due to malignancy can result from primary or epidural metastatic tumor extension into the neural foramina. Leptomeningeal disease is due to metastatic involvement of the leptomeninges from infiltrating cancer cells, and involvement of the cauda equina can be thought of as a lumbosacral polyradiculopathy. The most common primary cancers associated with leptomeningeal disease are breast, lung, gastric, melanoma, lymphomas, and leukemias.[3] Of the leukemias, leptomeningeal disease is most commonly seen in acute lymphocytic leukemia.[4,5]

Patients can present with an asymmetric array of symptoms resulting from radicular or polyradicular involvement, including focal and radicular pain, areflexia, paresthesias, and lower motor neuron weakness. In leptomeningeal disease, there may be associated findings of nuchal rigidity as well as upper motor neuron signs, especially if there is concomitant brain involvement. Cranial nerves can be involved as well, with the oculomotor, facial, and auditory nerves most commonly affected.

In radiculopathies, sensory responses should be normal on NCS, because the location of involvement is proximal to the dorsal root ganglion, thereby making the segment of sensory nerve fibers tested metabolically and histologically intact. Motor responses within the affected myotomes may be normal or reduced in amplitude, depending on severity. Needle EMG is the most sensitive electrodiagnostic test for evaluation of a radiculopathy. One should record neuropathic abnormalities in at least 2 muscles innervated by different peripheral nerves but sharing the same root innervation, including increased insertional activity, fibrillation potentials, reduced recruitment, and large, polyphasic motor unit potentials (MUPs). Because paraspinal muscles are innervated by the dorsal primary rami, branching directly off of the nerve root, abnormal neuropathic EMG findings noted in the paraspinals further support the diagnosis of radiculopathy. Electrodiagnostic studies in leptomeningeal disease can sometimes be consistent with a polyradiculopathy, with preserved SNAPs and abnormal paraspinal needle EMG findings. Absent F waves or prolonged F-wave latencies on NCS are thought to be an early indicator of nerve root involvement, but are not specific for either radiculopathy or leptomeningeal disease.[6]

PLEXOPATHY

Brachial plexopathies from neoplasms are usually the result of metastatic disease, with breast and lung being the most common primary sources.[7] Symptoms include pain, paresthesias, numbness, and weakness in the distribution of plexus involvement. Metastases can involve any portion of the brachial plexus, but usually involve the lower trunk preferentially, because of its proximity to axillary lymph nodes and the superior sulcus of the lung. Neoplastic lumbosacral plexopathies can also stem from metastatic disease, but are much more likely to be caused by direct extension of local tumor or perineural spread.[8] Common tumors involved in lumbosacral plexus injury include colon, gynecologic tumors, lymphomas, and sarcomas.

The primary differential diagnostic concern in a patient with cancer with a plexus injury is distinguishing between a neoplastic and radiation-induced cause. Occasionally, the 2 conditions can coexist. Classically, radiation-induced plexopathy is delayed in onset, pain is less common than in neoplastic plexopathy, and symptoms of weakness and paresthesias are usually progressive.[9,10] There is also more likely to be associated lymphedema in the involved limb. It has been reported that neoplastic brachial plexopathy tends to preferentially affect the lower trunk, and radiation plexopathy tends to preferentially affect the upper portion of the plexus; however, further studies suggest that plexus involvement may be more diffuse and with more overlap in both causes than previously suspected.[11]

The distribution of motor and sensory nerve conduction abnormalities is important in the localization of both brachial and lumbosacral plexopathies. For instance, upper extremity NCS in a lower trunk brachial plexopathy will demonstrate a characteristic pattern of normal median sensory nerve action potential (SNAP) amplitudes, reduced ulnar SNAP amplitudes, and reduced median and ulnar compound muscle action potential (CMAP) amplitudes. Abnormalities will also be noted in the medial antebrachial cutaneous SNAP. Findings on needle EMG will demonstrate fibrillation potentials, reduced recruitment, and large, polyphasic MUPs within the distribution of involvement. Needle EMG of the paraspinal muscles is normal in a pure plexopathy; however, one often sees both root and plexus involvement in a given patient, depending on the extent of disease. Documenting asymmetric findings on NCS and needle EMG can sometimes help distinguish a newer onset radiculopathy or plexopathy in the setting of an underlying chemotherapy-induced polyneuropathy.

Approximately 50% of all patients with cancer will undergo radiation therapy at some point during the course of their disease, and radiation therapy is involved in approximately one-quarter of all cancer cures.[12] As patients are living longer following cancer treatments, physicians are becoming more aware of late neuromuscular complications of therapy, especially radiation therapy. Side effects are essentially related to the dose of radiation and the volume of normal tissue that receives radiation.[13]

The pathognomonic EMG finding of radiation-induced neuropathic damage is the myokymic discharges, which are clusters of MUPs firing spontaneously with regular interburst and intraburst frequencies. The absence of myokymic discharges however does not exclude radiation damage, and although the presence of myokymic discharges and fasciculation potentials confirms a radiation-induced contribution to plexus injury, it does not exclude the possibility of tumor involvement.[10] Even in the setting of classic EMG findings, follow-up imaging of the brachial plexus with MRI is warranted to exclude a concomitant compressive or infiltrating lesion, which could be due to local recurrence or new metastases. In a patient with a history of prior radiation therapy to the axillary or supraclavicular lymph nodes, secondary radiation-induced neoplasms such as sarcomas should also be considered.

MONONEUROPATHY

Focal mononeuropathies directly related to cancer most often result from the external compression or invasion from tumor, such as an isolated radial neuropathy caused by a primary osteogenic sarcoma or a bone metastasis involving the spiral groove of the humerus. Malignant nerve sheath tumors arising from plexiform neurofibromas can also result in focal mononeuropathies. The presence of secondary sarcomas compressing or infiltrating nervous system structures, resulting from previous radiation therapy, needs to be excluded. NCS and needle EMG should correspond to clinical abnormalities, limited to the distribution of the individual nerve, involving both sensory and motor fibers, depending on the composition of the particular nerve involved.

Although uncommon, damage to the peripheral nervous system during the perioperative period can occur in the surgical patient with cancer. Because the nature of these procedures is likely to be more complex than in nononcologic surgeries, it is postulated that the likelihood of neuromuscular complications is greater in oncologic surgeries. There are no studies, however, comparing the incidence of unintentional nerve injury in the cancer surgery population to that in the general population. In addition, peripheral nerves are sometimes intentionally sacrificed in the cancer surgery patient in order to obtain local disease control, especially the spinal accessory nerve to the trapezius in radical or modified neck dissection for head and neck malignancies or in limb-salvage surgery for extremity sarcomas. The pattern and extent of neurologic involvement following surgery depends on the location of the tumor, patient positioning during surgery, and the patient's overall preoperative status and propensity to nerve injury.[14]

Perioperative neurapraxic injuries, resulting from either compression or traction of peripheral nerves, are well-recognized phenomena. It is thought that these injuries result from the patient's position during anesthesia and surgery or during the immediate postsurgical recovery period.[15] Common sites of injury and associated surgical procedures include brachial plexus injury during thoracotomy or mastectomy, given the abducted position of the involved upper extremity. Abduction of the upper extremity greater than 90° during surgery can cause the humeral head to sublux inferiorly, resulting in compression of the lower part and traction of the upper part of the brachial plexus. Patients upon awakening report varying degrees of pain, weakness, and numbness in both the upper and the lower trunk distribution. Complete, spontaneous recovery within weeks is common, even in cases of severe plegia. Ulnar neuropathies at the elbow, resulting from arm boards used to secure intravenous lines, and radial neuropathies at the spiral groove, resulting from prolonged time in the lateral decubitus position, are also noted following thoracic surgery. Findings of focal slowing, temporal dispersion, or conduction block across the level of injury can be demonstrated on motor NCS.

Compression of the femoral nerve or lumbar plexus can result from traction during pelvic surgery. Patients undergoing hip arthroplasty or acetabular reconstruction are especially susceptible to injury of the peroneal division of the sciatic nerve. Injuries to the superior gluteal, obturator, and femoral nerves have also been reported.[16] A patient with cancer having undergone a significant amount of weight loss may be more susceptible to a perioperative peroneal neuropathy at the fibular head, resulting from positioning following a prolonged surgery and postoperative recovery period. Finally, delayed postoperative hemorrhages and hematomas should be excluded in all patients who develop new neuropathic symptoms 24 to 48 hours after surgery.

Rapid weight loss is a common symptom of malignancy, and thus, there is a higher risk of focal compression neuropathy, especially the peroneal nerve at the level of the fibular head. The peroneal nerve in that location is no longer protected by soft tissue and is more easily compressed against bony structures. A history of habitual leg crossing is sometimes elicited. Focal slowing, temporal dispersion, and conduction block across the fibular head on peroneal motor NCS are characteristic findings. There may be additional predisposition to injury given exposure to neurotoxic chemotherapy.

POLYNEUROPATHY

Chemotherapy-induced peripheral neuropathy is a well-described and well-recognized phenomenon and is the most common neuromuscular condition associated with cancer. Side effects tend to be dose dependent, although it is important to recognize pre-existing subclinical neuropathies or a family history of neuropathy, such as in the case of the hereditary sensory and motor neuropathies. The neurotoxic effects of chemotherapy in these susceptible patients can occur earlier than expected in the treatment course, and symptoms can be severe and permanently disabling.[17–19] Although almost all agents have been associated with neuropathies, there are a select number of chemotherapeutics that are especially prone to causing neuropathy. These chemotherapeutics notably are the vinca alkaloids, the taxanes, and the platinum-based compounds.

The vinca alkaloids, such as vincristine, vinblastine, and vinorelbine, are used in the treatment of solid tumors, lymphomas, and leukemias. They are usually given in combination with other chemotherapeutic agents. The mechanism of action with the vinca alkaloids is to arrest dividing cells in metaphase by binding tubulin and preventing its polymerization into microtubules. Abnormal tubulin binding is also the proposed mechanism of inducing neuropathy, by inhibiting anterograde and retrograde transport via microtubules and causing axonal Wallerian degeneration. Taxanes such as paclitaxel and docetaxel are also used to treat solid tumors such as breast and ovarian cancer. As in the vinca alkaloids, the taxane-induced neuropathy results from damage to the axonal microtubule system.[20] Bortezomib, used in the treatment of multiple myeloma, is also highly associated with an axonal peripheral neuropathy.

Chemotherapy-induced axonal neuropathy generally is characterized by subacute onset, length-dependent, symmetric, sensory greater than motor deficits. NCS reveal normal or low-amplitude CMAPs and low-amplitude or absent SNAPs, with the lower extremities more affected than the upper extremities. Needle EMG findings include fibrillation potentials, reduced recruitment, and large, polyphasic MUPs in distal limb muscles, again more prominent in the lower limbs. The prognosis for neurologic recovery, upon discontinuation of the offending agent, is generally favorable but depends on the severity of symptoms.

Platinum-based compounds, such as cisplatin, carboplatin, and oxaliplatin, are used in the treatment of solid tumors, such as ovarian, testicular, and bladder cancer. Although platinum toxicity can also result in a distal, symmetric, sensorimotor polyneuropathy through microtubule disruption, it can also cause preferential apoptosis-related damage to the dorsal root ganglia, causing a pure sensory neuronopathy or ganglionopathy with clinical and electrodiagnostic features, including sensory ataxia and upper extremity SNAPs being more affected than in the lower extremities. CMAPs are preserved in a sensory neuronopathy, and needle EMG findings are normal, although patients may demonstrate poor volitional motor unit activation due to profound proprioceptive sensory loss. A "coasting phenomenon" may be noted, where symptoms can progress for months following discontinuation of the platinum-based agent. Prognosis for neurologic recovery in a sensory ganglionopathy is poor.[21]

Diffuse peripheral nerve infiltration directly from cancer, either in a distal symmetric pattern or in a mononeuritis multiplex pattern, is rare but has been reported in hematologic malignancies such as cutaneous T-cell lymphoma and chronic lymphocytic leukemia.[22,23] Amyloid deposition in systemic amyloidosis and multiple myeloma can also result in diffuse polyneuropathy as well as generalized proximal myopathies.[24,25] Neuropathies associated with paraproteinemias and plasma cell dyscrasias warrant special consideration, because there is a high association of neuropathies with these disorders and the presence of monoclonal proteins. These disorders include monoclonal gammopathy of unknown significance (MGUS), Waldenström macroglobulinemia, cryoglobulinemia, multiple myeloma, osteosclerotic myeloma, primary amyloidosis, non-Hodgkin lymphoma, and the chronic leukemias.[16] A diagnosis of MGUS should raise concern, because approximately 20% of these patients will at some point develop a malignant plasma cell disorder. Electrodiagnostic studies are usually consistent with an axonal process, although in the case of osteosclerotic myeloma and Polyneuropathy, Organomegaly, Endocrinopathy, M protein, Skin changes (POEMS syndrome), findings of both axonal loss and multisegmental demyelination can be seen. The electrodiagnostic findings in POEMS syndrome can be similar to those seen in chronic, inflammatory demyelinating polyradiculoneuropathy.[17] The monoclonal gammopathy in these disorders can involve immunoglobulin M (IgM), IgG, or IgA proteins, and there is some evidence to suggest that the type of paraproteinemia correlates to the clinical and electrophysiologic characteristics of the neuropathy.[26] That being the case, characterizing the pathophysiology of the neuropathy on NCS and needle EMG can help guide the hematologist/oncologist whether to initiate treatment.

Neuromuscular paraneoplastic syndromes cause damage to the peripheral nervous system as a result of remote effects from a malignant neoplasm or its metastases. Almost all tumor types have been associated with paraneoplastic syndromes, and any part of the nervous system can be affected. Although rare, it is important to recognize these syndromes. The clinical presentation is usually more rapidly progressive and severe than what would normally be expected in a noncancerous cause. They often precede the diagnosis of cancer, and early recognition may increase survival. Treatment of the underlying malignancy usually results in improvement of neurologic symptoms. In some disorders, neuronal antigens expressed by the tumor result in an autoimmune response against the tumor as well as healthy neural tissue, and identification of these markers can facilitate diagnosis of the primary tumor. For example, the presence of anti-Hu antibodies, sometimes detected in paraneoplastic sensory neuronopathies, has a strong association with small cell lung cancer, neuroblastoma, or prostate cancer.[27,28] Although some syndromes are associated with an identifiable neuro-oncologic autoantibody, frequently no such marker is detected.

Paraneoplastic sensory neuronopathy or ganglionopathy can present with either an acute or an insidious onset of pain and sensory loss. Clinical findings of sensory ataxia and pseudoathetosis are often present at various levels of severity. Both the clinical and the electrodiagnostic findings can be diffuse but commonly are more severe in the upper extremities and may be asymmetric. Motor dysfunction is usually absent; however, sensory neuronopathy can sometimes be seen along with a more diffuse paraneoplastic neurologic syndrome involving encephalomyelitis, autonomic neuropathy, and motor neuronopathy.[27] A pattern of more severe sensory abnormalities on NCS in the upper extremities compared with the lower extremities helps distinguish this entity from a length-dependent sensory neuropathy. Needle EMG is usually normal, although poor volitional activation of MUPs may be noted, because of the severity of sensory abnormalities. The most common associated neoplasm is small cell lung cancer; however, breast, prostate, renal, chondrosarcoma, and lymphoma have also been implicated.

The diagnosis of a true paraneoplastic distal, symmetric, sensorimotor polyneuropathy is difficult to confirm, because there are many more likely known causes that can cause this pattern of involvement, including diabetes mellitus, nutritional deficiencies, and toxic exposure such as chemotherapy. A subacute, sensorimotor polyneuropathy as a paraneoplastic syndrome is therefore a diagnosis of exclusion. Symptoms include pain, paresthesias, numbness, and weakness in a stocking-glove distribution, along with hyporeflexia. A more rapidly progressive course may be the only distinguishing factor differentiating a paraneoplastic syndrome from an idiopathic or diabetic cause. Electrodiagnostic findings are consistent with an axonal process, with reduction in motor and sensory amplitudes on NCS and the presence of fibrillation potentials and large, polyphasic MUPs in distal limb muscles on needle EMG. This syndrome has been associated with lung and breast cancer.[29] A peripheral neuropathy resembling a chronic inflammatory demyelinating polyradiculoneuropathy affects up to 50% of patients with the osteosclerotic form of plasmacytoma (the POEMS syndrome).[27] Motor fibers seem to be preferentially affected, with marked slowing of conduction velocities, prolonged distal latencies, and evidence of temporal dispersion on NCS.[30]

With regard to motor neuron disease syndromes, the anti-Hu–associated paraneoplastic encephalomyelitis/sensory neuronopathy/motor neuropathy syndrome has a strong link with small cell lung cancer. Subacute motor neuropathy and primary lateral sclerosis have been associated with lymphoma and breast cancer, respectively.[31,32] Sensory NCS in patients with pure motor neuron disease are normal. Motor responses will be either normal or reduced in amplitude. Needle EMG will demonstrate fibrillation and fasciculation potentials, reduced recruitment, and large, polyphasic, varying MUPs diffusely. There is no known association between cancer and amyotrophic lateral sclerosis; however, in newly diagnosed motor neuron disease, a screening for cancer should be part of the exclusionary diagnostic workup. Finally, a pattern of clinical and electrophysiologic involvement resembling mononeuritis multiplex may represent a paraneoplastic vasculitic neuropathy. This syndrome has been reported in association with small cell lung cancer and lymphoma.[33] The presence of an anti-Hu antibody can be seen with this syndrome as well.[34]

Autoimmune neuropathies have also been associated with chronic graft-versus-host disease (GVHD) and can present as either a distal symmetric sensorimotor polyneuropathy with characteristic electrodiagnostic findings or a multifocal demyelinating polyneuropathy with features similar to Guillain-Barré syndrome.

NEUROMUSCULAR JUNCTION DISORDERS

Lambert-Eaton myasthenic syndrome (LEMS) is a presynaptic disorder of neuromuscular transmission and is perhaps the best understood paraneoplastic neuromuscular syndrome. Clinically, patients present with fatigue, proximal weakness, hyporeflexia, and autonomic dysfunction. Repetitive strength testing may reveal a "warming-up" phenomenon, where one can display an initial increase in strength with repetition followed by eventual fatigue. Bulbar involvement is rare. LEMS can occur independent from cancer, but up to 40% to 60% of cases have been shown to be associated with small cell lung cancer.[7] LEMS has also been reported to be associated with lymphoma, breast, ovarian, pancreatic, and renal malignancies.

Electrodiagnostic studies are invaluable in the diagnosis of LEMS. Motor responses are reduced in amplitude at baseline. Repetitive stimulation of motor nerves at low frequency (2–3 Hz) demonstrates a further decrement in amplitude. Following brief isometric exercise, facilitation occurs, and CMAP amplitudes show at least a 100% increase.[35] This finding is essentially pathognomonic for LEMS. Sensory responses and needle EMG findings are usually normal, except for the presence of varying, unstable MUPs. Anti-voltage-gated calcium channel antibodies are seen in up to 92% of LEMS patients.[7]

Myasthenia gravis (MG) in the setting of chronic GVHD usually develops between 2 and 5 years after transplantation during tapering of immunosuppressive drug treatment.[36] Clinically and electrophysiologically, the findings are similar to typical autoimmune MG, with decrement of baseline CMAP amplitude noted with slow 2- to 3-Hz repetitive stimulation and repair of the decrement following brief isometric exercise. Needle EMG findings are similar to those seen in LEMS. Acetylcholine receptor antibodies may or may not be present. There has not been a reported association with thymoma in patients with GVHD-associated MG. Treatment regimens of GVHD-associated MG are similar to those of autoimmune MG, with equal efficacy.

MYOPATHIES

Focal myopathies from tumor involvement are rare and usually result from direct muscle infiltration from underlying bony metastases or local lymph node involvement, rather than from hematogenous spread. The findings of a symmetric, proximal myopathy on clinical examination and electrodiagnostic testing can also lead to the discovery of an undiagnosed cancer. Myopathic findings on needle EMG typically include fibrillation potentials and rapid recruitment of small-amplitude, short-duration, polyphasic MUPs. Complex repetitive discharges may be present. Findings are usually more pronounced in proximal versus distal muscles. NCS are usually normal. Although their classification as a true paraneoplastic syndrome is controversial, polymyositis and especially dermatomyositis are associated with an increased incidence of malignancy compared with the general population.[37] Breast, lung, and gynecologic malignancies are most frequently implicated.

Originally thought to be relatively radioresistant, it is now known that skeletal muscle is also susceptible to late onset effects of radiation therapy. The direct effect of radiation on muscle results in fibrosis and contracture.[26] There have been multiple reports of a late onset dropped head syndrome in patients who have received mantle field radiation therapy in the distant past as part of their treatment of Hodgkin lymphoma.[38,39] Clinical features include slowly progressive atrophy of neck and shoulder girdle musculature. Neck flexor and extensor muscles are markedly weak, with remarkably preserved motor function in the shoulder girdle and upper extremities. Affected muscles have a firm, fibrotic character on palpation. The head tends to be in a forward-flexed position, with a secondary kyphotic spinal posture, due to anterior cervical muscle contracture. Needle EMG demonstrates low-amplitude, short-duration, polyphasic MUPs in affected muscles, with normal or decreased insertional activity and rare, if any, fibrillation potentials. There may additionally be findings of a concomitant brachial plexopathy or cervical radiculopathy, depending on the extent of the prior treatment field.[40,41]

Polymyositis, and to a lesser extent, dermatomyositis are well-recognized but uncommon complications of chronic GVHD. The incidence of polymyositis in the GVHD population is greater than that of the general population.[42] The clinical presentation, electrodiagnostic findings, and pathologic findings in GVHD-associated polymyositis are identical to those found in idiopathic polymyositis.

SPECIAL CONSIDERATIONS

Hematopoietic stem cell transplantation is performed as part of the treatment of hematologic malignancies, such as leukemias, lymphomas, and multiple myeloma, as well as for select solid tumors and nonmalignant diseases. These patients will frequently receive additional chemotherapy and/or radiation therapy as part of their treatment regimen and are susceptible to related neurotoxic effects as described earlier. Metabolic derangements such as steroid-induced diabetes and malabsorption syndromes are also common following transplantation and can likewise result in secondary peripheral nervous system dysfunction. As mentioned previously, there are numerous autoimmune neuromuscular conditions associated with chronic GVHD, affecting any combination of peripheral nerves, muscles, or the neuromuscular junction.

Immunocompromised patients are at high risk for numerous infections and secondary complications. Sepsis with multisystem organ failure in the patient with cancer is a common reason for intensive care unit admission. Often these patients will be diagnosed with critical illness polyneuropathy and/or critical illness myopathy based on electrodiagnostic findings.[17] Other acute weakness syndromes, such as MG, LEMS, or steroid myopathy, should also be considered. Needle EMG of the diaphragm and phrenic motor NCS can help guide the critical care team with regards to the potential of weaning of ventilatory support, or determine whether interventions such as phrenic nerve pacing would be appropriate.

Certain medical conditions associated with cancer warrant special attention with regards to planning the needle EMG component of the electrodiagnostic study. Patients with lymphedema are thought to be at increased risk for cellulitis and are frequently cautioned to avoid needle puncture in the affected limb to prevent infection or worsening lymphedema. The actual risk of cellulitis associated with needle EMG in the setting of lymphedema however is unknown. Given this, reasonable caution should be exercised in performing needle examination, and physicians should balance the potential risks with the need to obtain the information gained.[45] Although there is no contraindication for performing NCS in the lymphedematous extremity, the need for adequate stimulus intensity to obtain an accurate nerve or muscle action potential may be greater depending on the limb volume and extent of fibrosis, and therefore, could result in more discomfort for the patient.

Patients with cancer often receive therapeutic agents that adversely affect platelet counts, or are anticoagulated for treatment of associated deep venous thromboses, all of which increase the likelihood of bleeding. Mild reduction in platelet counts (<50,000/mm^3) increases the chance of bleeding, and more severe thrombocytopenia (<20,000/mm^3) markedly increases the risk.[46] There is a scant evidence base to guide the electromyographer in these clinical scenarios. As with balancing the potential risks and benefits of performing needle EMG in the lymphedema patient, clinical judgment is warranted in the patient with cancer with increased bleeding risk. Careful selection and minimal exploration of easily compressible, superficial compartment muscles are recommended.

REFERENCES

1. Garzon-Rodriguez G, Leonidas L, Gayoso LO, et al. Cancer-related neuropathic pain in out-patient oncology clinics: a European survey. BMC Palliat Care 2013; 12:41–52.
2. Shelerud RA, Paynter KS. Rarer causes of radiculopathy: spinal tumors, infections, and other unusual causes. Phys Med Rehabil Clin N Am 2002;13:646–96.
3. Stubgen JP. Neuromuscular disorders in systemic malignancy and its treatment. Muscle Nerve 1995;18:636–48.
4. Demopoulous A, DeAngelis LM. Neurologic complications of leukemia. Curr Opin Neurol 2002;15:691–9.
5. Argov Z, Siegal T. Leptomeningeal metastases: peripheral nerve and root involvement—clinical and electrophysiologic study. Ann Neurol 1985;17:593–6.
6. Breinberg HR, Amato AA. Neuromuscular complications of cancer. Neurol Clin N Am 2003;21:141–65.
7. Ladha SS, Spinner RJ, Suarez GA, et al. Neoplastic lumbosacral radiculoplexopathy in prostate cancer by direct perineural spread: an unusual entity. Muscle Nerve 2006;34:659–65.
8. Kori SH, Foley KM, Posner JB. Brachial plexus lesions in patients with cancer: 100 cases. Neurology 1981;31:45–50.
9. Younger D, Dalmau J, Inghirami G, et al. Anti-Hu-associated peripheral nerve and muscle microvasculitis. Neurology 1994;44:181–3.
10. Amato AA, Barohn RJ, Sahenk Z, et al. Polyneuropathy complicating bone marrow and solid organ transplantation. Neurology 1993;43:1513–8.
11. Wen PY, Alyea EP, Simon D, et al. Guillain-Barré syndrome following allogenic bone marrow transplantation. Neurology 1997;49:1711–4.
12. Younger DS. Motor neuron disease and malignancy. Muscle Nerve 2000;23: 658–60.
13. Oh SJ. Paraneoplastic vasculitis of the peripheral nervous system. Neurol Clin 1997;15:849–63.
14. Kelly JJ, Kyle RA, Miles JM, et al. The spectrum of peripheral neuropathy in myeloma. Neurology 1981;31:24–31.
15. Rubin DI, Hermann RC. Electrophysiologic findings in amyloid myopathy. Muscle Nerve 1999;22:355–9.
16. Ropper AH, Gorson KC. Neuropathies associated with paraproteinemias. N Engl J Med 1998;338:1601–7.
17. Sliwa JA. Acute weakness syndromes in the critically ill patient. Arch Phys Med Rehabil 2000;81(3 Suppl):S45–52.
18. Vissink A, Jansma J, Spijkervet FK, et al. Oral sequelae of head and neck radiotherapy. Crit Rev Oral Biol Med 2003;14:199–212.
19. Darnell RB, Posner JB. Paraneoplastic syndromes involving the nervous system. N Engl J Med 2003;349:1543–54.
20. Posner JB. Paraneoplastic syndromes. In: Posner JB, editor. Neurologic complications of cancer. 1st edition. Philadelphia: F.A. Davis; 1995. p. 353–85.
21. Dispenzieri A. POEMS syndrome. Hematology 2005;1:360–7.
22. Harper CM, Thomas JE, Cascino TL, et al. Distinction between neoplastic and radiation-induced brachial plexopathy, with emphasis on the role of EMG. Neurology 1989;39:502–6.

23. Boyaciyan A, Oge AE, Yazici J, et al. Electrophysiological findings in patients who received radiation therapy over the brachial plexus: a magnetic stimulation study. Electroencephalogr Clin Neurophysiol 1996;101:483–90.
24. Hauer-Jensen M, Fink LM, Wang J. Radiation injury and the protein C pathway. Crit Care Med 2004;32(5 Suppl):S325–30.
25. Pan CC, Hayman JA. Recent advances in radiation oncology. J Neuro-opthalmol 2004;24:251–7.
26. Krouwer HGJ, Wijdicks EFM. Neurologic complications of bone marrow transplantation. Neurol Clin N Am 2003;21:319–52.
27. Posner JB. Neurotoxicity of surgical and diagnostic procedures. In: Posner JB, editor. Neurologic complications of cancer. 1st edition. Philadelphia: F.A. Davis; 1995. p. 338–52.
28. Dawson DM, Krarup C. Perioperative nerve lesions. Arch Neurol 1989;46: 1355–60.
29. DeHart MM, Riley LH Jr. Nerve injuries in total hip arthroplasty. J Am Acad Orthop Surg 1999;7:101–11.
30. Graf WD, Chance PF, Lensch MW, et al. Severe vincristine neuropathy in Charcot-Marie-Tooth disease type 1A. Cancer 1996;77:1356–62.
31. Kelly JJ, Karcher DS. Lymphoma and peripheral neuropathy: a clinical review. Muscle Nerve 2005;31:301–13.
32. Amato AA, Dumitru D. Acquired neuropathies. In: Dumitru D, Amato AA, Zwarts MD, editors. Electrodiagnostic medicine. 2nd edition. Philadelphia: Hanley and Blefus; 2002. p. 937–1041.
33. Chauvenet AR, Shashi V, Selsky C, et al. Vincristine-induced neuropathy as the initial presentation of Charcot-Marie-Tooth disease in acute lymphoblastic leukemia: a Pediatric Oncology Group study. J Pediatr Hematol Oncol 2003;25: 316–20.
34. Chaudhry V, Chaudhry M, Crawford TO, et al. Toxic neuropathy in patients with pre-existing neuropathy. Neurology 2003;60:337–40.
35. Peltier AC, Russell JW. Recent advances in drug-induced neuropathies. Curr Opin Neurol 2002;15:633–8.
36. Al-Shekhlee A, Shapiro BE, Preston DC. Iatrogenic complications and risk of nerve conduction studies and needle electromyography. Muscle Nerve 2003; 27:517–26.
37. Stubblefield MD, Burstein HJ, Burton AW, et al. NCCN task force report: management of neuropathy in cancer. J Natl Compr Canc Netw 2009;7(Suppl 5):S1–26.
38. Yazici Y, Kagen LJ. The association of malignancy with myositis. Curr Opin Rheumatol 2000;12:498–500.
39. Portlock CS, Boland P, Hays AP, et al. Nemaline myopathy: a possible late complication of Hodgkin's disease therapy. Hum Pathol 2003;34:816–8.
40. Rowin J, Cheng G, Lewis SL, et al. Late appearance of dropped head syndrome after radiotherapy for Hodgkin's disease. Muscle Nerve 2006;34:666–9.
41. Stevens AM, Sullivan KM, Nelson JL. Polymyositis as a manifestation of chronic graft-versus-host disease. Rheumatology (Oxford) 2003;42:34–9.
42. American Association of Neuromuscular & Electrodiagnostic Medicine. Needle EMG in certain uncommon clinical contexts. Muscle Nerve 2005;31:398–9.

Index

Note: Page numbers of article titles are in **boldface** type.

http://dx.doi.org/10.1016/S1047-9651(16)30111-5
1047-9651/17

Moving?

Make sure your subscription moves with you!

To notify us of your new address, find your **Clinics Account Number** (located on your mailing label above your name), and contact customer service at:

Email: journalscustomerservice-usa@elsevier.com

800-654-2452 (subscribers in the U.S. & Canada)
314-447-8871 (subscribers outside of the U.S. & Canada)

Fax number: 314-447-8029

Elsevier Health Sciences Division
Subscription Customer Service
3251 Riverport Lane
Maryland Heights, MO 63043

*To ensure uninterrupted delivery of your subscription, please notify us at least 4 weeks in advance of move.

Printed and bound by CPI Group (UK) Ltd, Croydon, CR0 4YY

03/10/2024

01040395-0004